Fractures: Evidence-Based Management

Fractures: Evidence-Based Management

Edited by Brandon Gomez

AMERICAN
MEDICAL PUBLISHERS
www.americanmedicalpublishers.com

American Medical Publishers,
41 Flatbush Avenue,
1st Floor, New York,
NY 11217, USA

Visit us on the World Wide Web at:
www.americanmedicalpublishers.com

ISBN: 978-1-63927-394-2

Cataloging-in-Publication Data

Fractures : evidence-based management / edited by Brandon Gomez.
p. cm.
Includes bibliographical references and index.
ISBN 978-1-63927-394-2
1. Fractures. 2. Fractures--Diagnosis. 3. Fractures--Treatment.
4. Bones--Wounds and injuries. I. Gomez, Brandon.
RD101 .F73 2022
617.15--dc23

Table of Contents

Preface

Over the recent decade, advancements and applications have progressed exponentially. This has led to the increased interest in this field and projects are being conducted to enhance knowledge. The main objective of this book is to present some of the critical challenges and provide insights into possible solutions. This book will answer the varied questions that arise in the field and also provide an increased scope for furthering studies.

The continuity of a bone may break in response to a trauma, injury or stress. This condition is called a bone fracture. In orthopedic medicine, bone fractures are classified on the basis of the mechanism by which the fracture has been incurred, soft-tissue involvement, fracture pattern, anatomical location, etc. Some of its various types are skull fracture, spinal fracture, complete fracture, spiral fracture, impacted fracture, pathologic fracture, periprosthetic fracture, etc. A bone fracture is assessed on the basis of a physical examination and the medical history. Radiographic imaging of the bone and nearby joints helps to determine dislocations and fracture-dislocations if any. In certain cases, MRI and CT scans may also be required. Bone fractures can be treated surgically or non-surgically. Non-surgical strategies comprise of immobilization, pain management and stabilization. In cases where absence of operative interventions may result in prolonged immobilization and complications such as deep vein thrombosis, pulmonary embolism, pressure sores and chest infections, surgery is a recommended strategy. From theories to research to practical applications, case studies related to all contemporary topics of relevance in the diagnosis and management of bone fractures have been included in this book. It presents researches and studies performed by experts across the globe. Doctors and students actively engaged in orthopedics will find this book full of crucial and unexplored concepts.

I hope that this book, with its visionary approach, will be a valuable addition and will promote interest among readers. Each of the authors has provided their extraordinary competence in their specific fields by providing different perspectives as they come from diverse nations and regions. I thank them for their contributions.

Editor

1

The impact of hip fracture on mortality in Estonia: a retrospective population-based cohort study

Mikk Jürisson[1*], Mait Raag[1], Riina Kallikorm[2,3], Margus Lember[2,3] and Anneli Uusküla[1]

Abstract

Background: Estimates of hip fracture mortality in Eastern Europe are scarce. We aimed to estimate the magnitude and duration of excess mortality after hip fracture in Estonia.

Methods: Retrospective, population-based 10-year study of persons aged ≥50 in two cohorts: with hip fracture and an age- and sex-matched (in a 1:4 ratio) random sample from the national health insurance fund database for comparison. Cumulative risks, excess risks and relative risks of death were estimated using Poisson regression with 95% bootstrap confidence intervals (CI). Risks were adjusted for age and Charlson comorbidity index.

Results: We identified 8298 (2383 men, 5915 women) incident hip fracture patients from 2005 to 2013 and 33,191 (9531 men, 23,660 women) individuals for the reference group. 5552 (1564 men, 3988 women) cases and 14,037 (3514 men, 10,523 women) reference individuals died during the 10-year follow-up period. Among hip fracture patients we observed a pronounced and durable excess risk of death that was highest within 3–6 months after fracture and persisted for the full 10-year follow-up period. After adjustment for age and Charlson index, hip fracture was associated with a 21.1% (95% CI 20.0–22.5%) 10-year cumulative excess risk of death (RR 1.37, 95% CI 1.35–1.40). We found a high immediate excess risk of death in older age groups (≥80 years) and gradually accumulating excess risk in younger age groups (50–79 years). The excess risk was more pronounced among men than women.

Conclusions: By the end of the 10-year follow-up, 1 in 4 deaths in the hip fracture group was attributable to the hip fracture. The results indicate a high attributable impact of hip fracture as an independent risk factor for death.

Keywords: Hip fracture, Excess mortality, Eastern Europe, Estonia

Background

Patients who have a hip fracture are at considerable risk for premature death [1, 2]. A recent report of osteoporosis in the European Union estimated that mortality related to low-impact trauma hip fracture is greater than road traffic accidents and equivalent to breast cancer [3]. This mortality burden will increase over the next few decades commensurate with the aging of the population [3]. Targeted interventions among at-risk groups may contribute to mortality reductions [1], thus, a contemporary epidemiology of hip fracture mortality would be useful in developing risk profiles and estimates of potential lives saved. To this end, country-specific mortality data should be collected to refine estimates of the longitudinal burden of hip fracture and conduct economic evaluations of hip fracture prevention and treatment measures [4].

The data describing excess mortality after hip fracture are well established in developed Western European and North American countries [1, 5]. In a systematic analysis, the documented cumulative excess risk (i.e., exceeding mortality rates among non-hip fracture or community control populations) during the first year after hip fracture varied widely from 8.4% to 36% [1]. Studies of short- vs. long-term mortality almost always note increased mortality soon after the fracture, within the first 3–6 months [1, 2, 5–9]. Although the relative risk decreases in subsequent years, it does not return to that of age- and sex-matched reference groups

* Correspondence: mikkjurisson@gmail.com
[1]Institute of Family Medicine and Public Health, University of Tartu, Ravila st 19, 50411 Tartu, Estonia

even 10 years post-fracture [5]. The excess risk increases with advancing age, although this differential becomes less pronounced over the following years due to increased mortality, unrelated to hip fracture, in the reference populations [1, 5]. The excess risk is also higher among men than women [1, 5], notably among the oldest age categories (≥80 years) in the first months and years after fracture [5].

Estimates of hip fracture mortality in Eastern Europe are scarce [10, 11]. However, the data in this region suggests a sex-specific difference in the incidence of hip fractures between Eastern and Western Europe [12–14], and the age and sex-specific all-cause mortality rates in Eastern Europe differ from those in Western countries [15]. Longitudinal data is needed to quantify the change in excess mortality after hip fracture by temporal, clinical and geographic characteristics. This study estimates the impact of hip fracture on 10-year all-cause mortality among Estonian men and women ≥50 years of age.

Methods

Overview

This was a population-based retrospective cohort study to examine the excess all-cause mortality after hip fracture in Estonia. The data on all-cause mortality in men and women aged ≥50 years with incident hip fracture (cases) were compared with randomly selected age- and sex-matched subjects from the reference group with no known history of hip fracture prior to the index date (defined below). The excess mortality risk related to the hip fracture over a 10-year follow-up period was evaluated using Poisson regression and adjusting for demographic and clinical characteristics.

Setting, data source, and participants

The population of Estonia is approximately 1,315,000 residents, of whom 479,000 are aged 50 years or more (197,000 men and 282,000 women) (2015 data) [16], and universal public health insurance covers >94% of the population [17]. Since its inception in the early 2000s, the Estonian Health Insurance Fund (EHIF) has maintained a complete record of inpatient and outpatient health care services. The EHIF electronic database contains information on characteristics of the person (sex, age at health care service utilization), health care utilization (date of service, primary and other diagnoses, treatment type (in- or outpatient), a specialty of the provider), and the date of death. For the current study we ascertained study subjects' demographic characteristics, clinical characteristics, and outcome data. Although the EHIF database captures provision of healthcare services country-wide, loss to follow-up upon emigration from Estonia is possible, albeit rare, among those 50 years or older (estimated to be less than 0.5% per year) (2015 data) [16].

The sample frame included all publicly insured individuals, including those with no record of health care services provided from January 1, 2004 – December 31, 2013. Health care utilization data on all patients (aged ≥50 years) hospitalized with incident hip fractures during the period January 1, 2005-December 31, 2013 were identified (case group). The hip fracture patients were matched by sex and age (year of birth) in a 1:4 ratio to the reference group. By definition, reference group subjects were alive and without evidence of hip fracture prior to the case patient's index date of fracture. Study subjects were assigned a unique identifier decoupled from personal identification information to enable longitudinal tracking of care and mortality while maintaining patient privacy. We followed all study subjects (belonging to the case and reference groups) until the study closure May 4, 2016, or the date of death.

Identification of incident hip fracture

The case definition of hip fracture was based on the following specific diagnosis codes (The International Classification of Diseases, Tenth Revision (ICD-10): S72.0 - fracture of femoral neck, S72.1 - pertrochanteric fracture and S72.2 - subtrochanteric fracture). These codes must have been listed as the primary diagnosis on the electronical inpatient health care claim submitted to the EHIF. The index date of diagnosis was defined as the first day of care indicated in the claim; patients with a diagnostic code primary for hip fracture and no previous evidence of hip fracture according to EHIF records were selected for inclusion. The validity of this case definition (i.e., incident hip fracture case) from a population-based administrative database has been demonstrated [18].

Identification of pre-fracture comorbidity

Clinical characteristics and comorbidities were captured for the 365-day period prior to the index date for case patients and their matched controls. The comorbidity status for both groups was computed using the Charlson comorbidity index (CCI) [19]. We used the revised coding algorithm described by Quan, et al., and subsequently validated for estimating comorbidity using ICD-10 coded administrative data [20]. We also updated disease weighting to reflect advances in chronic disease management and treatment outcomes since the introduction of the original Charlson index in 1984 [21]. The updated Charlson index has demonstrated comparable predictive utility for mortality using ICD-10 coded administrative data [21] and has been validated among hip fracture patients [22].

Comorbidities were defined as secondary or other diagnoses coded at the index hip fracture claim and/or diagnoses of any type on hospital or outpatient health care claims during the year preceding the index date [22, 23]. We applied a restriction to outpatient claims, such that a comorbid condition could be flagged during the preceding period only if it appeared two or more times at least 7 days apart [7, 23].

The primary outcome for the study was death from any cause. The dates of death were obtained from the EHIF database.

Statistical analysis

The hip fracture group and the reference group were described by group size, mean age, age range and 10-year groups, CCI mean score and range; 95% Wald confidence intervals for mean differences of age and CCI were calculated. To capture the rapid and extensive changes in mortality during the first 3–6 months following a hip fracture [1, 5], we divided our 10-year follow-up period into graduated discrete intervals as follows: using shorter periods close to the index date and wider intervals later with cut-points at 0.5, 1, 1.5, ..., 3, 4, ..., 12, 15, ..., 24, 30, ..., 48, 60, ..., 120 months after the index date. Subsets defined by age group and sex were analyzed separately, the results were aggregated by weighting by group sizes when necessary. Within each subset Poisson regression was used to estimate mortality rates for each of those intervals. Two regression models were considered: crude (unadjusted), containing only the interaction between hip fracture and follow-up time interval besides main effects of both and the logarithm of time at risk as an offset term, and adjusted, including main effects of hip fracture, CCI, age, follow-up time interval, and logarithm of time at risk in the respective follow-up time interval as an offset term as well as interactions between hip fracture and follow-up time interval, hip fracture and CCI, hip fracture and age, follow-up time interval and age. Interval-specific mortality rates were transformed to probabilities which were used to calculate cumulative risks. Age adjustment within age groups was used to account for residual confounding [24]. Excess risks and risk ratios (RR) were calculated using cumulative risks. Bootstrap with bias correction was used to compute 95% confidence intervals (CI) for cumulative and excess risks, and the bootstrap percentile method was used to calculate 95% CIs for risk ratios.

All analyses were performed in R (versions 3.1.1 to 3.3.1) [25–32].

The study procedures were conducted in accordance with local data protection regulations. The study was approved by the Tartu University Research Ethics Committee.

Results

Characteristics of hip fracture patients and reference group subjects

From the EHIF database we identified 8298 (2383 men, 5915 women) incident hip fracture patients and 33,191 (9531 men, 23,660 women) individuals for the reference group between 2005 and 2013 (Table 1). There were only three reference individuals available for one 100-year old man with hip fracture, therefore the total size of age- and sex-matched reference (non-hip fracture) group was 33,191. Similar numbers of hip fractures occurred each year in 2005—2013. Most of the fractures (71%) occurred in women. On average, men were 8.2 years (95% CI 7.7—8.7) younger than women at hip fracture, over 70% of men were younger than 80 years at hip fracture while 60% of women were 80 years or older.

Mean Charlson comorbidity index was 0.28 points lower (95% CI 0.24—0.31) among the reference group (mean 0.66, SD 1.12) than in the hip fracture group (mean 0.94, SD 1.36), this difference was similar both among men and women (Table 1).

Absolute risk of death

The average follow-up time was 4.3 years (3.4 years among hip fracture patients and 5.0 among the reference group. 5552 cases (1564 men, 3988 women) and 14,037 reference individuals (3514 men, 10,523 women) died during the 10-year follow-up period. The crude cumulative risk of death in the hip fracture group was high compared to reference patients: at 3 months 17.5% (95% CI 16.8–18.1%) vs 2.0% (95% CI 1.9–2.1%), respectively, in 1 year 28.3% (95% CI 27.6–29.0%) vs 7.8% (95% CI 7.6–8.0%), in 5 years 54.4% (53.6–55.2%) vs 29.8% (95% CI 29.4–30.1%), and in 10 years 78.2% (95% CI 77.2–79.2%) vs 55.6% (95% CI 55.0–56.2%), respectively. When stratified by sex, women experienced an elevated crude cumulative 10-year risk of all-cause death among both the hip fracture and reference groups (both $p < 0.0001$). The adjusted cumulative 10-year risk of all-cause death was 77.6% (95% CI 76.7–78.8%) in the hip fracture group and 56.5% (95% CI 56.0–57.3%) in the reference group. The adjusted sex-specific cumulative risks in both study groups are presented in Fig. 1, and the adjusted age-specific cumulative risks are presented in Fig. 2.

Excess (attributable) risk of death

We observed a pronounced and durable excess risk of death after a hip fracture that was highest within 3–6 months after fracture and persisted for the full 10-year follow-up period. Compared with reference group individuals, those with hip fracture experienced 22.6% (95% CI 21.4–23.8%) crude excess risk, and 21.1% (95% CI 20.0–22.5%) adjusted excess risk in 10-year cumulative mortality. The proportion of deaths in the hip fracture group attributable to the exposure (attributable risk fraction) in 10 years from fracture was 27.2% (95% CI 25.9–28.5%). Consequently, by the end of the 10-year follow-up, one in four deaths in the case group was attributable to the patient's hip fracture. 10-year attributable fraction varied widely across the age and sex groups: in the 50–59-year age group

Table 1 Characteristics of hip fracture patients and reference group subjects aged 50 years or more in Estonia, January 1, 2005, to December 31, 2013

Characteristic	Hip fracture group				Reference group			
	Men		Women		Men		Women	
	n	%	n	%	n	%	n	%
N	2383	29%	5915	71%	9531	29%	23,660	71%
Age, mean (sd)	72.2 (11.4)		80.4 (9.1)		72.2 (11.4)		80.4 (9.1)	
Age range	50–102		50–103		50–102		50–103	
Age groups								
50–59	401	17%	202	3%	1604	17%	808	3%
60–69	561	24%	484	8%	2244	24%	1936	8%
70–79	724	30%	1689	29%	2896	30%	6756	29%
80–89	564	24%	2749	46%	2256	24%	10,996	46%
90+	133	6%	791	13%	531	6%	3164	13%
Charlson index, mean (sd)	0.88 (1.38)		0.96 (1.36)		0.59 (1.11)		0.69 (1.13)	
Charlson index range	0–9		0–9		0–9		0–10	

it was 67.5% (95% CI 61.1—73.1%) in men and 78.0% (95% CI 61.5—87.6%) in women, in the 70–79-year group 38.8% (95% CI 34.7—42.3%) and 39.2% (95% CI 35.8—42.6%), whereas in over 90-year old group it was only 13.0% (95% CI 7.4—20.3%) in men and 11.1% (95% CI 8.9—13.2%) in women.

The age- and CCI-adjusted excess cumulative risk of death for hip fracture group patients is presented in Fig. 3. In stratified analysis, the adjusted excess risk was extensive within 3 months of the fracture (13.7%, 95% CI 12.9–14.9% in men, 14.5%, 95% CI 13.8–15.3% in women), and increased by 1 year to 18.7% (95% CI 17.8–20.2%) in men and 19.2% (95% CI 18.3–20.2%) in women. The excess risk was highest by the seventh year after hip fracture in men (28.5%, 95% CI 26.8–30.3%) and by the fifth in women (21.9%, 95% CI 19.5–21.9%).

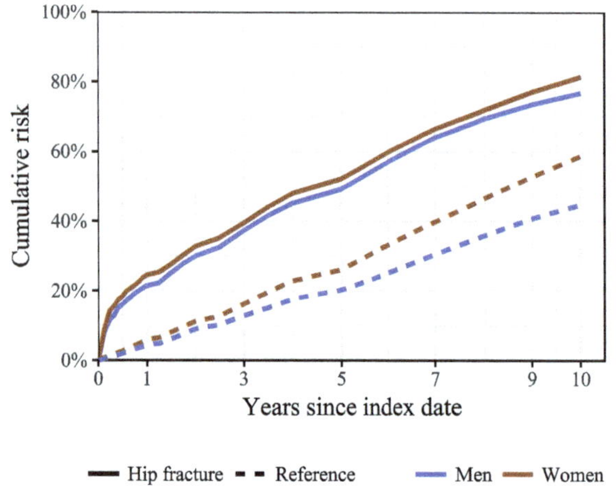

Fig. 1 Sex-specific cumulative 10-year risk of all-cause mortality (adjusted for age and Charlson index score) by study group in men and women ≥50 years in Estonia, January 1, 2005-May 4, 2016

After 3 years of the hip fracture, men were at significantly greater excess risk of death than women.

The adjusted excess risk of mortality in the hip fracture group increased exponentially with age immediately after fracture (Fig. 4). For example, in the 60–69-year-olds, the 3-month excess risk was moderate (men 8.1%, 95% CI 6.5–9.9%; women 4.6% (95% CI 3.3–6.2%), whereas in the ≥90-year group the risk was 45.1% (95% CI 38.7–52.7%) in men and 24.2% (95% CI 21.8–26.7%) in women. However, over the study period the excess risk accumulated differentially by age. In older patients (≥80 years) the excess risk decreased over the observation period, but in younger age groups (50–79 years) the excess risk increased in a linear fashion over the 10-year follow-up period. For example, in the 60–69-year group the excess risk increased to 30% in 10 years (men 32.8%, 95% CI 28.0–38.1%, and women 31.5%, 95% CI 26.1–37.6%). In all age- and sex-specific groups, the excess risk of mortality due to hip fracture was present until the end of the follow-up period, and in any given age group the excess risk was higher in men.

Relative risk of death

The adjusted relative risk of all-cause death among hip fracture patients versus age- and sex-matched controls is presented in Table 2. At 1 year, the hip fracture patients were between two and 10 times more likely to die than their age- and gender-matched reference subjects, depending on age and sex. The long-term relative risk was higher in younger age groups (women greater than men) where the absolute risk in the respective reference groups was lower and decreased with advancing age. The relative risk remained elevated over 10 years in all age- and sex-specific comparisons.

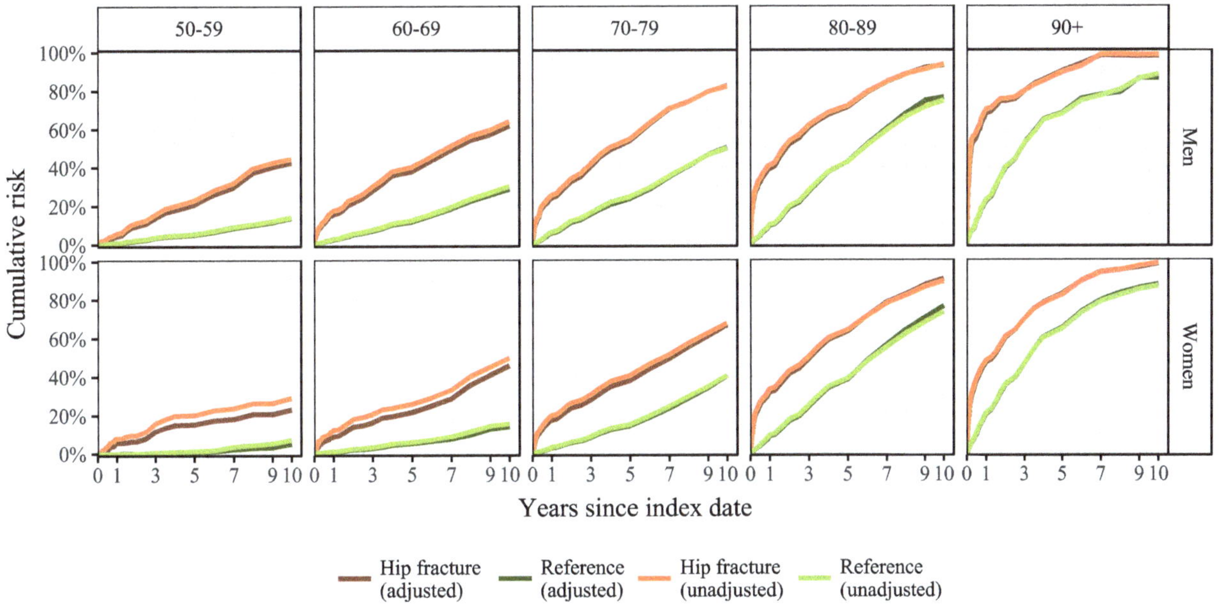

Fig. 2 Age group-specific cumulative risk of all-cause mortality (adjusted for age and Charlson index score) by study group in men and women ≥50 years in Estonia, January 1, 2005-May 4, 2016

Discussion

Our study assessed the impact of hip fracture on the all-cause risk of death over 10 years among people 50 years of age or older in Estonia. We observed a pronounced and sustained excess mortality risk after a hip fracture that was highest within 6–12 months after the fracture and persisted for the full 10-year follow-up period. After adjustment for age and pre-fracture comorbidities (CCI), hip fracture was associated with a 21.1% (95% CI 20.0–22.5%) 10-year cumulative excess risk of death (RR 1.37, 95% CI 1.35–1.40). Even after 10 years following the hip fracture, more than 1 in 4 deaths among hip fracture patients was attributable to the initial injury. The 1-year average relative all-cause excess mortality (4.1 in men, 3.4 in women) after hip fracture was comparable to that of dementia, cancer, and heart failure [21], mental disorders [33], and higher than that for diabetes [34].

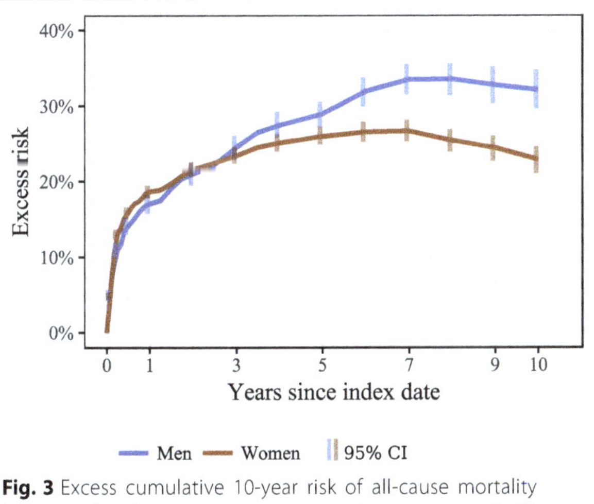

Fig. 3 Excess cumulative 10-year risk of all-cause mortality following hip fracture among men and women age ≥ 50 years (adjusted for age and Charlson index score) in Estonia, January 1, 2005-May 4, 2016

The excess risk of death differed by the duration of follow-up time after the hip fracture, by sex, and according to age at the time of fracture. We found a high immediate excess risk of death in older age groups (≥80 years) and a gradually increasing excess risk in younger age groups (50–79 years) that was more pronounced in men than in women. In the elderly, hip fracture has an immediate devastating impact on mortality that lasts for years. For example, in the group of men ≥90 years old, the excess risk of death 3 months after fracture was 45%, and the risk of dying was 8 times higher than in men who had not had a fracture. Consequently, over half of the men in that group had died within 3 months of the fracture, and within 12 months over two-thirds of the men had died. It is important to note that the excess risk among the elderly (aged 80 years or more) persisted throughout the 10-year follow-up period and did not disappear in any age- or sex-specific group. In contrast, the excess risk in younger age groups increased in a linear fashion over the follow-up period. For example, in the 60–69-year group the excess risk increased with time to a maximum of 30%. Thus, 6 out of 10 men with a hip fracture and 1 in 2 women in that age group died during the 10-year follow-up period. The risk of death was 2–3 times higher in the fracture group than in the reference group even 10 years after the fracture.

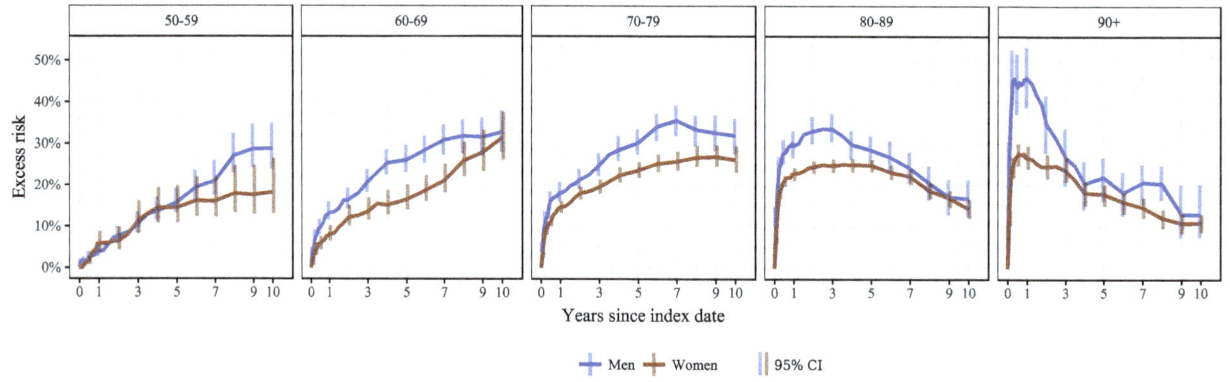

Fig. 4 Age group-specific 10-year cumulative excess risk of death following hip fracture among those ≥50 years old (adjusted for age and Charlson index score), men and women in Estonia, January 1, 2005-May 4, 2016

Previous studies have demonstrated an immediate elevated risk of mortality after hip fracture [1, 2, 5, 6, 35–39], however, the evidence of persistence is not universal [1, 7, 9, 40, 41]. Overall, our results are in line with the meta-analysis suggesting that the excess mortality after hip fracture in patients over 50 years is extensive already in the first months after fracture and persists for at least 10 years [5]. Notably, the relative risk of all-cause mortality within the 3 months after hip fracture was as high as 9.5 in men and 8.3 in women, comparable to that in the meta-analysis [5]. However, compared to the pooled estimates [5] the excess risk of death in Estonian men and women in younger (50–79 years) age groups was rather high, particularly in the first months and years after fracture. For example, in the 70–79-year-old men the excess risk in our study reached as high as 18% within 1 year, and 30% within 5 years, whereas in the meta-analysis the respective estimates were lower (11% and 20%). Likewise, in women of the same age we found the excess risk to be 14% in 1 year and 24% in 5 years, versus 5% and 13% in the meta-analysis. It is difficult to explain the reasons for increased mortality in these groups, but insufficient case management upon discharge and low utilization of rehabilitation, nursing care, and social care [42] could be potential contributors. In addition, it is possible that not all comorbid conditions were diagnosed and recorded in these patients (especially men), and their impact on mortality therefore could not be adjusted in the models. Finally, excess mortality study results are difficult to compare due to differences in study design and sources of data, ascertainment of cases and controls, determination of death, differences in follow-up time, presentation of results, and adjustment for confounding [1, 5].

A number of confounding factors, such as advanced age, male sex, poor preoperative health status and multiple comorbidities have been associated with excess mortality following hip fractures [43]. Our results are in

Table 2 Age group specific and average 10-year relative risk (risk ratio (RR) comparing hip fracture cases to reference group) of all-cause death after hip fracture in men and women ≥50 years, adjusted for age and Charlson index score

Sex	Age group	3 months		1 year		5 years		10 years	
		RR	95% CI	RR	95% CI	RR	95% CI	RR	95% CI
Men	50–59	*		5.6	3.3–10.2	4.0	3.2–4.9	3.1	2.6–3.7
	60–69	10.6	7.3–18.1	5.9	4.8–7.5	3.2	2.9–3.6	2.1	1.9–2.4
	70–79	10.0	7.8–13.2	3.9	3.4–4.5	2.3	2.1–2.4	1.6	1.5–1.7
	80–89	9.9	8.2–12.4	4.0	3.6–4.6	1.7	1.6–1.8	1.2	1.2–1.3
	90+	8.0	6.3–11.0	3.1	2.7–3.7	1.3	1.3–1.4	1.2	1.1–1.3
	Weighted average	9.5	8.4–10.9	4.1	3.8–4.4	2.0	2.0–2.1	1.6	1.5–1.6
Women	50–59	*		*		14.6	7.7–44.0	4.6	2.6–8.1
	60–69	14.6	8.6–34.8	9.8	6.8–15.0	4.1	3.4–5.0	3.3	2.8–3.9
	70–79	14.9	11.5–19.3	6.0	5.3–6.8	2.6	2.5–2.8	1.6	1.6–1.7
	80–89	9.1	8.2–10.1	3.5	3.3–3.7	1.7	1.6–1.7	1.2	1.2–1.2
	90+	5.3	4.6–6.1	2.3	2.1–2.5	1.3	1.2–1.3	1.1	1.1–1.2
	Weighted average	8.3	7.7–9.0	3.4	3.3–3.6	1.7	1.7–1.8	1.3	1.3–1.3

*Respective risk ratios had too high variance and were not reliable

line with the collective evidence confirming that excess mortality increases with age, and is higher in men than in women in all age groups [1, 5]. The average excess risk among men in our study did not exceed that among women during 3 years following the fracture; this may be explained by the different age distribution of fractures in men and women in our study. We know that most hip fractures in Estonian men occur at a younger age (50–79 years) due to the elevated incidence of hip fractures in that age [14] and low life expectancy in men (15.1 years at age 65, 2014 data) [16], whereas over half of fractures in women occur among those ≥80 years [14]. Due to the considerable age difference between sexes in our study (8.2 years) women experienced an elevated crude cumulative 10-year risk of all-cause death among both the hip fracture and reference groups (see Fig. 1), and the weighted average excess risk in both study groups (see Fig. 3) was influenced by the higher-weighted age groups, with younger groups in men and older groups in women.

Numerous studies have reported that the presence of pre-fracture concomitant medical conditions are negative predictors for survival [35, 36, 43–46], whereas the extent to which underlying conditions contribute to the excess mortality associated with hip fracture is still unclear [1]. In our study the hip fracture patients had higher CCI score than the age- and sex-matched reference subjects. However, because the sample in our study was matched for age and sex, and the risks were adjusted for major confounders, we believe that the results strongly suggest that hip fracture is an independent and attributable risk factor for death. This implies that preventative efforts and post fracture rehabilitation and social care are essential to reduce the excess risk of death.

The possible reasons for the greater mortality risk in men than in women following hip fracture are still poorly understood [1]. Previously described risk factors in older men include multi-morbidity, smoking, lower dietary protein, greater height combined with the use of antidepressants leading to a greater impact upon falling, whereas the traditional risk factors in women (rheumatoid arthritis, use of benzodiazepines and corticosteroids) were not related to hip fractures in men [47]. It has also been suggested that men have higher rates of pneumonia and septicemia than women [48], or more severe medical comorbidities prior to the hip fracture [49, 50]. However, in our study the CCI score was lower in men than in women in both study groups, suggesting that men were healthier than women. It is possible that the lower CCI score in men was related to their younger age compared to women. Our study adjusted for CCI, yet the excess risk was higher in men than in women.

We acknowledge the limitations of our study. Our objective was strictly aligned with assessing the impact of hip fracture on mortality, thus, we did not assess the impact of hip fracture complications on excess mortality, or the causes of death. Nursing home or facility residence, poor preoperative walking capacity, poor activities of daily living and poor mental state have been identified as strongly predictive factors for the excess mortality [43] suggesting that frail and disabled elderly are at higher immediate risk of death after hip fracture [7, 46]. It is possible that the level of functional impairment in our study was higher among hip fracture patients. We used data from the (administrative) health insurance database that covers the overwhelming majority of the Estonia's population. However, we are not aware of any data documenting the completeness of the database. Furthermore, the data on additional useful indicators (sociodemographic factors such as income, education, occupation, social deprivation, and other health/lifestyle indicators (BMI, smoking, alcohol consumption)) [6, 43, 46, 51] were not available. Finally, we did not account for changes in hip fracture mortality in the population over time.

We also did not analyze in detail the impact of comorbidities on excess mortality in detail. We used the CCI as a well-accepted comorbidity burden index for adjusting for concomitant diseases [22, 23, 44, 45, 52, 53]. We chose the CCI because of its adaptability to large population databases using diagnostic codes from the ICD-10 [44]. It has also been documented that excess deaths among hip fracture patients can mainly be explained by the conditions predominantly responsible for mortality in the general population, i.e. those represented in the CCI [54]. However, we know that as a composite index it does not discriminate well between diseases, i.e. it equates the entities. Models incorporating comorbidities as individual variables perform better in predicting mortality than the weighted index [22]. The CCI ignores most of the disorders known to cause secondary osteoporosis [54], and it does not include hyperthyroidism or Parkinson's disease which are known to increase the propensity to falls [47]. Furthermore, it does not allow for risk stratification based on disease severity [22, 44]. Further research is needed to identify the specific diseases most responsible for the excess mortality.

It is possible that the excess risk of death in our analysis was slightly overestimated due to measurement bias. Our data collection started from 2004, and some subjects with unascertained fractures before 2004 might have been misclassified as incident cases (fracture group) or non-fracture patients (reference group). This misclassification might have resulted in slightly overestimating mortality in both groups. However, as the risk for further hip fracture after previous hip fracture is over 2-fold [3, 55] and a subsequent fracture is associated with increased mortality risk [56], the overestimation would have been higher in the fracture group, resulting in a slightly overestimated excess mortality.

The comorbidity data for both groups were collected at the time of, and for 1 year before, the index dates of a hip fracture cases. We are aware that by using hospitalization data as a part of index case definition we might have introduced differential misclassification into assessing comorbidity. However, we believe that people with severe life-threatening conditions would have received health care, and in including data from hospitalization episodes (including primary and secondary diagnoses) within the 12-months recall period into CCI for individuals in the reference group might mitigate some of this bias. Further, we speculate that potential differential misclassification described above might lead to overestimating the effect of comorbid conditions on mortality and thus support our main finding of hip fracture as a major independent risk factor for death.

To our knowledge, this is the first population-based observational study to estimate the impact of hip fracture on mortality in Eastern Europe. The strength of our analysis lies in the use of a data source with nationwide coverage (EHIF data). We had a large sample size of a representative population (given the >94% population coverage of the EHIF), long follow-up, and standardized recording of health events across the period of observation, which avoids problems related to imperfect recall and incomplete records. The large sample size provided a high number of events (deaths) to derive precise estimates over the long follow-up period, and the high frequency of observations allowed for assessment of rapid and extensive changes during the first months after fracture. We believe that our study provides informative results allowing inferences to other Eastern European hip fracture populations ≥50 years of age.

Conclusion

This population-based study is a contemporary evaluation of the impact of hip fractures on mortality in Eastern Europe and adds to the rather scant data previously available. By the end of the 10-year follow-up, 1 in 4 deaths in the hip fracture group was attributable to the hip fracture. We found a high immediate excess risk of death in older age groups (≥80 years) and gradually accumulating excess risk in younger age groups (50–79 years), that was more pronounced in men than in women. Compared to the pooled estimates, the excess risk of death in younger (50–79 years) Estonian men and women was higher, particularly in the first months and years after fracture. The results indicate an attributable impact of hip fracture as a major independent risk factor for death, and suggest that preventive efforts and post fracture rehabilitation and social care are essential to reduce the excess risk of death. To reduce the excess mortality following hip fracture, research should focus on refining country- or region-specific prognostic indicators.

Abbreviations

CCI: Charlson Comorbidity Index; EHIF: Estonian Health Insurance Fund; ICD-10: The International Classification of Diseases, Tenth Revision; SD: Standard deviation

Acknowledgements

We thank Prof. Esa Läärä from the University of Oulu for his help with methodology, and Allison Krug and Elizabeth Wager for editorial contribution.

Funding

The work was supported by the Estonian Science Foundation [grant number 9368] and the Estonian Ministry of Education and Research [grant numbers IUT 34–17, IUT 2–8]. The funders had no role in study design, data collection and analysis, decision to publish, or preparation of the manuscript.

Authors' contributions

All authors, MJ, MR, RK, ML, and AU, participated in the design of the study, in the interpretation of the results, in the elaboration of the manuscript, and approved the final draft. MR performed the statistical analysis. MJ wrote the manuscript. All authors read and approved the final manuscript.

Competing interests

The authors declare that they have no competing interests.

Consent for publication

Not applicable.

Author details

[1]Institute of Family Medicine and Public Health, University of Tartu, Ravila st 19, 50411 Tartu, Estonia. [2]Institute of Clinical Medicine, University of Tartu, L. Puusepa st 8, 51014 Tartu, Estonia. [3]Internal Medicine Clinic, Tartu University Hospital, L. Puusepa st 8, 51014 Tartu, Estonia.

References

1. Abrahamsen B, van Staa T, Ariely R, Olson M, Cooper C. Excess mortality following hip fracture: a systematic epidemiological review. Osteoporos Int. 2009;20:1633–50. doi:10.1007/s00198-009-0920-3.
2. Johnell O, Kanis JA, Odén A, Sernbo I, Redlund-Johnell I, Petterson C, et al. Mortality after osteoporotic fractures. Osteoporos Int. 2004;15:38–42. doi:10.1007/s00198-003-1490-4.
3. Hernlund E, Svedbom A, Ivergård M, Compston J, Cooper C, Stenmark J, et al. Osteoporosis in the European Union: medical management, epidemiology and economic burden. A report prepared in collaboration with the International Osteoporosis Foundation (IOF) and the European Federation of Pharmaceutical Industry Associations (EFPIA). Arch Osteoporos. 2013;8:136. doi:10.1007/s11657-013-0136-1.
4. Kanis JA, Hiligsmann M. The application of health technology assessment in osteoporosis. Best Pract Res Clin Endocrinol Metab. 2014;28:895–910. doi:10.1016/j.beem.2014.04.001.

5. Haentjens P, Magaziner J, Colón-Emeric CS, Vanderschueren D, Milisen K, Velkeniers B, et al. Meta-analysis: excess mortality after hip fracture among older women and men. Ann Intern Med. 2010;152:380–90. doi:10.1059/0003-4819-152-6-201003160-00008.Meta-analysis.
6. Vestergaard P, Rejnmark L, Mosekilde L. Increased mortality in patients with a hip fracture-effect of pre-morbid conditions and post-fracture complications. Osteoporos Int. 2007;18:1583–93. doi:10.1007/s00198-007-0403-3.
7. Tosteson ANA, Gottlieb DJ, Radley DC, Fisher ES, Melton LJ. Excess mortality following hip fracture: the role of underlying health status. Osteoporos Int. 2007;18:1463–72. doi:10.1007/s00198-007-0429-6.
8. Forsen L, Søgaard AJA, Meyer HE, Forsén L, Edna T-H, Kopjar B. Survival after hip fracture: short-and long-term excess mortality according to age and gender. Osteoporos Int. 1999;10:73–8. doi:10.1007/s001980050197.
9. Michaëlsson K, Nordström P, Nordström A, Garmo H, Byberg L, Pedersen NL, et al. Impact of hip fracture on mortality: a cohort study in hip fracture discordant identical twins. J Bone Miner Res. 2014;29:424–31. doi:10.1002/jbmr.2029.
10. Kurtinaitis J, Dadonienė J, Kvederas G, Porvaneckas N, Butėnas T. Mortality after femoral neck fractures: a two-year follow-up. Medicina (Kaunas). 2012;48:145–9. http://www.ncbi.nlm.nih.gov/pubmed/22588346. Accessed 6 Mar 2015
11. Sebestyén A, Boncz I, Sándor J, Nyárády J. Effect of surgical delay on early mortality in patients with femoral neck fracture. Int Orthop. 2008;32:375–9. doi:10.1007/s00264-007-0331-z.
12. Wilk R, Skrzypek M, Kowalska M, Kusz D, Wielgórecki A, Horyniecki M, et al. Standardized incidence and trend of osteoporotic hip fracture in Polish women and men: a nine year observation. Maturitas. 2013;77:59–63. doi:10.1016/j.maturitas.2013.09.004.
13. Icks A, Arend W, Becker C, Rapp K, Jungbluth P, Haastert B. Incidence of hip fractures in Germany, 1995-2010. Arch Osteoporos. 2013;8:140. doi:10.1007/s11657-013-0140-5.
14. Jürisson M, Vorobjov S, Kallikorm R, Lember M, Uusküla A. The incidence of hip fractures in Estonia, 2005-2012. Osteoporos Int. 2015;26:77–84. doi:10.1007/s00198-014-2820-4.
15. Eurostat. Eurostat. 2011. http://ec.europa.eu/eurostat/web/population-demography-migration-projections/population-data/database. Accessed 24 Jan 2017.
16. Statistics Estonia/Statistikaamet. http://www.stat.ee/database. Accessed 15 Oct 2016.
17. Estonian Health Insurance Fund - Eesti Haigekassa. https://www.haigekassa.ee/en/annual-reports. Accessed 29 Apr 2016.
18. Lix L, Azimaee M, Osman B. Osteoporosis-related fracture case definitions for population-based administrative data. BMC Public Health. 2012;12:301. https://bmcpublichealth.biomedcentral.com/articles/10.1186/1471-2458-12-301. Accessed 5 Feb 2014
19. Charlson ME, Pompei P, Ales KL, MacKenzie CR, Medical C. A new method of classifying prognostic comorbidity in longitudinal studies: development and validation. J Chronic Dis. 1987;40:373–83. doi:10.1016/0021-9681(87)90171-8.
20. Quan H, Sundararajan V, Halfon P, Fong A. Coding algorithms for defining comorbidities in ICD-9-CM and ICD-10 administrative data. Med Care. 2005;43:1130–9. https://www.ncbi.nlm.nih.gov/pubmed/16224307. Accessed 4 Jul 2014
21. Quan H, Li B, Couris CM, Fushimi K, Graham P, Hider P, et al. Updating and validating the Charlson comorbidity index and score for risk adjustment in hospital discharge abstracts using data from 6 countries. Am J Epidemiol. 2011;173:676–82. doi:10.1093/aje/kwq433.
22. Toson B, Harvey LA, Close JCT. The ICD-10 Charlson Comorbidity Index predicted mortality but not resource utilization following hip fracture. J Clin Epidemiol. 2015;68:44–51. doi:10.1016/j.jclinepi.2014.09.017.
23. Radley DC, Gottlieb DJ, Fisher ES, Tosteson ANA. Comorbidity risk-adjustment strategies are comparable among persons with hip fracture. J Clin Epidemiol. 2008;61:580–7. doi:10.1016/j.jclinepi.2007.08.001.
24. Sjölander A, Greenland S. Ignoring the matching variables in cohort studies - When is it valid and why? Stat med. 2013;32:4696–708. doi:10.1002/sim.5879.
25. R Core Team. R: the R project for statistical computing. R Foundation for Statistical Computing, Vienna, Austria. 2015. https://www.r-project.org/. Accessed 22 Mar 2016.
26. Carstensen B, Plummer M, Laara E, Hills M. Epi: a package for statistical analysis in epidemiology. R package version 2.7. 2016. http://cran.r-project.org/package=Epi. Accessed 9 Mar 2017.
27. Dowle M, Srinivasan A, Gorecki J, Short T, Lianoglou S, Antonyan E. data.table: extension of data.frame. R package version 1.9.8. 2016. https://cran.r-project.org/package=data.table. Accessed 9 Mar 2017.
28. Wickham H, Francois R. A grammar of data manipulation. R package dplyr version 0.5.0. 2016. https://cran.r-project.org/package=dplyr. Accessed 9 Mar 2017.
29. Canty A, Ripley B. boot: Bootstrap R (S-Plus) functions. R package version 1.3–18. 2016. https://cran.r-project.org/web/packages/boot. Accessed 9 Mar 2017.
30. Calaway R, RevolutionAnalytics, Weston S. Foreach: provides Foreach looping construct for R. R package version 1.4.3. 2015. https://cran.r-project.org/package=foreach. Accessed 9 Mar 2017.
31. Calaway R, RevolutionAnalytics, Weston S, Tenenbaum D. doParallel: Foreach parallel adaptor for the "parallel" package. R package version 1.0.10. 2015. https://cran.r-project.org/package=doParallel. Accessed 9 Mar 2017.
32. Wickham H. ggplot2: elegant graphics for data analysis: Springer; 2009. https://link.springer.com/book/10.1007%2F978-0-387-98141-3.
33. Nordentoft M, Wahlbeck K, Hällgren J, Westman J, Ösby U, Alinaghizadeh H, et al. Excess mortality, causes of death and life expectancy in 270,770 patients with recent onset of mental disorders in Denmark, Finland and Sweden. PLoS One. 2013;8:e55176. doi:10.1371/journal.pone.0055176.
34. Tancredi M, Rosengren A, Svensson A-M, Kosiborod M, Pivodic A, Gudbjörnsdottir S, et al. Excess mortality among persons with type 2 diabetes. http://www.nejm.org/doi/full/10.1056/NEJMoa1504347#t=article; 2015. doi:10.1056/NEJMOA1504347.
35. Kannegaard PN, van der Mark S, Eiken P, Abrahamsen B. Excess mortality in men compared with women following a hip fracture. National analysis of comedications, comorbidity and survival. Age Ageing. 2010;39:203–9. doi:10.1093/ageing/afp221.
36. Kanis JA, Oden A, Johnell O, De Laet C, Jonsson B, Oglesby AK. The components of excess mortality after hip fracture. Bone. 2003;32:468–73. doi:10.1016/S8756-3282(03)00061-9.
37. Omsland TK, Emaus N, Tell GS, Magnus JH, Ahmed LA, Holvik K, et al. Mortality following the first hip fracture in Norwegian women and men (1999–2008). A NOREPOS study. Bone. 2014;63C:81–6. doi:10.1016/j.bone.2014.02.016.
38. Klop C, Welsing PMJ, Cooper C, Harvey NC, Elders PJM, Bijlsma JWJ, et al. Mortality in British hip fracture patients, 2000–2010: a population-based retrospective cohort study. Bone. 2014;66:171–7.
39. Klop C, van Staa TP, Cooper C, Harvey NC, de Vries F. The epidemiology of mortality after fracture in England: variation by age, sex, time, geographic location, and ethnicity. Osteoporos Int. 2017;28:161–8. doi:10.1007/s00198-016-3787-0.
40. Rapp K, Becker C, Lamb SE, Icks A, Klenk J. Hip fractures in institutionalized elderly people: incidence rates and excess mortality. J Bone Miner Res. 2008;23:1825–31. doi:10.1359/jbmr.080702.
41. LeBlanc ES, Hillier TA, Pedula KL, Rizzo JH, Cawthon PM, Fink HA, et al. Hip fracture and increased short-term but not long-term mortality in healthy older women. Arch Intern Med. 2011;171:1831. doi:10.1001/archinternmed.2011.447.
42. Jürisson M, Pisarev H, Kanis J, Borgström F, Svedbom A, Kallikorm R, et al. Quality of life, resource use, and costs related to hip fracture in Estonia. Osteoporos Int. 2016;27:2555–66. doi:10.1007/s00198-016-3544-4.
43. Hu F, Jiang C, Shen J, Tang P, Wang Y. Preoperative predictors for mortality following hip fracture surgery: a systematic review and meta-analysis. Injury. 2012;43:676–85. doi:10.1016/j.injury.2011.05.017.
44. Hindmarsh D, Loh M, Finch CF, Hayen A, Close JCT. Effect of comorbidity on relative survival following hospitalisation for fall-related hip fracture in older people. Australas J Ageing. 2014;33:E1–7. doi:10.1111/j.1741-6612.2012.00638.x.
45. Luise C, Brimacombe M, Pedersen L, Sørensen HT, de Luise C. Comorbidity and mortality following hip fracture: a population-based cohort study. Aging Clin Exp Res. 2008;20:412–8. doi:10.1007/BF03325146.
46. Cenzer IS, Tang V, Boscardin WJ, Smith AK, Ritchie C, Wallhagen MI, et al. One-year mortality after hip fracture: development and validation of a prognostic index. J am Geriatr Soc. 2016;64:1863–8. doi:10.1111/jgs.14237.
47. Cauley JA, Cawthon PM, Peters KE, Cummings SR, Ensrud KE, Bauer DC, et al. Risk factors for hip fracture in older men: the osteoporotic fractures in men study (MrOS). J Bone Miner Res. 2016;31:1810–9. doi:10.1002/jbmr.2836.
48. Wehren LE, Hawkes WG, Orwig DL, Hebel JR, Zimmerman SI, Magaziner J. Gender differences in mortality after hip fracture: the role of infection. J Bone Miner Res. 2003;18:2231–7. doi:10.1359/jbmr.2003.18.12.2231.
49. Endo Y, Aharonoff G, Zuckerman J, Egol K, Koval K. Gender differences in patients with hip fracture: a greater risk of morbidity and mortality in men. J Orthop Trauma. 2005;19:29–35. https://www.ncbi.nlm.nih.gov/pubmed/15668581. Accessed 10 Mar 2016
50. Holt G, Smith R, Duncan K, Hutchison JD, Gregori A. Gender differences in epidemiology and outcome after hip fracture: evidence from the Scottish

hip fracture audit. J Bone Joint Surg Br. 2008;90:480–3. doi:10.1302/0301-620X.90B4.20264.
51. Thorne K, Johansen A, Akbari A, Williams JG, Roberts SE. The impact of social deprivation on mortality following hip fracture in England and Wales: a record linkage study. Osteoporos Int. 2016;27:2727–37. doi:10.1007/s00198-016-3608-5.
52. Neuhaus V, King J, Hageman MG, Ring DC. Charlson comorbidity indices and in-hospital deaths in patients with hip fractures. Clin Orthop Relat Res. 2013;471:1712–9. doi:10.1007/s11999-012-2705-9.
53. Smith T, Pelpola K, Ball M, Ong A, Myint PK. Pre-operative indicators for mortality following hip fracture surgery: a systematic review and meta-analysis. Age Ageing. 2014;43:464–71.
54. Melton LJ, Atkinson EJ, St. Sauver JL, Achenbach SJ, Therneau TM, Rocca WA, et al. Predictors of excess mortality after fracture: a population-based cohort study. J Bone Miner Res. 2014;29:1681–90. doi:10.1002/jbmr.2193.
55. Klotzbuecher CM, Ross PD, Landsman PB, Abbott TA, Berger M. Patients with prior fractures have an increased risk of future fractures: a summary of the literature and statistical synthesis. J Bone Miner Res. 2010;15:721–39. doi: 10.1359/jbmr.2000.15.4.721.
56. Bliuc D, Nguyen ND, Milch VE, Nguyen TV, Eisman JA, Center JR. Mortality risk associated with low-trauma osteoporotic fracture and subsequent fracture in men and women. JAMA. 2009;301:513–21. doi:10.1001/jama.2009.50.

2

Clavicle fractures: epidemiology, classification and treatment of 2 422 fractures in the Swedish Fracture Register; an observational study

Caroline Kihlström[1*], Michael Möller[2], Katarina Lönn[1] and Olof Wolf[1]

Abstract

Background: Large multi-centre studies of clavicle fractures have so far been missing. The aim of this observational study was to describe the epidemiology, classification and treatment of clavicle fractures in the The Swedish Fracture Register (SFR) that collects national prospective data from large fracture populations.

Methods: Data were retrieved from the SFR on all clavicle fractures sustained by patients ≥ 15 years of age in 2013–2014 ($n = 2\ 422$) with regards to date of injury, cause of injury, fracture classification and treatment.

Results: Sixty-eight per cent of the clavicle fractures occurred in males. The largest subgroup was males aged 15–24 years, representing 21% of clavicle fractures. At the ages of 65 years and above, females sustained more clavicle fractures than males. Same-level falls and bicycle accidents were the most common injury mechanisms. Displaced midshaft fractures constituted 43% of all fractures and were the most frequently operated fractures. Seventeen per cent of the patients underwent operative treatment within 30 days of the injury, where plate fixation was the choice of treatment in 94% of fractures.

Conclusion: The largest patient group was young males. Displaced midshaft fractures were the most common type of clavicle fracture as well as the most frequently operated type of fracture.

Keywords: Clavicle fracture, Epidemiology, Classification, Treatment, The Swedish Fracture Register

Background

Fractures of the clavicle, which primarily occur in young males, constitute 2.6–4% of all fractures in adults [1, 4]. A male dominance of approximately 70% has been reported [1–4]. The most frequent injury mechanism is a direct fall on the shoulder [2–4]. Fractures are often sustained during sports activities or traffic accidents [1–4].

The majority (69–82%) of fractures occur in the midshaft of the clavicle, followed by 12–26% in the lateral part and 2–6% in the medial part [1–4]. This can be anatomically explained by the fact that the medial and lateral parts of the clavicle are firmly secured by strong ligaments and muscles, whereas the middle part of the clavicle lacks any strong attachments and thus is more vulnerable to trauma. The muscle attachments often cause a dislocation of the major fragments in clavicle fractures and a shortening of the clavicle, particularly in midshaft fractures [5].

Traditionally, clavicle fractures have been treated almost exclusively non-operatively, regardless of the type of fracture. Studies in the 1960s described good functional results for non operatively treated midshaft clavicle fractures and a lower nonunion rate compared to fractures treated with primary open reduction [6, 7]. In contrast, several more recent studies have reported opposite results with newer methods of fracture fixation [8–14], which may have contributed to the 705% increase in operative treatment of clavicle fractures in Sweden between 2001 and 2012 [15]. Optimal treatment of clavicle fractures however remains a debated subject.

* Correspondence: caroline.kihlstrom@akademiska.se
[1]Department of Orthopaedics, Institute of Surgical Sciences, Uppsala University Hospital, SE-751 85 Uppsala, Sweden

Simple slings, collar 'n' cuffs and figure-of-eight-bandages are commonly used to immobilise the fracture during the first weeks in non-operatively treated fractures [16], which often include medial fractures, most lateral fractures and midshaft fractures without displacement [17].

The most commonly used operative method today is open reduction and internal plate fixation; a smaller number of fractures are treated with intramedullary nails, pins or wires [14, 17].

Because the treatment of clavicle fractures is a debated question and because there are no national guidelines in place for it in Sweden, treatment can vary between different departments, with regards both to which fractures are operated and operative method chosen ([18]).

Previous studies on clavicle fractures have generally been limited to one specific orthopaedic department at a time and thus to a limited patient material [2–4] with susceptibility to local treatment traditions that may not adequately reflect a more general treatment routine. Multi-centre studies that include conformed data from a large number of departments have so far been missing. The largest study populations in epidemiological studies are also at least 20 years old [2–4]. Much has happened in the area of treatment of clavicle fractures since then, especially with the rate of operative treatment having increased substantially even with an absence of studies showing compelling evidence to support this [15]. An updated study on the current epidemiology, classification and treatment of clavicle fractures in a more generalised setting would hopefully create a framework for contextual aid for future analysis of the best treatment for clavicle fractures. The aim of this study was therefore to describe the modern epidemiology, classification and treatment of clavicle fractures in Sweden, with a secondary aim of assessing the presence of polytrauma in patients with clavicle fractures.

Methods

Data collection and study population

In the Swedish Fracture Register (SFR), started in 2011, information about fractures of the extremities, pelvis and spine is registered locally in affiliated departments, building up a national database of the epidemiology, classification and treatment of different fractures [19]. Affiliated departments are hospital-based and include university hospitals, district general hospitals and general hospitals since 2013, creating a mixed catchment population. At the end of 2013, there were 7 registering departments (1 university hospital, 5 general hospitals and 1 district general hospital). The number had increased to 22 at the end of 2014 (3 university hospitals, 11 general district hospitals and 8 district hospitals). The number of orthopaedic departments that treat fractures in Sweden is approximately 55. Hence apprixmately 44% of Sweden's orthopaedic departments reported to the SFR at the end of the study period. Due to lack of full national coverage, the SFR can not provide numbers on incidence of fractures but a recent study [15] showed that the incidence of clavicle fractures in Sweden increased from 35.6 per 100,000 person-years in 2001 to 59.3 per 100,000 person-years in 2012. Clavicle fractures have been registered since April 2012 [19–21].

Data collected in the SFR include date of injury, cause of injury, fracture classification and treatment. Inclusion requires the patient to have a permanent Swedish personal identity number and a radiographically verified fracture. Fractures need also to have occurred in Sweden. Fractures that have occurred abroad are excluded from registration [19]. Completeness of registrations of clavicle fractures has yet to be investigated. We have used data from the SFR to construct an observational descriptive register study, employing a cross-sectional design. Selection criteria were all registered clavicle fractures sustained in 2013–2014 and patients had to be at least 15 years of age. No additional exclusion criteria were applied.

Medical records and radiographs were also reviewed for the presence of polytrauma in a subset local population comprising all clavicle fractures that were treated at the authors' own orthopaedic department at Uppsala University Hospital during the selected period. The selection of department was made so as to allow for full access to medical records and radiographs. This subpopulation was very similar to the overall population with regards to age, sex and fracture type distribution and is as such representative of the overall study population.

Variables

Injury mechanism

Four main categories were constructed for injury mechanism – falls, transport accidents, non-traumatic fractures and others. Falls were further sub-categorised into falls on the same level, falls from a level and unspecified falls. Transport accidents were sub-categorised into bicycle accidents, motorcycle accidents and other transport accidents. Pathological fractures, spontaneous fractures and stress fractures were grouped together and labeled non-traumatic fractures. The other-category included patients who had sustained their clavicle fractures for example from having been pushed to the ground or having suffered a direct impact from a person or object. Many sporting injuries sort into this category.

The registering doctor in the SFR classifies the energy level of the injury. The SFR has no strict guidelines for how to make the distinction between high- and low energy injuries, making the distinction rather subjective. Examples on how to classify the energy level are however presented in the registration module. Examples of high-energy injuries are traffic accidents, falls from heights and work place accidents with crushing injuries. Low-energy injuries are exemplified as falls on the same level and similar traumas.

Fracture classification

Clavicle fractures were classified according to Robinson's classification system for registration in the SFR (Fig. 1) [3].

Primary treatment

Operative treatment methods were divided into fixation with anatomical plates, standard plates, hook plates, intramedullary fixations and other methods. Who performed the operation was also taken into account, i.e. a consultant orthopaedic trauma surgeon, a consultant orthopaedic surgeon or a resident. For the non-operatively treated patients no information was provided on the type of sling received for short-term immobilisation or on the application of physiotherapy. Operative treatment was divided into an acute stage and an early stage. Acute stage operations are defined as such when they are registered in the SFR as the first type of treatment for a particular fracture. Early operations are defined as operations where non-operative treatment was the first registered choice of treatment but was abandoned early on for secondary operative treatment, typically after an X-ray follow-up 7–10 days after the injury shows a worsened fracture position. An upper cut-off value of 30 days was applied to filter out seemingly faulty registrations. Fractures being treated operatively after more than 30 days post-injury were considered to have been treated non-operatively as the first choice of treatment.

Polytrauma

Polytrauma was defined as having multiple radiographically verified concurrent fractures in addition to a clavicle fracture. All fracture types except for rib fractures were included, because they are usually radiographically diagnosed only if a trauma computed tomography scan has been performed and typically not seen on clavicular projections with conventional x-rays, making their frequency difficult to assess.

Statistical analysis

Data was summarised for fracture occurence with groupings of sex, age with subgroupings of both 10-year intervals and groupings of young (15–24 year-olds), mature (25–64 year-olds) and old (over 65 year-olds), time

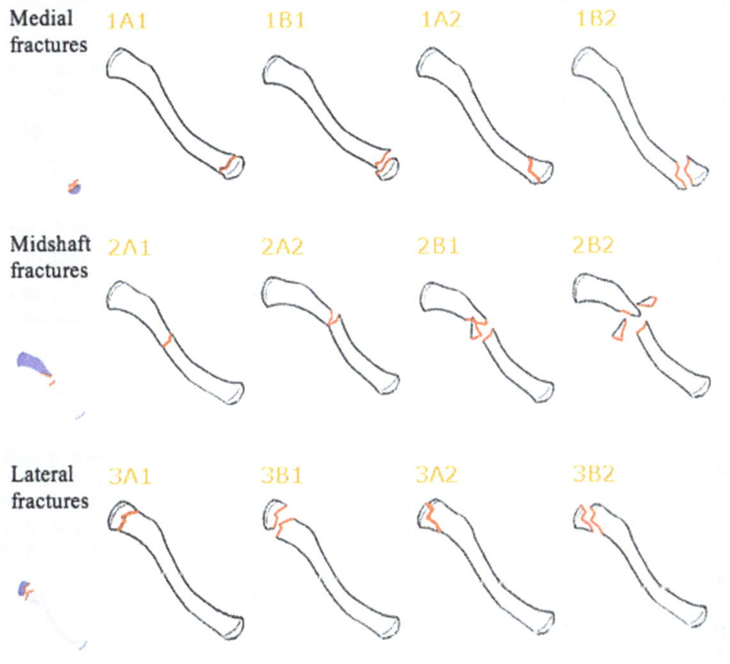

Fig. 1 Robinson's classification system for clavicle fractures as presented in the SFR's online registration module (18). *1A1* Medial, undisplaced, extra-articular. *1B1* Medial, displaced, extra-articular. *1A2* Medial, undisplaced, intra-articular. *1B2* Medial, displaced, intra-articular. *2A1* Midshaft, cortical alignment, undisplaced. *2A2* Midshaft, cortical alignment, angulated. *2B1* Midshaft, displaced, simple or wedge comminuted. *2B2* Midshaft, displaced, isolated or comminuted segmental. *3A1* Lateral, cortical alignment, extra-articular. *3B1* Lateral, displaced, extra-articular. *3A2* Lateral, cortical alignment, intra-articular. *3B2* Lateral, displaced, intra-articular. The use of the figure in this study has been approved by the SFR

of year and day of the week. Because of the descriptive nature of the study, formal testing of potential differences between subgroups was not made. Calculations of means, first and third quartiles and standard deviations (SD) were made.

A minority of the registrations (4%, *n* = 87) were incomplete and lacked one or more types of particular data, such as injury mechanism (1%, *n* = 24), energy level of injury (1%, *n* = 33) or type of treatment (2%, *n* = 41). In these cases data analysis of percentages is based on the total of each completely registered sub-data set.

Results

Epidemiology

We found 2 422 registered clavicle fractures in 2013–2014; 1 056 in 2013, 1 366 in 2014. Sixty-eight per cent (*n* = 1 654) of the clavicle fractures occurred in males and 32% (768) in females, creating a male:female ratio of 2.2:1. Mean age was 48 years (SD 23 years). Mean age was higher in females (mean 59 years, SD 23 years) than in males (mean 43 years, SD 21 years). The fractures occurred more often in younger than in older individuals (Fig. 2), with 15–24 year-olds representing 21% (*n* = 517) of the study population. Males in this age group represented 17% (*n* = 420) of the total fracture burden. As many as 45% of the females (*n* = 348) but only 17% (*n* =283) of the males were 65 years or older, creating a male:female ratio of 0.8:1 (*n* = 283:348) within the age group.

Fractures more frequently occurred during weekends, particularly on Saturdays, and had a peak occurrence in the summer months of May to August (Figs. 3 and 4).

Injury mechanism

The most common cause of injury was either a fall, generally on the same level, or a transport accident (Table 1). Bicycle accidents were by far the most common cause among the transport accidents, followed by motorcycle accidents. Males and younger patients most commonly sustained their clavicle fractures from transport accidents in comparison to females and older patients who more often sustained their clavicle fractures from a fall.

High-energy trauma was reported as the type of injury in 28% (*n* = 668) of the fractures. Males sustained more high-energy injuries than females: males 35% (*n* = 538) versus females 17% (*n* = 130). The mean age for high-energy injuries was also lower (41 years, SD 18 years) than that for low-energy injuries (51 years, SD 24 years).

Non-traumatic fractures included pathological fractures (*n* = 10), spontaneous fractures (*n* = 5) and stress fractures (*n* = 2).

Fracture classification

Fifty-two per cent (*n* = 1 271) of the clavicle fractures occurred on the left side. Four patients sustained simultaneous bilateral fractures and another 11 sustained multiple clavicle fractures on the same or opposite side at separate times of injury during the 2-year period. Only 0.7% (*n* = 16) of clavicle fractures were open fractures.

The most frequent fracture location was the midshaft of the clavicle. Among the midshaft fractures, 90% (*n* = 1 424) had some type of angulation or displacement (2A2, 2B1, 2B2) (Table 2). The most common fractures of all were the midshaft simple displaced or wedge comminuted 2B1 fractures. Medial fractures were uncommon. Ninety per cent (*n* = 649) of the lateral fractures were extra-articular. Lateral fractures were slightly more often displaced than undisplaced.

Displaced midshaft fractures (2B1 and 2B2) were found in 47% (*n* = 779) of the male patients versus 35% (*n* = 265) of the female patients. Conversely, lateral fractures were more frequent in females than in males. Medial and lateral fractures were much more common in the higher age groups while younger patients typically sustained midshaft clavicle fractures.

The majority of the high-energy injuries resulted in displaced midshaft clavicle fractures.

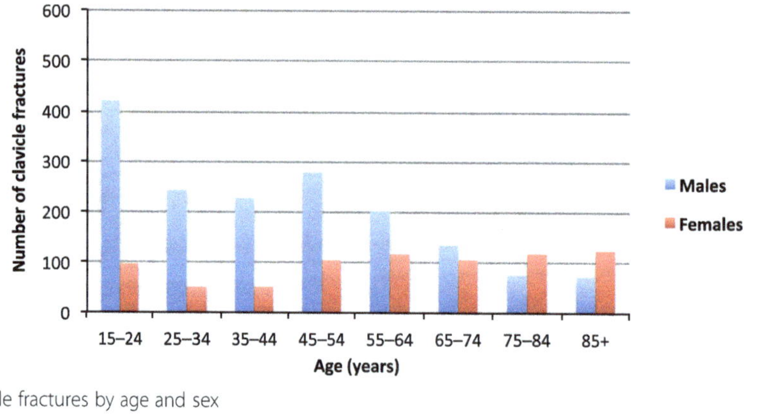

Fig. 2 Distribution of clavicle fractures by age and sex

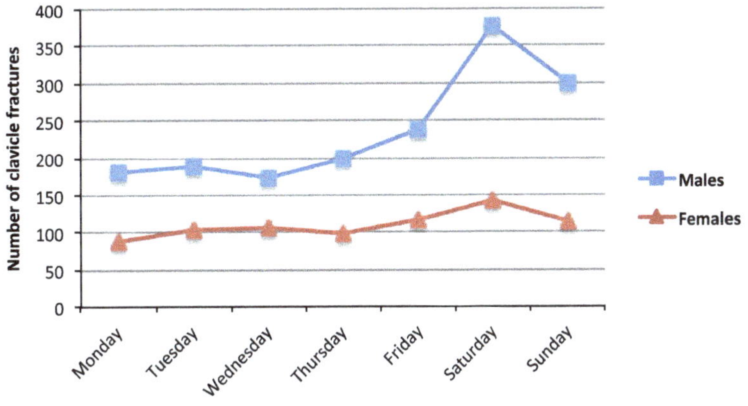

Fig. 3 Daily distribution of clavicle fractures by sex

Primary treatment

Eleven per cent ($n = 270$) of all fractures were treated operatively in the acute stage as the first choice of treatment after a median of 5 days (interquartile range 4–10 days). An additional 6% ($n = 138$) of the fractures were treated operatively after non-operative treatment had been abandoned at an early stage, after a median of 14 days (interquartile range 11–17 days).

Males, in comparison with females, were more likely to undergo operative treatment in the acute or early stages: 20% ($n = 323$) of the males versus 11% ($n = 85$) of the females. The mean age for operative treatment was 36 years (SD 15 years). The mean age for non-operative treatment was 51 years (SD 23 years).

Eighty percent of the operatively treated fractures were midshaft fractures (Table 3). The most frequently operated fractures were the fully displaced 2B1 and 2B2 midshaft fractures. Together, these two fracture types accounted for 73% ($n = 296/408$) of the operatively treated fractures. A fair few of the lateral displaced 3B1 and 3B2 fractures were also treated operatively but since they were not very frequent to begin with, they accounted for less than 20% of the total number of operated fractures. Few of the midshaft and lateral fractures without full displacement (2A1, 2A2, 3A1, 3A2) and none of the medial fractures were treated operatively.

Anatomical plates were by far the most common choice of operative treatment. Hook plates were used mainly for the lateral displaced extra-articular 3B1 fractures while intramedullary nailing was used mainly for the angulated midshaft 2A2 and simple displaced or wedge comminuted 2B1 fractures.

Consultant orthopaedic trauma surgeons performed 56% ($n = 227$) of the operations, consultant orthopaedic surgeons 35% ($n = 142$) and residents 7% ($n = 27$) (2% of surgeons were undefined).

Polytrauma

In the locally reviewed population of 321 clavicle fractures at Uppsala University Hospital 21% of patients ($n = 66$) had multiple radiographically verified concurrent fractures in addition to their clavicle fracture. The most prevalent concurrent fractures were those of the vertebral column, scapula, cranium and forearm (Table 4).

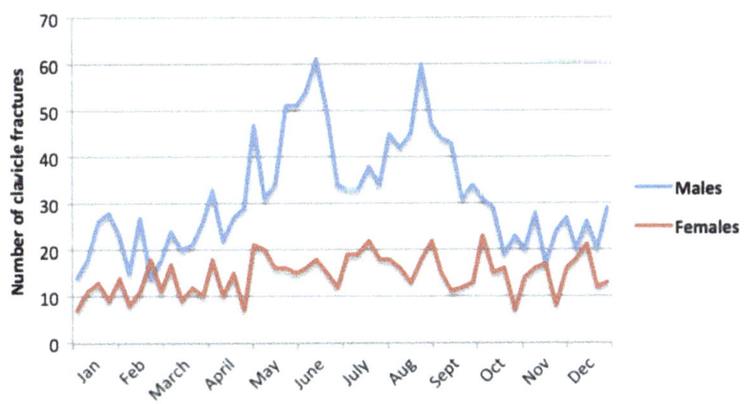

Fig. 4 Monthly distribution of clavicle fractures by sex

Table 1 Injury mechanism by sex, age and high-energy injuries

	Total, *n* (%)	Males, *n* (%)	Females, *n* (%)	Young, *n* (%)	Mature, *n* (%)	Old, *n* (%)	High-energy (%)
Fall	**1 175 (49.0)**	**663 (40.5)**	**512 (67.5)**	**200 (39.0)**	**467 (37.0)**	**508 (81.5)**	**101 (15.2)**
Fall on the same level	817 (34.1)	469 (28.6)	348 (45.8)	169 (32.9)	303 (24.0)	345 (55.4)	41 (6.2)
Fall from a height	210 (8.8)	117 (7.1)	93 (12.3)	10 (1.9)	101 (8.0)	99 (15.9)	55 (8.3)
Unspecified fall	148 (6.2)	77 (4.7)	71 (9.4)	21 (4.1)	63 (5.0)	64 (10.3)	5 (0.8)
Transport accident	**996 (41.5)**	**803 (49.0)**	**193 (25.4)**	**203 (39.6)**	**705 (55.9)**	**88 (14.1)**	**539 (81.1)**
Bicycle	492 (20.5)	404 (24.6)	88 (11.6)	58 (11.3)	394 (31.2)	40 (6.4)	183 (27.5)
Motorcycle	309 (12.9)	298 (18.2)	11 (1.4)	95 (18.5)	198 (15.7)	16 (2.6)	233 (35.0)
Other transport accident	195 (8.1)	101 (6.2)	94 (12.4)	50 (9.7)	113 (9.0)	32 (5.1)	123 (18.5)
Non-traumatic fractures	**17 (0.7)**	**7 (0.4)**	**10 (1.3)**	**0 (0)**	**6 (0.5)**	**11 (1.8)**	**0 (0)**
Other	**210 (8.8)**	**166 (10.1)**	**44 (5.8)**	**110 (21.4)**	**84 (6.7)**	**16 (2.6)**	**25 (3.8)**
Total	**2 398**	**1 639**	**759**	**513**	**1 262**	**623**	**665**

Young = 15–24 years of age, Mature = 25–64 years old, Old = 65+ years of age. Main groups of injury mechanisms are presented in bold letters, followed by subgroups in normal letters

Discussion

Main findings

In this observational study of clavicle fractures in Sweden, the largest patient group was males younger than 25 years of age and the most frequent causes of injury were same-level falls, bicycle and motorcycle accidents. Displaced midshaft fractures were the most common type of fracture. These fractures, together with extra-articular displaced lateral fractures, were also the most frequently operated fractures. Seventeen per cent of the fractures underwent operative treatment within 30 days of the injury, most commonly with plate fixation.

Comparisons with other studies

The sex-related distribution of clavicle fractures is in line with that reported in previous studies [1–4]. The mean age of our population of 48 years is actually higher than several other studies of adults, where the mean age ranged from 29 to 34 years. However, the youngest age for inclusion has varied between these studies. As in previous studies, we found that the mean age was highest for fractures occurring in the medial part of the clavicle and lowest for midshaft fractures and that the mean age was higher in females than in males [1–4].

Table 2 Fracture classification by sex, age and high-energy injuries

	Total, *n* (%)	Males, *n* (%)	Females, *n* (%)	Young, *n* (%)	Mature, *n* (%)	Old, *n* (%)	High energy, *n* (%)
Medial	**109 (4.5)**	**68 (4.1)**	**41 (5.3)**	**8 (1.5)**	**30 (2.4)**	**71 (11.3)**	**16 (2.4)**
1A1	49 (2.0)	33 (2.0)	16 (2.1)	4 (0.8)	15 (1.2)	30 (4.8)	7 (1.0)
1A2	16 (0.7)	9 (0.5)	7 (0.9)	1 (0.2)	5 (0.4)	10 (1.6)	3 (0.4)
1B1	33 (1.4)	18 (1.1)	15 (2.0)	3 (0.6)	7 (0.5)	23 (3.6)	3 (0.4)
1B2	11 (0.5)	8 (0.5)	3 (0.4)	0 (0)	3 (0.2)	8 (1.3)	3 (0.4)
Midshaft	**1 584 (65.4)**	**1 168 (70.6)**	**416 (54.2)**	**439 (84.9)**	**889 (69.8)**	**256 (40.6)**	**550 (82.3)**
2A1	160 (6.6)	113 (6.8)	47 (6.1)	62 (12.0)	70 (5.5)	28 (4.4)	50 (7.5)
2A2	380 (15.7)	276 (16.7)	104 (13.5)	161 (31.1)	158 (12.4)	61 (9.7)	107 (16.0)
2B1	676 (27.9)	489 (29.6)	187 (24.3)	161 (31.1)	387 (30.4)	128 (20.3)	232 (34.7)
2B2	368 (15.2)	290 (17.5)	78 (10.2)	55 (10.6)	274 (21.5)	39 (6.2)	161 (24.1)
Lateral	**719 (29.7)**	**410 (24.8)**	**309 (40.2)**	**68 (13.2)**	**351 (27.6)**	**300 (47.5)**	**100 (15.0)**
3A1	291 (12.0)	144 (8.7)	147 (19.1)	25 (4.8)	126 (9.9)	140 (22.2)	25 (3.7)
3A2	29 (1.2)	20 (1.2)	9 (1.2)	1 (0.2)	14 (1.1)	14 (2.2)	6 (0.9)
3B1	358 (14.8)	215 (13.0)	143 (18.6)	34 (6.6)	189 (14.8)	135 (21.4)	63 (9.4)
3B2	41 (1.7)	31 (1.9)	10 (1.3)	8 (1.5)	22 (1.7)	11 (1.7)	6 (0.9)
Not classified	**10 (0.4)**	**8 (0.5)**	**2 (0.3)**	**2 (0.4)**	**4 (0.3)**	**4 (0.6)**	**2 (0.3)**
Total	**2 422**	**1 654**	**768**	**517**	**1 274**	**631**	**668**

Young = 15–24 years of age, Mature = 25–64 years old, Old = 65+ years of age. Main groups of fracture classification are presented in bold letters, followed by subgroups in normal letters

Table 3 Operatively treated clavicle fractures in an acute or early stage by fracture classification including operative method

	Total, *n* (%)	Anatomical plate, *n* (%)	Hook plate, *n* (%)	Standard plate, *n* (%)	Intramedullary fixation, *n* (%)	Other method, *n* (%)
Midshaft	**326 (79.9)**	**281 (88.6)**	**1 (2.4)**	**24 (96.0)**	**19 (100.0)**	**1 (20)**
2A1	2 (0.5)	2 (0.6)	0 (0)	0 (0)	0 (0)	0 (0)
2A2	26 (6.4)	20 (6.3)	0 (0)	3 (12.0)	3 (15.8)	0 (0)
2B1	158 (38.7)	134 (42.3)	0 (0)	11 (44.0)	13 (68.4)	0 (0)
2B2	140 (34.3)	125 (39.4)	1 (2.4)	10 (40.0)	3 (15.8)	1 (20)
Lateral	**82 (20.1)**	**36 (11.4)**	**41 (97.6)**	**1 (4.0)**	**0 (0)**	**4 (80.0)**
3A1	4 (1.0)	1 (0.3)	2 (4.8)	0 (0)	0 (0)	1 (20.0)
3A2	0 (0)	0 (0)	0 (0)	0 (0)	0 (0)	0 (0)
3B1	68 (16.7)	33 (10.4)	33 (78.6)	1 (4.0)	0 (0)	1 (20.0)
3B2	10 (2.5)	2 (0.6)	6 (14.3)	0 (0)	0 (0)	2 (40.0)
Not classified	**0 (0)**	**0 (0)**	**0 (0)**	**0 (0)**	**0 (0)**	**0 (0)**
Total	**408**	**317**	**42**	**25**	**19**	**5**

Medial fractures are not included in the table because none of the medial fractures were treated operatively. Main groups of fracture classification are presented in bold letters, followed by subgroups in normal letters

Clavicle fractures occurred more frequently during the weekends and during the summer months. The finding is consistent with previous Swedish studies [2, 4] but in contrast with the findings of an Italian study [1]. Inasmuch as clavicle fractures are closely related to physical activities, the difference in frequency is possibly due in large part to an increase in outdoor activities during summer and weekends in Sweden.

Same-level falls have been reported as the most common cause of clavicle fractures not only in this but in previous studies as well [2, 3]. An Italian study reported the most common cause of fractures to be accidental falls in elderly but traffic accidents in young adults [1], which is not far off from the results of this study.

The finding that bicycle accidents were the second most common cause of clavicle fractures is in agreement with another Swedish epidemiological study demonstrating that bicycle accidents caused 45% of the clavicle fractures in females and 26% in males aged 15 years and above [2]. It is however in contrast with the findings of a Scotland-based epidemiological study [3], where only 11% of clavicle fractures were sustained through bicycle accidents, suggesting bicycle accidents are a more common cause of clavicle fractures in Sweden than in Scotland. The Scottish study population was however younger than ours, with a mean age of 34 and a lower age limit for inclusion of 13.

Table 4 Concurrent fractures within each fracture group in addition to a patient's clavicle fracture in patients seen at Uppsala University Hospital

Concurrent fracture location	Fractures, *n* (%)
Vertebral column	19 (18)
Scapula (including 2 floating shoulders)	15 (15)
Cranium	13 (13)
Radius and/or ulna	11 (11)
Hand	10 (10)
Humerus	7 (7)
Sternum	7 (7)
Pelvis	6 (6)
Femur	5 (5)
Tibia and/or fibula	5 (5)
Contralateral clavicle, foot or patella	5 (5)
Total	103

As in previous studies, left-sided fractures were slightly more common than right-sided fractures [2, 4, 5, 10], whereas bilateral clavicle fractures and open fractures were uncommon [1, 2, 14].

The distribution of fracture types is consistent with previous results [1–4]. Sociodemographic variations such as age or sports involvement among the population as well as injury mechanism should reasonably affect the distribution, suggesting similarities in these areas between our nationally collected data with previous single-department studies.

Clavicle fractures were the single most common fracture type in polytrauma patients at the Orthopaedic Department, Sahlgrenska University Hospital (Möller M., Sahlgrenska University Hospital 2016, personal communication February 13). The reported frequency of concomitant orthopaedic injuries has varied somewhat between different studies in the past. Robinson [3] reported that among his population of 1 000 patients, 142 required inpatient care, and out of these, 75 had other orthopaedic injuries. A Swedish study [2] reported that only 5% of 185 patients had another extremity fracture with an additional 20% having rib fractures. In comparison to these studies, we had a large proportion of orthopaedic multiple trauma patients in our local population. This observation might be explained with the argument that Uppsala University Hospital is a regional referral centre for polytraumatised patients in need of orthopaedic and neurosurgical treatment.

Our rate of operative treatment was lower than that reported in a meta-analysis of 2 144 midshaft fractures [14], where as many as 47% of the total number of fractures and 79% of the displaced midshaft fractures were treated operatively. The most commonly operated fractures, the displaced midshaft ones, occurred more often in males than in females, which can help explain why the rate of operative treatment was higher in males than in females. In the meta-analysis [14] intramedullary fixation was more common (17%) than in our material (5%). Previous studies have shown similar results with regards to epidemiology and classification of clavicle fractures, which might otherwise have helped to explain the discrepancies in treatment. It therefore seems like treatment decisions are influenced much by local traditions and surgeon preferences, a notion that is supported in the literature [15]. Since convincing evidence to support the selection of one or the other type of treatment (operative versus non-operative treatment, plate fixation versus intramedullary nailing etc.) is missing, this is hardly surprising.

Strengths of the study

One of the strengths of the present study is that using data from the SFR provides a very large database of clavicle fractures. Data on 2 422 clavicle fractures were uniformly recorded in the SFR according to a pre-specified standard. The material describes national prospective data, reducing the bias of local differences in epidemiology, sociodemographics and treatment traditions. A validation study of the SFR showed high accuracy in classification of tibia fractures when comparing registered data to a gold standard, as well as good inter-observer agreement [22]. Another strength of this observational study is that all data were collected during a recent short period of only 2 years, whereas data collection in earlier studies has often been conducted for many years [1, 3, 13]. This provides an up-to-date overview of epidemiology, classification and treatment of clavicle fractures in recent time. Our minimum age (15 years) was higher than that of many other studies [1, 3, 13], which in our opinion creates a better platform for analysis of an adult population because of the clinically significant high remodelling capacity of clavicle fractures in children and adolescents [23].

Limitations of the study

The SFR's coverage at the end of the study period was, with 22 participating departments, approximately 44% of Sweden's orthopaedic departments. Although more representative of the national population of clavicle fractures than singe-centre studies, the incomplete coverage is a limitation. Completeness has not yet been investigated in the area of clavicle fracture registrations in the SFR. The classification of clavicle fractures in the SFR has not yet been validated.

Implications and future research

This study is unique in the sense that it assesses uniformly registered data on epidemiology, classification and treatment of clavicle fractures from a large number of orthopaedic departments. The best treatment for clavicle fractures is a debated subject. In order to know how best to treat them, we must first know what and whom we are treating. This study serves as an up-to-date overview of modern clavicle fractures that will hopefully provide a framework for future research on the treatment of clavicle fractures. Future studies should focus on outcome aspects of the treatment of clavicle fractures in order to obtain better guidelines for treatment.

Conclusions

In conclusion, we have described the epidemiology of clavicle fractures that were registered over a 2-year period in the prospective national SFR for injury mechanism, fracture classification and treatment. The largest patient group was young males. Displaced midshaft fractures were the most common type of clavicle fracture as well as the most frequently operated type of fracture.

Abbreviations

SFR: The Swedish Fracture Register

Acknowledgements

Not applicable.

Funding

No external sources of funding have been used.

Authors' contributions

CK analysed the data and wrote the manuscript with close guidance from OW, constructed tables and figures and compiled references. MM helped with data collection and revised the manuscript. KL provided general input and support along the way. OW planned the outline of the project, collected data and revised the manuscript. All authors read and approved the final manuscript.

Authors' information

Not applicable.

Competing interests

The authors declare that they have no competing interests.

Consent for publication

Not applicable.

Author details
[1]Department of Orthopaedics, Institute of Surgical Sciences, Uppsala University Hospital, SE-751 85 Uppsala, Sweden. [2]Department of Orthopaedics, Sahlgrenska University Hospital Gothenburg/ Mölndal, SE-431 80 Mölndal, Sweden.

References

1. Postacchini F, Gumina S, De Santis P, Albo F. Epidemiology of clavicle fractures. J Shoulder Elbow Surg. 2002;11(5):452–6.
2. Nowak J, Mallmin H, Larsson S. The aetiology and epidemiology of clavicular fractures. A prospective study during a 2-year period in Uppsala, Sweden. Injury. 2000;31(5):353–8.
3. Robinson CM. Fractures of the clavicle in the adult. Epidemiology and classification. J Bone Joint Surg Br. 1998;80(3):476–84.
4. Nordqvist A, Petersson C. The incidence of fractures of the clavicle. Clin Orthop Relat Res. 1994;300:127–32.
5. Smekal V, Oberladstaetter J, Struve P, Krappinger D. Shaft fractures of the clavicle: current concepts. Arch Orthop Trauma Surg. 2009;129(6):807–15.
6. Neer 2nd CS. Nonunion of the clavicle. J Am Med Assoc. 1960;172:1006–11.
7. Rowe CR. An atlas of anatomy and treatment of midclavicular fractures. Clin Orthop Relat Res. 1968;58:29–42.
8. Virtanen KJ, Remes V, Pajarinen J, Savolainen V, Bjorkenheim JM, Paavola M. Sling compared with plate osteosynthesis for treatment of displaced midshaft clavicular fractures: a randomized clinical trial. J Bone Joint Surg Am. 2012;94(17):1546–53.
9. Altamimi SA, McKee MD. Nonoperative treatment compared with plate fixation of displaced midshaft clavicular fractures. Surgical technique. J Bone Joint Surg Am. 2008;90(Suppl 2 Pt 1):1–8.
10. Lazarides S, Zafiropoulos G. Conservative treatment of fractures at the middle third of the clavicle: the relevance of shortening and clinical outcome. J Shoulder Elbow Surg. 2006;15(2):191–4.
11. McKee MD, Pedersen EM, Jones C, Stephen DJ, Kreder HJ, Schemitsch EH, et al. Deficits following nonoperative treatment of displaced midshaft clavicular fractures. J Bone Joint Surg Am. 2006;88(1):35–40.
12. Nowak J, Holgersson M, Larsson S. Sequelae from clavicular fractures are common: a prospective study of 222 patients. Acta Orthop. 2005;76(4):496–502.
13. Robinson CM, Court-Brown CM, McQueen MM, Wakefield AE. Estimating the risk of nonunion following nonoperative treatment of a clavicular fracture. J Bone Joint Surg Am. 2004;86-a(7):1359–65.
14. Zlowodzki M, Zelle BA, Cole PA, Jeray K, McKee MD. Treatment of acute midshaft clavicle fractures: systematic review of 2144 fractures: on behalf of the Evidence-Based Orthopaedic Trauma Working Group. J Orthop Trauma. 2005;19(7):504–7.
15. Huttunen TT, Launonen AP, Berg HE, Lepola V, Fellander-Tsai L, Mattila VM. Trends in the Incidence of Clavicle Fractures and Surgical Repair in Sweden: 2001–2012. J Bone Joint Surg Am. 2016;98(21):1837–42.
16. Andersen K, Jensen PO, Lauritzen J. Treatment of clavicular fractures. Figure-of-eight bandage versus a simple sling. Acta Orthop Scand. 1987;58(1):71–4.
17. van der Meijden OA, Gaskill TR, Millett PJ. Treatment of clavicle fractures: current concepts review. J Shoulder Elbow Surg. 2012;21(3):423–9.
18. Ban I, Nowak J, Virtanen K, Troelsen A. Overtreatment of displaced midshaft clavicle fractures. Acta Orthop. 2016;87(6):541–5.
19. Wennergren D, Ekholm C, Sandelin A, Möller M. The Swedish fracture register: 103,000 fractures registered. BMC Musculoskelet Disord. 2015;16:338.
20. The SFR. Annual report 2013 in English. https://stratum.registercentrum.se/#!page?id=1525. Accessed 15 Mar 2016.
21. The SFR's home web page. https://stratum.registercentrum.se/#!page?id=1094. Accessed 15 Mar 2016.
22. Wennergren D, Ekholm C, Sundfeldt M, Karlsson J, Bhandari M, Moller M. High reliability in classification of tibia fractures in the Swedish Fracture Register. Injury. 2016;47(2):478–82.
23. O'Neill BJ, Molloy AP, Curtin W. Conservative management of paediatric clavicle fractures. Int J Pediatr. 2011;2011:172571.

Biomechanical efficacy of AP, PA lag screws and posterior plating for fixation of posterior malleolar fractures: a three dimensional finite element study

Adeel Anwar[1], Zhen Zhang[1*], Decheng Lv[1*], Gang Lv[2], Zhi Zhao[3], Yanfeng Wang[2], Yue Cai[4], Wasim Qasim[5], Muhammad Umar Nazir[6] and Ming Lu[1]

Abstract

Background: Clinically there are different fixation methods used for fixation of the posterior malleolar fractures (PMF), but the best treatment modality is still not clear. Few studies have concentrated on this issue, least of all using a biomechanical comparison. The purpose of this study was to carry out a computational comparative biomechanics of three different commonly used fixation constructs for the fixation of PMF by finite element analysis (FEA).

Methods: Computed tomography (CT) images were used to reconstruct three dimensional (3D) model of the tibia. Computer aided design (CAD) software was used to design 3D models of PMF. Finally, 3D models of PMF fixed with two antero-posterior (AP) lag screws, two postero-anterior (PA) lag screws and posterior plate were simulated through computational processing. Simulated loads of 500 N, 1000 N and 1500 N were applied to the PMF and proximal ends of the models were fixed in all degrees of freedom. Output results representing the model von Mises stress, relative fracture micro-motion and vertical displacement of the fracture fragment were analyzed.

Results: The mean vertical displacement value in the posterior plate group (0.52 mm) was lower than AP (0.68 mm) and PA (0.69 mm) lag groups. Statistically significant low amount of the relative micro-motion ($P < 0.05$) was observed in the posterior plate group.

Conclusions: It was concluded that the posterior plate is biomechanically the most stable fixation method for fixation of PMF.

Keywords: Posterior malleolar fracture, Fixation, Biomechanical, Three dimensional, Finite element analysis

Background

The posterior malleolar fractures account for 7%–44% among the ankle fractures [1–5]. Ankle fractures involving the posterior malleolus have worse prognostic outcomes compared with ankle injuries without involvement of the posterior malleolus [1]. The treatment recommendations for the medial and lateral malleolar fractures are well recognized, but the guidelines for surgical fixations used for posterior malleolar fractures remain unclear [6–8], and there is an ongoing debate on this issue. Though most of the researchers agreed that the posterior malleolar fractures of > 25% articular involvement should be fixed surgically, but several studies have argued the importance of smaller size fractures and evaluated the critical role of posterior malleolus fixation for syndesmotic stabilization [9–14]. Different surgeons approach differently to treat the posterior malleolar fractures. By using the indirect anterior approach, it can be reduced through ligamentotaxis

* Correspondence: zhangzhendmu@163.com; doctorzz@126.com; lvdecheng_dmu@163.com; lvdecheng55@126.com
[1]Department of Orthopaedic Surgery, The First Affiliated Hospital of Dalian Medical University, 222 Zhongshan road, 116011 Dalian, Liaoning, People's Republic of China

and fixation can be achieved by antero-posterior (AP) lag screws. Conversely, fracture can be reduced by using direct approach (postero-lateral), in which internal fixation is maintained either by postero-anterior (PA) lag screws or by posterior plating. Less attention has focused on the prognosis of the different fixation constructs. A sound knowledge of comparative biomechanical efficiency of the different fixation constructs is essential for trauma surgeons to choose the optimal fixation method in ankle fractures involving the posterior malleolus and for improved clinical outcomes. Highly variable fracture patterns of the posterior malleolar fractures were classified by Haraguchi et al. [15] into three distinct categories. Among these three types, the type 2 (29.8% of the tibial plafond involvement) meet the current fixation indications. The aim of this study was to evaluate the biomechanical efficiency of AP lag screws, PA lag screws and posterior buttress plate for the fixation of posterior malleolar fractures of > 25% size. This size was selected because at present most of the trauma surgeons are agreed to fix the fractures of more than 25% size. Finite element analysis (FEA) was conducted to compare the stress and displacement patterns in different load conditions.

Methods

Three dimensional (3D) modeling

CT scan images of the right ankle of a volunteer in the neutral unloaded position were used to reconstruct the three dimensional (3D) model of the ankle joint. There was no past history of trauma or anatomical abnormality. This research work was approved and in accordance with the Medical Research Ethics Committee of the author's hospital. Experimental work was performed in accordance with the Helsinki Declaration. CT scan data in Dicom form was then imported into Mimics 10.1 software (Materialise, Leuven, Belgium) to reconstruct the surface geometry of the bones. Then structure of the each bone in igs format was transferred to Geomagics 11.0 software (Raindrop Company, USA). Processing in Geomagics was done to obtain the volumes of the bones. Stp files of bone's volume were imported into Pro E (CREO 3.0 PTC Corp., USA). Finally, the solid objects representing the bones were assembled within Pro E to make 3D foot-ankle complex (Fig. 1 a). The coordination axes of the 3D assembled model were assigned as; X-axis pointed posteriorly (toe to heel), Y-axis pointed upward (heel to knee) and Z-axis pointed laterally (medial to lateral malleolus). To obtain the geometry of posterior malleolar fracture of > 25% size, the postero-lateral margin of the ankle was modeled in Pro E Fig. 1 (c). In this study, an exact fit fracture model was illustrated; there was no fracture gap between the fracture fragment and the remaining bone. However, the posterior fragment can move in relation to the un-fractured bone with an assigned friction coefficient of 0.3 [16]. Three different fixation modalities; two AP lag screws, two PA lag screws and posterior malleolar anatomic plate were adapted to fix the fracture models as shown in Fig. 2. The 3D models of the implants were designed using the computer aided design (CAD) software (ProE CREO 3.0 PTC Corp., USA)). All the assembled models were meshed using the HyperMesh 11.0 software (Altair Engineering, Inc., USA). Fig. 1(b).

Finite element (FE) modeling and material properties

3D models of tibia with associated fixation implants in ing files were then imported into finite element analysis software Abaqus 6.14 (Simulia Corp., USA). In Abaqus, interaction between different parts of the models was performed. Bone was assumed to behave as

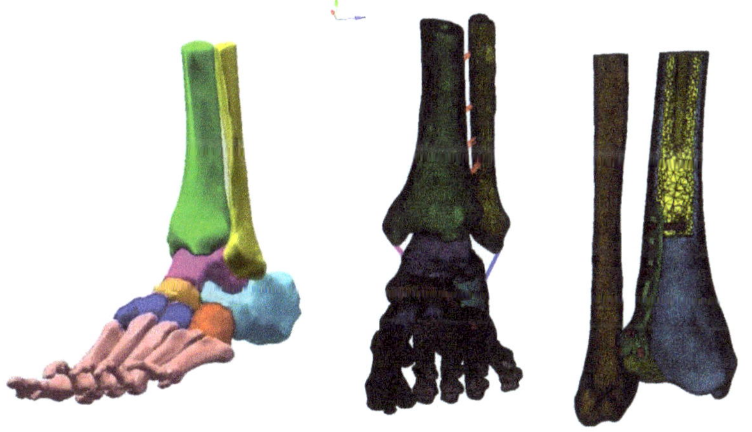

(a) (b) (c)

Fig. 1 3D ankle model (**a**) Initial 3D modeling, (**b**) Meshing of the processed model, (**c**) Finite element model showing cortical and cancellous portions of the bone

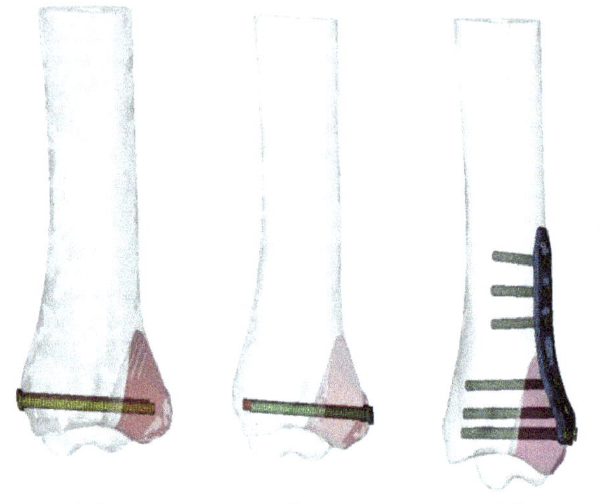

Fig. 2 Model of posterior malleolar fracture showing three different fixation strategies. **a** Two AP lag screws, **b** Two PA lag screws, **c** Posterior plate

homogeneous, isotropic and linearly elastic material. The cortical and cancellous portions of the distal tibia were modeled with Young's modulus (E) of 7300 and11100 MPa and Poisson ratio (y) of 0.3 and 0.26 respectively [17, 18]. Fixation implants including screws and plate were assigned an elastic modulus and Poisson's ratio of 110,000 MPa and 0.3 respectively [19]. The effect of gravity was considered as negligible in the model. Material properties are given in Table 1.

Boundary conditions and validation of model

3D model is validated as it has cortical shell and inner cancellous bone and material properties were assigned accordingly [17, 18]. The proximal end of the tibia was fixed in all degrees of freedom as shown in Fig. 3. In this experiment, the force was applied to the fracture fragment in the direction of fracture mechanism [20]. Three different magnitudes of axial force i.e.; 500 N, 1000 N and 1500 N were simulated according to previous study [21]. The analysis was done using finite element software Abaqus 6.14 (Simulia Corp., USA). In put units of KPa, seconds and mm were used for elastic modulus, time and displacement in this analysis respectively. Von Mises stress output unit was KPa, and final stress values are represented using MPa. For easy interpretation of the results, we divided the 3D models in three groups; model using two lag screws in antero-posterior direction was assigned as AP lag group and models with postero-anterior screws and posterior plate were named PA lag and plate groups respectively as shown in Fig. 3.

Table 1 Material properties used in finite element models

Material	Young's modulus (E)	Poisson ratio (y)	References
Cortical bone	7300	0.3	[17]
Cancellous bone	1100	0.26	[18]
Fixation constructs	110,000	0.3	[19]

Statistics

Statistical analysis was done using SPSS 16.0 (SPSS Inc., Chicago IL). Descriptive statistics were used to determine means and standard deviations. One way ANOVA (Post Hoc/LSD) was used for multi comparisons.

Results

The total number of nodes were 71,970, 57,342 and 85,825 in AP, PA and plate models respectively and total number of elements were 333,768, 273,181 and 412,913 for AP, PA and plate respectively.

Von Mises stress (VMS) patterns

Von Mises Stress (VMS) distributions in the three models using different magnitudes of the load are shown in Fig. 4. Over all stress patterns showed more concentrated stress in upper anterior and posterior portions of tibia (Fig. 5). The bone model with AP lag screws showed the highest peak values. Higher stress values were observed in AP and PA lag screws. The stress distribution was concentrated in the screw area near the fracture line. In plate group stress areas were also observed in the upper three screws and plate junctions.

Model displacement

Analysis of the model displacement shows that AP lag group shows the highest amount of displacement. Whereas, PA lag and plate groups show nearly same amount of displacement. In AP and PA lag models, mainly the fracture fragment is displaced, but displacement is also prominent in the tibial plafond in posterior plate model (See Fig. 6). In X-axis (posterior component of displacement), the highest displacement was observed in AP lag model (1.27, 3.12, 4.28 mm). PA lag model with displacement values of 1.12, 2.45, 4.08 mm shows better fixation power than AP group. The posterior plate group had slight higher displacement values (4.45, 4.29, 4.19 mm). Y-axis represents the vertical displacement in direction of the applied load. This vertical movement is higher in AP group followed by PA and plate groups. The largest VD values were noted in the 1500 N loading. In this loading condition, PA lag showed 1.46 times more VD than posterior plating and PA lag showed 1.4 times higher displacement than plate group. Key

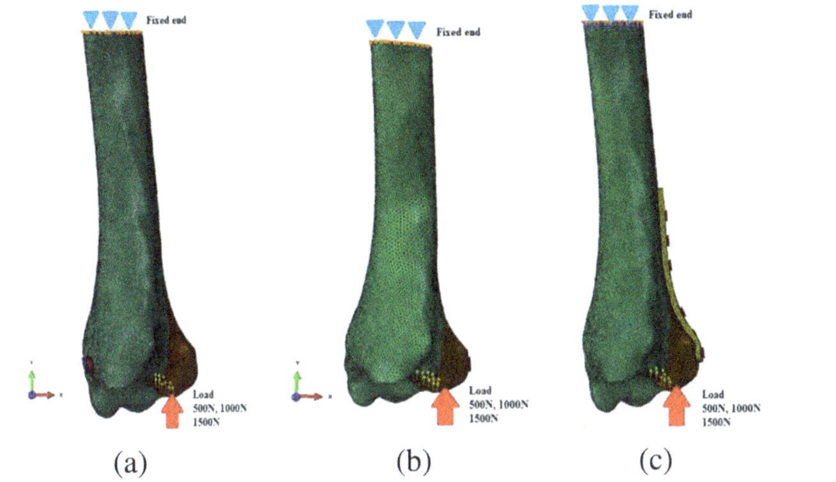

Fig. 3 Finite element model showing boundary conditions and load direction. **a** AP lag group, **b** PA lag group, **c** Plate group

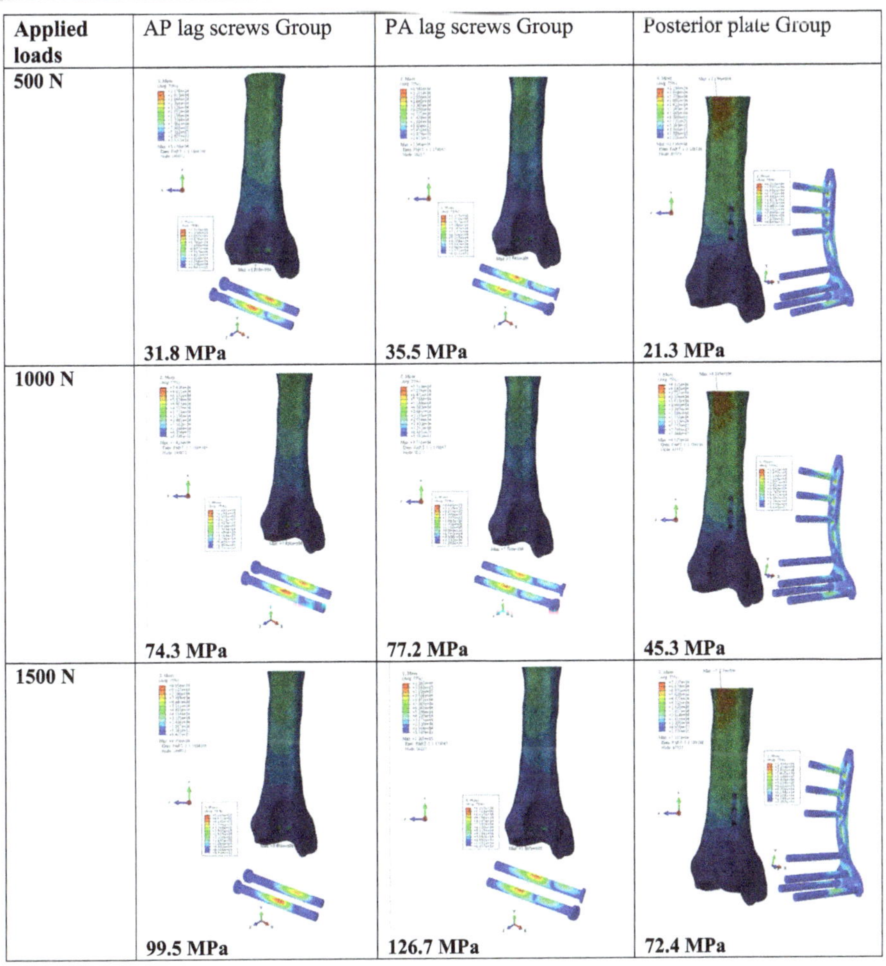

Fig. 4 Von Mises Stress (VMS) pattrens in three models with loads of three different magnitudes

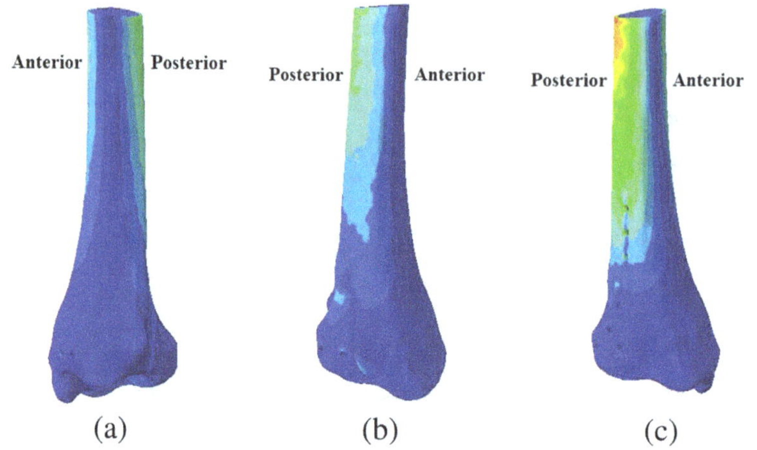

Fig. 5 Peak von Mises Stress (VMS) stress distribution in models using three different fixation strategies. **a** AP, **b** PA, **c** Posterior plate models

movement of fracture in three co-ordinate axes using 1500 N compressive force is given in Fig. 7. Z-axis (lateral movement), plate shows the greater amount of distal tibia. Table 2 shows the displacement values in three axes.

Relative micro-motion (RM)

The fracture micro-motion analysis demonstrated that the mean RM in the plate group (0.03 mm) was lowest among the three models. Whereas the mean relative motions in AP and PA lag models were 0.60 mm and 0.39 mm respectively (Table 3). When magnitude of the applied load increased, the RM in the individual group was also increased. The detailed values of RM in each group are summarized in Figs. 8 and 9.

Discussion

To our knowledge, this is the first computational study comparing the biomechanical efficiency of practically used three different fixation modalities (AP lag screws, PA lag screws and posterior plating) in which the force is applied in the direction of fracture mechanism. According to the findings of this finite element study, the fixation of the posterior malleolar fractures with the posterior buttress plating is most stable fixation construct than the AP and PA lag screws. This was represented by the lowest relative fracture displacement in the posterior plate group. In this study we simulated the posterior malleolar fracture of greater than 25% size of the tibial plafond. Though in recent literature there is no consensus about the indications for surgical interventions, but most of the clinicians recommended the

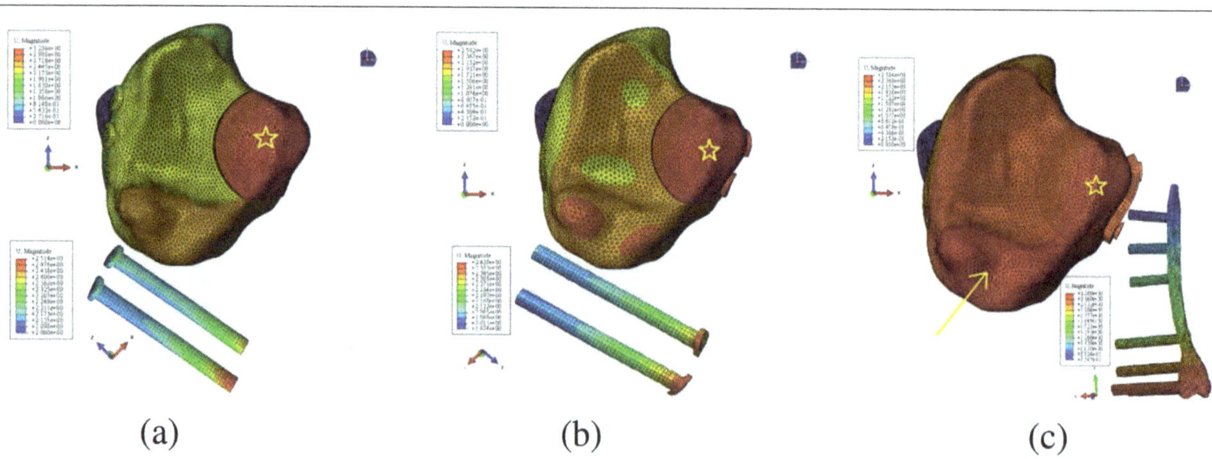

Fig. 6 Tibial plafond showing the model and implant displacements (mm). Star represents the displacemnt of fracture fragment only. Arrow represnts the movement of medial malleolus. **a** AP lag, **b** PA lag, **c** Posterior plate models

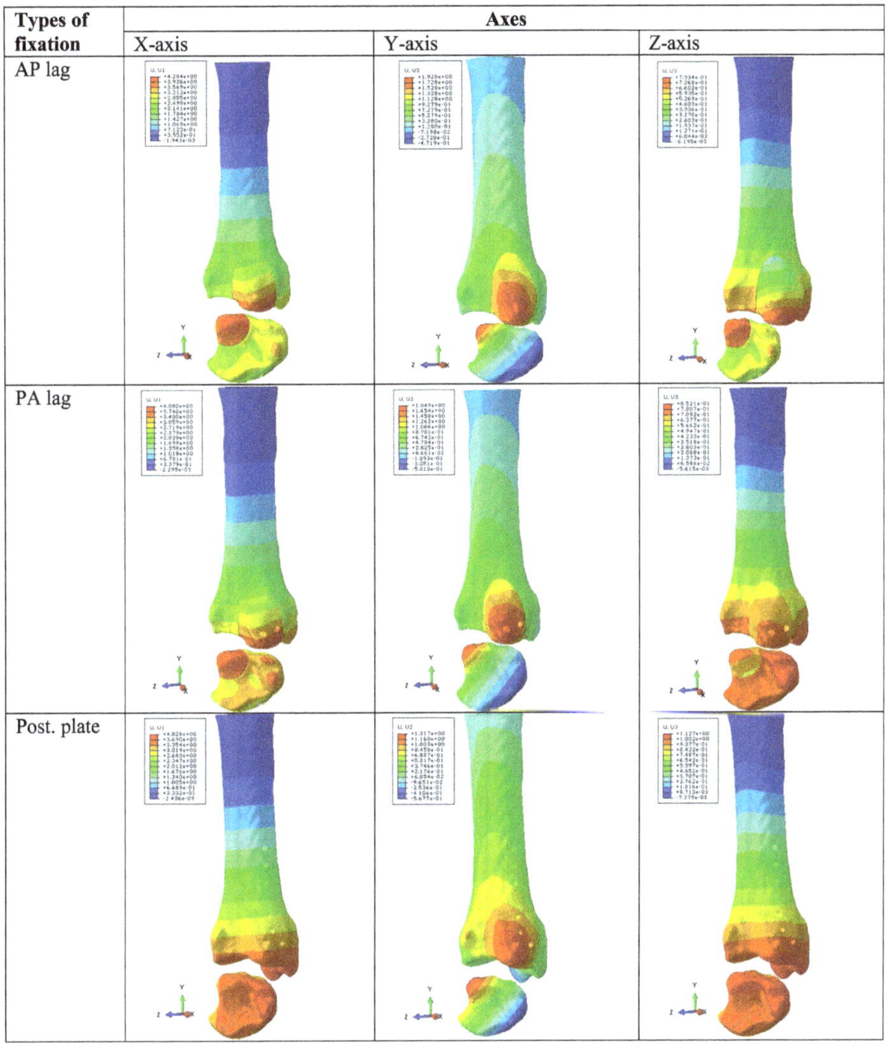

Fig. 7 Representation of displacement patterns in X,Y and Z axes in the higest load group (1500 N)

Table 2 Displacement values (mm) in X, Y and Z axes

Loads	Fixation methods	Axes		
		X-axis	Y-axis	Z-axis
500 N	AP lag screw	1.27	0.57	0.26
	PA lag screw	1.12	0.52	0.23
	Posterior plate	1.16	0.37	0.30
1000 N	AP lag screw	3.12	1.40	0.61
	PA lag screw	2.45	1.14	0.51
	Posterior plate	2.49	0.86	0.67
1500 N	AP lag screw	4.28	1.93	0.81
	PA lag screw	4.08	1.85	0.85
	Posterior plate	4.03	1.32	1.13

posterior malleolar fracture of >25% size should fix surgically [22–24]. Furthermore, biomechanical research has evaluated that the posterior malleolus plays an important role in the tibiotalar load propagation. It also prevents the posterior displacement of the talus [25, 26]. With the increasing size of the posterior fragment, the risk of posterior talar subluxation increase especially when the fracture size is greater than 25% [22].

The von Mises stress (VMS) analysis of the tibia showed the higher stress areas both in anterior and posterior side (See Fig. 5). These stress distribution patterns were different from the previously described finding [27]. The difference was due to the fact that the direction of the applied force used this study was in the opposite direction and the force was concentrated only to the fracture fragment in this analysis. Though the displacement analysis of PA and plate

Table 3 Mean and standard deviation (SD) values of relative micro-motion and vertical displacement

Variables	Groups	Magnitude of applied force			Mean	SD	*P*-value*
		500 N	1000 N	1500 N			
Relative micro-motion (RM)	AP lag (1)	0.23	0.58	0.99	0.60	0.38	
	PA lag (2)	0.16	0.36	0.67	0.39	0.25	
	Post. Plate (3)	0.01	0.03	0.05	0.03	0.02	0.039 (3–1)
Vertical displacement(VD)	AP lag	0.57	1.40	1.93	1.30	0.68	
	PA lag	0.52	1.14	1.85	1.19	0.69	
	Post. Plate	0.37	0.86	1.32	0.88	0.52	

**P*-value is significant at < 0.05

groups showed nearly the same amounts of displacement, but it should be noted that in PA lag model, the displacement was limited mainly to the fracture fragment to which load was applied with a negligible amount of displacement in the rest of model (Fig. 6, b). But in case of posterior plate, the displacement was also prominent in the tibial plafond (Fig. 6, c). This combined displacement of the distal tibia along with the fracture fragment signifies that the fixation strength of the plate is better than AP and PA lag screws. Due to better anchorage power of the posterior plate, it resisted the vertical displacement and the resulted displacement (Fig. 6, c) was also demonstrated in the rest of distal tibia. The model displacement comparison between AP and PA lag groups showed that the biomechanical fixation strength of PA lag screws was superior to AP lag screws, because in case of AP lag screws mainly the fracture fragment was displaced (Fig. 6, a) whereas in PA lag model a slight displacement was also observed in the tibial plafond.

In this study, the lowest vertical displacement (Y component of the displacement) was observed in the plate group which can be easily explained by the fact that the plate resisted the upward displacement more effectively than AP and PA lag screws. AP lag group with the largest VD values was the biomechanically least stable fixation construct in this study. The relative fracture micro-motion in AP lag group was also higher than other constructs.

Posterior plate with the minimum amount of RM represented that it offered the best fixation strength among the three groups. Fixation by the AP lag screws showed nearly 23 times more RM (0.23 mm) than the posterior plate (0.01 mm) and PA lag screws showed 16 times more RM (0.16 mm) as compared to the posterior plate (0.01 mm) by applying 500 N force. These inter-fragmentary motions even became more prominent when we increased the applied force to 1500 N. Clinically the less stable fixation constructs with large amounts of relative micro motion may result in implant loosening and mimics the reduction stability. The resulted loss of fracture reduction (secondary to the less stable fixation constructs) can cause successive increase in the focal contact pressure which ultimately leads to the formation of degenerative osteoarthritis [24, 28].

The previous studies have reported the outcomes of posterior plating and documented that the posterior plating is superior in achieving the fracture reduction. But these studies compared only the two fixation methods. In one of these biomechanical studies comparison was done between AP screws and posterior buttress plate and in another study, the analysis was done

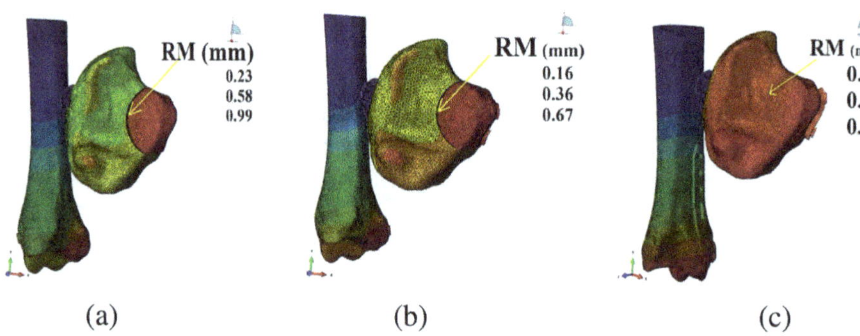

Fig. 8 Relative micro-motion (RM) of the fracture in (**a**) AP, (**b**) PA and (**c**) posterior plate models

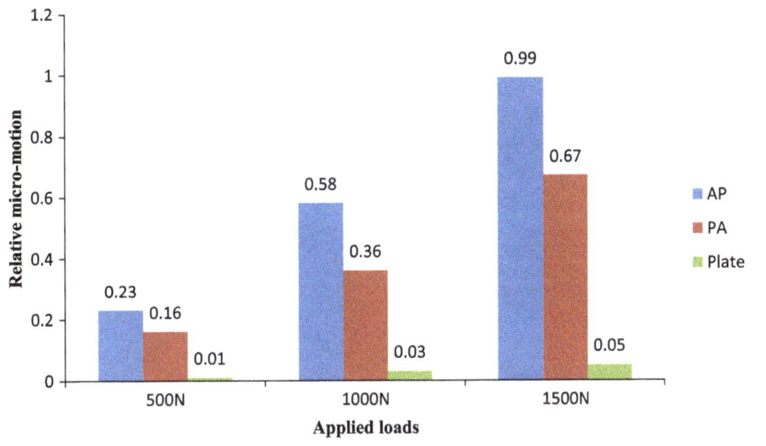

Fig. 9 Graphical representation of Relative micro-motion (RM) of the fracture in three different fixation models

for PA lag screw and posterior plate [20, 29]. Here we have compared the three different fixation modalities. Our computational findings are consistent with previous biomechanical and clinical studies. In a recent biomechanical study, Bennett et al. [20] has compared the fixation strength of one-third tubular posterolateral plate and AP lag screws in the cadaveric models of posterior malleolar fractures. The results of this study advocated the less displacement using the posterior buttress plating than AP lag screws during cyclical loading. Another study published in Chinese literature, documented that the fixation of posterior malleolus with distal radius plate is more stable than PA lag screws [29]. A retrospective clinical study carried out by O'Connor et al. [30] demonstrated the improved clinical and radiographic outcomes at follow up in 27 patients treated with posterior plate compared with AP screws fixation. In our FEA though the posterior plate still remained the strongest implant for fixation of the posterior malleolus, it also showed that PA lag screws are the second most stable construct.

This work has several limitations. Firstly, soft tissues such as ligaments and syndesmosis were not simulated in this study, and only the ability of the used implants to resist the displacements and stress changes were calculated. So the stability offered by the surrounding soft tissues was ignored. But, this technical limitation affected all the groups equally and it didn't question the validity of our findings. Secondly, it is a static simulated study and further studies are needed to explore the cyclic loading conditions.

Conclusions

FEA of 3D posterior malleolar fracture model shows that posterior buttress plating with minimum amount of the relative fracture micro-motion and vertical displacement is biomechanically the most stable fixation implant. The second most stable construct is PA lag, whereas AP lag group with the largest RM and VD values is the least stable fixation method. Surgeons should consider the findings of this computational exploration study when selecting a fixation strategy for posterior malleolar fractures.

Abbreviations

3D: Three dimensional; AP: Antero-posterior; CAD: Computer aided design; CT: Computed tomography; FEA: Finite element analysis; i.e.: That is; PA: Postero-anterior; PMF: Posterior malleolar fracture; RM: Relative micro-motion; VD: Vertical displacement

Acknowledgements

Not applicable.

Funding

There is no source of funding related to this work.

Author's contributions

AA, ZZ and LDC drafted the article and conceived of the study. AA, MUN, WQ and LM were also responsible for data collection and statistical analysis. AA, LDC and MUN participated in the design of the study. AA and CY participated in computational process. LG, ZZ and WYF helped to revise the manuscript. All authors read and approved the final manuscript.

Consent for publication

Not applicable.

Competing interests

The authors declare that they have no competing interest.

Author details

[1]Department of Orthopaedic Surgery, The First Affiliated Hospital of Dalian Medical University, 222 Zhongshan road, 116011 Dalian, Liaoning, People's Republic of China. [2]Department of Orthopaedic Surgery, The First Affiliated Hospital of China Medical University, 155 Nanjing north street, 110001 Shenyang, Liaoning, People's Republic of China. [3]Department of Orthopaedic Surgery, The Second Affiliated Hospital of Dalian Medical University, 456

Zhongshan road, 116027 Dalian, Liaoning, People's Republic of China. [4]Department of Automation, School of Electrical Engineering, Dalian Jiaotong University, 794 Huanghe road, 116028 Dalian, Liaoning, People's Republic of China. [5]Department of General Surgery, The Second Affiliated Hospital of Dalian Medical University, 456 Zhongshan road, 116027 Dalian, Liaoning, People's Republic of China. [6]Department of Respiratory Medicine, The Second Affiliated Hospital of Dalian Medical University, 456 Zhongshan road, 116027 Dalian, Liaoning, People's Republic of China.

References

1. Jaskulka RA, Ittner G, Schedl R. Fractures of the posterior tibial margin: their role in the prognosis of malleolar fractures. J Trauma. 1989;29:1565–70.
2. Court-Brown CM, McBirnie J, Wilson G. Adult ankle fractures-an increasing problem? Acta Orthop Scand. 1998;69:43–7.
3. Boggs LR. Isolated posterior malleolar fractures. Am J Emerg Med. 1986;4:334–6.
4. Broos PL, Bisschop AP. Operative treatment of ankle fractures in adults: correlation between types of fracture and final results. Injury. 1991;22:403–6.
5. Koval KJ, Lurie J, Zhou W, Sparks MB, Cantu RV, Sporer SM, Weinstein J. Ankle fractures in the elderly: what you get depends on where you live and who you see. J Orthop Trauma. 2005;19:635–9.
6. van den Bekerom MPJ, Haverkamp D, Kloen P. Biomechanical and clinical evaluation of posterior malleolar fractures. A systematic review of the literature. J Trauma. 2009;66:279–84.
7. Gardner MJ, Streubel PN, McCormick JJ, Klein SE, Johnson JE, Ricci WM. Surgeon practices regarding operative treatment of posterior malleolus fractures. Foot Ankle Int. 2011;32:385–93.
8. Odak S, Ahluwalia R, Unnikrishnan P, Hennessy M, Platt S. Management of Posterior Malleolar Fractures: a systematic review. J Foot Ankle Surg. 2016;55:140–5.
9. Langenhuijsen JF, Heetveld MJ, Ultee JM, Steller EP, Butzelaar RM. Results of ankle fractures with involvement of the posterior tibial margin. J Trauma. 2002;53:55–60.
10. Miller AN, Carroll EA, Parker RJ, Helfet DL, Lorich DG. Posterior malleolar stabilization of syndesmotic injuries is equivalent to screw fixation. Clin Orthop Relat Res. 2009;468:1129–35.
11. Papachristou G, Efstathopoulos N, Levidiotis C, Chronopoulos E. Early weight bearing after posterior malleolar fractures: an experimental and prospective clinical study. J Foot Ankle Surg. 2003;42:99–104.
12. Ebraheim NA, Elgafy H, Padanilam T. Syndesmotic disruption in low fibular fractures associated with deltoid ligament injury. Clin Orthop Relat Res. 2003;409:260–7.
13. Gardner MJ, Brodsky A, Briggs SM, Nielson JM, Lorich DG. Fixation of posterior malleolar fractures provides greater syndesmotic stability. Clin Orthop Relat Res. 2006;447:165–71.
14. Ebraheim NA, Lu J, Yang H, Rollins J. The fibular incisure of the tibia on CT scan: a cadaver study. Foot Ankle Int. 1998;19:318–21.
15. Haraguchi N, Haruyama H, Toga H, Kato F. Pathoanatomy of posterior malleolar fractures of the ankle. J Bone Joint Surg Am. 2006;88:1085–92.
16. Chen WP, Tai CL, Shih CH, Hsieh PH, Leou MC, Lee MS. Selection of fixation devices in proximal femur rotational osteotomy: clinical complications and finite element analysis. Clin Biomech. 2004;19:255–62.
17. Qiu TX, Teo EC, Yan YB, Lei W. Finite element modeling of a 3D coupled foot-boot model. Med Eng Phys. 2011;33:1228–33.
18. Kim H-J, Kim S-H, Chang S-H. Bio-mechanical analysis of a fractures tibia with composite bone plates according to the diaphyseal oblique fracture angle. Compos B: Eng. 2011;42:666–74.
19. Fan Y, Xiu K, Duan H, Zhang M. Biomechanical and histological evaluation of the application of biodegradable poly- L -lactic cushion to the plate internal fixation for bone fracture healing. Clin Biomech (Bristol, Avon). 2008; 23(Suppl 1):7–16.
20. Bennett C, Behn A, Daoud A, Nork S, Sangeorzan B, Dikos G, Bishop J. Buttress plating versus anterior-to-posterior lag screws for fixation of the posterior malleolus: a biomechanical study. J Othop. Trauma. 2016;30:664–9.
21. Zhang W, Luo CF, Putnis S, Sun H, Zeng ZM, Zeng BF. Biomechanical analysis of four different fixations for the posterolateral shearing tibial plateau fracture. Knee. 2012;19:94–8.
22. McDaniel WJ, Wilson FC. Trimalleolar fractures of the ankle. An end result study. Clin Orthop Relat Res. 1977;122:37–45.
23. De Vries JS, Wijgman AJ, Sierevelt IN, Schaap GR. Long-term results of ankle fractures with a posterior malleolar fragment. J Foot Ankle Surg. 2005;44:211–7.
24. Hartford JM, Gorczyca JT, McNamara JL, Mayor MB. Tibiotalar contact area. Contribution of posterior malleolus and deltoid ligament. Clin Orthop Relat Res. 1995;320:182–7.
25. Raasch WG, Larkin JJ, Draganich LF. Assessment of the posterior malleolus as a restraint to posterior subluxation of the ankle. J Bone Joint Surg Am. 1992;74:1201–6.
26. Scheidt KB, Stiehl JB, Skrade DA, Barnhardt T. Posterior malleolar ankle fractures: an in vitro biomechanical analysis of stability in the loaded and unloaded states. J Orthop Trauma. 1992;6:96–101.
27. Raja Izaham RM, Abdul Kadir MR, Abdul Rashid AH, Hossain MG, Kamarul T. Finite element analysis of Puddu and Tomofix plate fixation for open wedge high tibial osteotomy. Injury. 2012;43:898–902.
28. Macko VW, Matthews LS, Zwirkoski P, Goldstein SA. The joint-contact area of the ankle. The contribution of the posterior malleolus. J Bone Joint Surg Am. 1991;73:347–51.
29. Li YD, Liu SM, Jia JS, Zhou JL. Choice of internal fixation methods for posterior malleolus fracture in both biomechanics and clinical application [in Chinese]. Beijing Da Xue Xue Bao. 2011;43:718–23.
30. O'Connor TJ, Mueller B, Ly TV, Jacobson AR, Nelson ER, Cole PA. "A to p" screw versus posterolateral plate for posterior malleolus fixation in trimalleolar ankle fractures. J Orthop Trauma. 2015;29:e151–6.

4

Treatment of thoracolumbar burst fractures by short-segment pedicle screw fixation using a combination of two additional pedicle screws and vertebroplasty at the level of the fracture: a finite element analysis

Jen-Chung Liao[1], Weng-Pin Chen[2*] and Hao Wang[2]

Abstract

Background: Traditional one-above and one-below four-screw posterior short-segment instrumentation is used for unstable thoracolumbar burst fractures. However, this method has a high rate of implant failure and early loss of reduction. The purpose of this study was to use finite element (FE) analysis to determine the effect of treating thoracolumbar burst fractures by short-segment pedicle screw fixation using a combination of two additional pedicle screws and vertebroplasty at the level of the fracture.

Methods: An intact T11-L1 spine FE model was created from the computed tomography images of a male subject. Four fixation models with posterior fusion devices (pedicle screws, rods, cross-link) were established to simulate an unstable thoracolumbar fracture with different fusion surgeries: short-segment fixation with: 1) a link (S-L); 2) intermediate bilateral screws (S-I); 3) a link and calcium sulfate cement (S-L-C); 4) intermediate bilateral screws and calcium sulfate cement (S-I-C). Different loading conditions (flexion, extension, lateral bending, and axial rotation) were applied on the models and analyzed with a FE package. The range of motion (ROM), and the maximum value and distribution of the implant stress, and the stress in the facet joint, were compared between the intact and fixation models.

Results: The ROM in flexion, extension, axial rotation, and lateral bending was the smallest in the S-I-C model, followed by the S-I, S-L-C, and S-L models. Maximum von Mises stress values were larger under lateral bending and axial rotation loadings than under flexion and extension loading. High stress was concentrated at the crosslink and rod junctions. Maximal von Mises stress on the superior vertebral body for all loading conditions was larger than that on the inferior vertebral body. The maximal von Mises stress of the pedicle screws during all states of motion were 265.3 MPa in S-L fixation, 192.9 MPa in S-I fixation, 258.4 MPa in S-L-C fixation, and 162.3 MPa in S-I-C fixation.

Conclusions: Short-segment fixation with two intermediate pedicle screws together with calcium sulfate cement at the fractured vertebrae may provide a stiffer construct and less von Mises stress of the pedicle screws and rods as compared to other types of short-segment fixation.

Keywords: Thoracolumbar burst fracture, Posterior instrumentation, Vertebroplasty, Finite element analysis

* Correspondence: wpchen@ntut.edu.tw
[2]Department of Mechanical Engineering, National Taipei University of Technology, 1, Sec. 3, Chung-Hsiao E. Rd, Taipei 10608, Taiwan

Background

Burst fractures account for approximately 20% of thoracolumbar fractures, and occur due to an axial loading force that results in failure to support the anterior and middle column [1, 2]. Surgery is usually indicated when there is a severe deformity, and/or neurologic deficit. Whether anterior or posterior surgery is the most effective treatment for burst fractures remains controversial. Some authors advise anterior surgery to remove retropulsed fragments [3, 4], but posterior surgery is popular because it is an easier approach and allows clearance of the spinal canal by ligamentotaxis.

One-above and one-below posterior short-segment instrumentation with fusion has been widely used for unstable thoracolumbar burst fractures for the past 3 decades [5]. Pedicular instrumentation enables kyphotic correction, indirect reduction of canal encroachment, and early mobilization. However, this method has a high rate of implant failure, and early loss of reduction because of loss of anterior support [6]. Over the past decade, some studies have demonstrated that augmentation of the fractured vertebra with absorbable bone cement could enhance fracture union and prevent implant failure. Liao et al. [7] and Korovessis et al. [8] demonstrated that injectable calcium sulfate cement or injectable calcium phosphate cement used as a transpedicular grafting material in thoracolumbar fractures could obtain clinical and radiographic results equal to autogenous cancellous bone graft.

In recent years, biomechanical and clinical studies have suggested that two additional screws inside the fractured vertebra could improve stability and provide better kyphotic correction. In a biomechanical study, Norton et al. [9] showed that two additional screws in the fractured vertebra (a six-screw construct) of an unstable thoracolumbar burst fracture could increase the stiffness of the implant, and reduce stress on each pedicle screw, as compared to a four-screw construct. However, there have been no studies examining the effect of augmentation by a combination of screws and bone cement at the fractured vertebra, and comparing the effect of this fixation method with other types of posterior short-segment instrumentation for thoracolumbar burst fractures.

We hypothesize that posterior short-segment instrumentation with fractured vertebra augmentation by a combination of vertebroplasty and two additional screws can provide a stronger construct than other types of posterior short-segment instrumentation for thoracolumbar burst fractures. In the current study, we established a finite element (FE) model of thoracolumbar burst fractures, and four posterior short-segment fixation methods were tested. The purpose was to determine the most optimal methods for the treatment of thoracolumbar burst fractures.

Methods

Models

Four fixation models with posterior fusion devices (pedicle screws, rods, cross-link) were established to simulate an unstable thoracolumbar fracture with different fusion surgeries: short-segment fixation with: 1) a link (S-L); 2) intermediate bilateral screws (S-I); 3) a link and calcium sulfate cement (S-L-C); 4) intermediate bilateral screws and calcium sulfate cement (S-I-C). Radiographs representing these four types of fixation are shown in Fig. 1.

Establishment of FE model of an intact normal thoracolumbar spine

A FE model of an intact normal spine was developed based on 1-mm-interval cross-sectional computed tomography (CT) spine images of a 55-year-old male provided by the US National Library of Medicine (NLM; NIH, Bethesda, MD). The FE model of the thoracolumbar section from T10 to L2 was established as follows. 1) A series of CT scans were imported into Amira 4.1 software (Visage Imaging, Carlsbad, CA). The vertebral boundaries as regions of interest (ROI) were identified on multiple images to form a three-node triangular surface model. 2) The surface model was imported into SolidWorks (SOLIDWORKS Corporation, Boston, MA), to further reconstruct a three-dimensional solid model

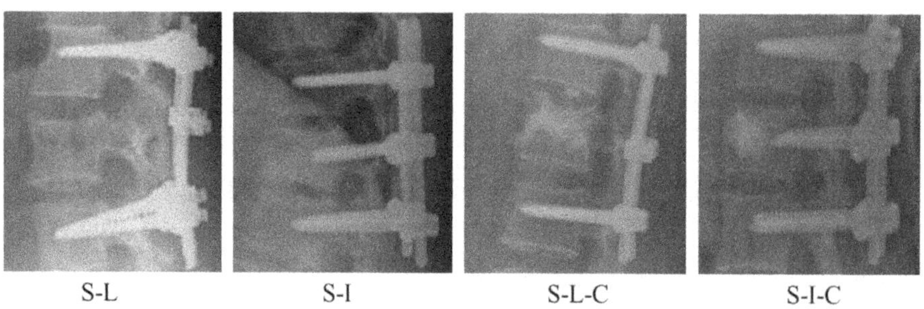

Fig. 1 Four types of fixation. S-L: four screws with a link. S-I: six-screw construct. S-L-C: four screws with a link, and calcium sulfate bone cement vertebroplasty. S-I-C: six screws with calcium sulfate bone cement vertebroplasty

of the thoracolumbar spine. 3) The solid model of the thoracolumbar spine was imported into HyperWorks 10.0 (Altair Engineering, Inc., Troy, MI) to form an eight-node hexahedral FE model. Since CT scanning does not provide the soft tissue contours of the intervertebral discs, the geometric characteristics of intervertebral discs were created as previously described [10]. The volume ratio of the annulus fibrosus to the nucleus pulposus was set to 6:4, the thickness of the cortical bone was set to 1 mm, and the endplate was set to 0.5 mm [10]. 4) The final FE model was imported into Abaqus FE analysis software (Abaqus/CAE v.6.10; Simulia Corp., Providence, RI) for analysis (Fig. 2).

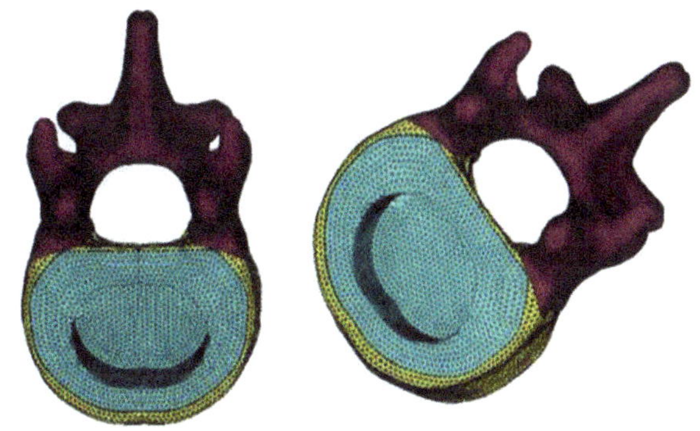

Fig. 3 T12 injured vertebrae finite element model

Establishment of FE models of injured vertebra

In this study, the vertebral resection (corpectomy) method was used to simulate a vertebra fracture. Briefly, one-half of the sponge bone of the T12 vertebra was removed to weaken the vertebral strength; the structure of the posterior portion was reserved to establish a FE model of an unstable thoracolumbar fracture (Fig. 3).

Establishment of solid internal fixator models

Pedicle screw system

The pedicle screw system in this study was modeled based on the SmartLoc Spinal Fixation System (A-SPINE Asia Co., Ltd.). Using physical measurements and 3D reverse engineering, a solid model was created using Solidworks. The length of the screw was 45 mm, the radius was 2.4 mm, and the cross-sectional area was 18.1 mm^2. The length of the vertical connecting rod was 80 mm, the radius was 2 mm, and the cross-sectional area was 12.6 mm^2. The horizontal connecting rod was 35 mm long, 7 mm wide, and 5 mm high. In order to shorten the FE analysis time, the screw thread part and the vertical connecting rod middle connection part of the structure were neglected. After the solid models of the implants were created, they were imported into HyperWorks to generate the FE meshes. The four-vertebral pedicle screw plus transverse connecting rod FE mesh model is shown in Fig. 4a, and the six-vertebral pedicle screw model is shown in Fig. 4b.

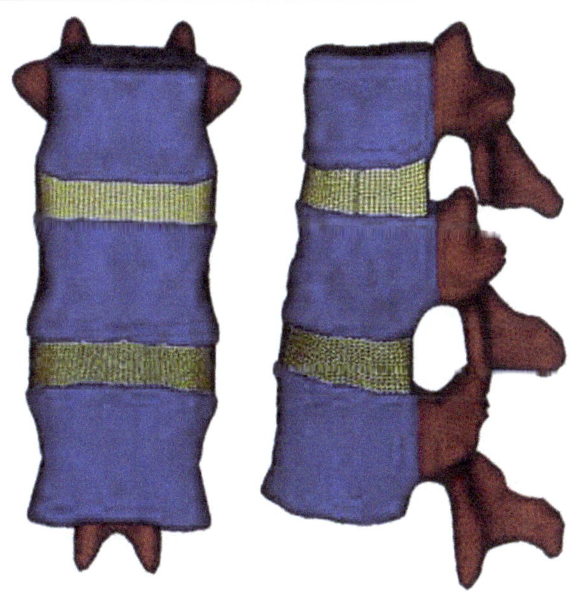

Fig. 2 T11-L1 finite element model

Four fixation models

The internal fixators were placed in the thoracolumbar models as described by Park et al. [11]. Four fixation models were used for comparison in this study: S-L, S-I, S-L-C, S-I-C. FE models of these four fixation types are shown in Fig. 5.

Material parameter settings

The material parameters (Young's moduli and the Poisson's ratios of cortical bone, cancellous bone, posterior bone element, endplate, and intervertebral disc) of the thoracolumbar models were set based on the work of Qiu et al. [12]. The models were assumed to be homogeneous,

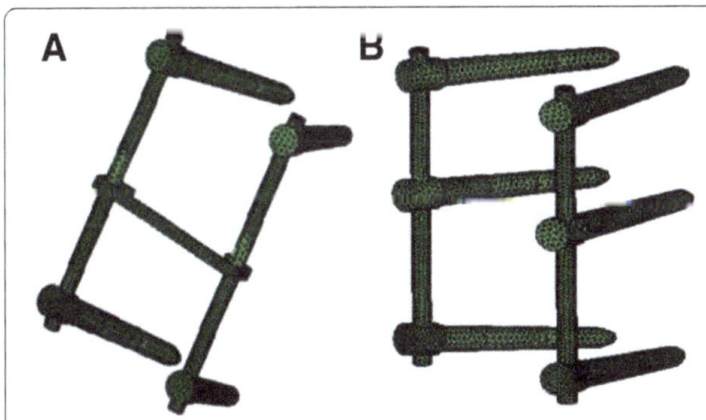

Fig. 4 Finite element models of internal fixations. **a**: Four screws with a link. **b**: Six-screw construct

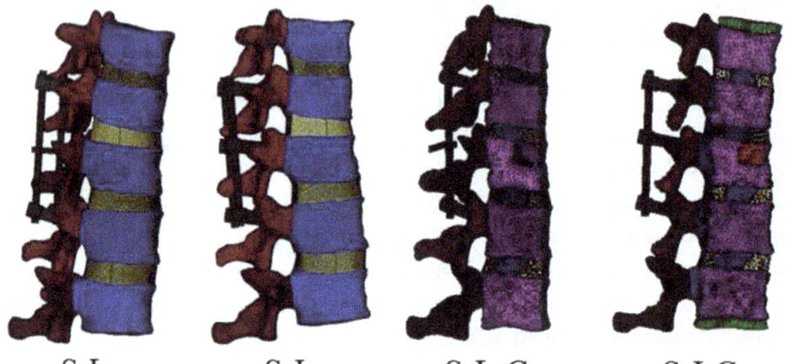

Fig. 5 Four-screw fixation finite element model with T11-L1 spine segments. S-L, short-segment pedicle screw fixation with a link; S-I, short-segment pedicle screw fixation with two intermediate screws; S-C, short-segment pedicle screw fixation with cement vertebroplasty; S-I-C, short-segment pedicle screw fixation with two intermediate screws plus cement vertebroplasty

isotropic, and linearly elastic. Material parameters are summarized in Table 1.

Loading and boundary conditions, and friction coefficient settings

The loading and boundary conditions of the FE analysis were based on the work of Qiu et al. [13]. Flexion, extension, lateral bending, and axial rotation were applied to the rigid plane above the T11 vertebra, respectively, and the load was applied as a set in a progressive manner (2.5 Nm, 5.0 Nm, 7.5 Nm of bending moment), respectively, and all degrees of freedom on the bottom nodes of L1 were constrained. To simulate a real contact setting, the friction coefficient of the contact surface of the facet joint was set to 0.1. This study simulated bone fusion following surgery, therefore, the interfaces between the screw and vertebrae were set to be perfectly bonded.

Table 1 The material properties of the finite element model

Component name	Young's modulus (Mpa)	Poisson ratio, y	Element type
Cortical bone	12,000	0.3	tetrahedral
Cancellous bone (normal)	345	0.2	tetrahedral
Cancellous bone (osteoporosis)	70	0.2	tetrahedral
Cement (Calcium sulfate)	147	0.3	tetrahedral
Posterior element	3500	0.25	tetrahedral
Endplate	12,000	0.3	tetrahedral
Disc-annulus	4.2	0.45	Prism
Disc-nucleus	6	0.499	Prism
Annuls fiber	500	0.3	tri
Rigid body	10,000,000	0.4	tetrahedral
Titanium	110,000	0.3	tetrahedral

Assessment indexes

By evaluating the range of motion (ROM) of T11-L1, the maximum von Mises stress on the pedicle screw root, and stress distribution of the pedicle screws and rods of the four fixation FE models under flexion, extension, left/right lateral bending, and left/right axial rotation, the biomechanical differences between the four fixation models could be compared.

Results

Validation of the intact T11-L1 FE model

After establishment of the normal T11-L1 FE model, moments of 7.5 Nm in six directions were obtained. The ROM of the T11-T12 segment were: flexion (3.0°), extension (3.1°), left bending (3.3°), right bending (3.8°), left rotation (2.2°), and right rotation (2.0°). The ROM of the T12-L1 segment were: flexion (3.3°), extension (3.7°), left bending (4.0°), right bending (3.6°), left rotation (1.3°), and right rotation (1.4°) (Table 2). The ROM results were similar to those reported by Panjabi et al. [14].

ROM of the four FE fixation models

The moments of 7.5 Nm in six directions were applied to the four fixation models. The ROM of the T11-L1 segment were: S-L group: flexion (1.03°), extension (1.05°), left bending (2.92°), right bending (2.80°), left rotation (2.60°), right rotation (2.60°); S-I group: flexion (0.95°), extension (0.98°), left bending (2.67°), right bending (2.54°), left rotation (2.32°), right rotation (2.32°); S-L-C group: flexion (0.98°), extension (1.00°), left bending (2.75°), right bending (2.61°), left rotation (2.46°), right rotation (2.46°); S-I-C group: flexion (0.87°), extension (0.92°), left bending (2.57°), right bending (2.51°), left rotation (2.23°), right rotation (2.23°) (Table 3).

Table 2 Comparison between the present intact model and that of Panjabi et al. [12]

Loading mode	T11-T12		T12-L1	
	Panjabi study	Present study	Panjabi study	Present study
Flexion (7.5 Nm)	2.7° ± 1.3°	3.0°	2.9° ± 1.4°	3.3°
Extension (7.5 Nm)	2.4° ± 1.3°	3.1°	3.9° ± 1.4°	3.7°
Left bending (7.5 Nm)	3.5° ± 1.1°	3.3°	3.7° ± 1.1°	4.0°
Right bending (7.5 Nm)	3.5° ± 1.1°	3.8°	3.7° ± 1.1°	3.6°
Left rotation (7.5 Nm)	1.8° ± 0.7°	2.2°	1.2° ± 0.7°	1.3°
Right rotation (7.5 Nm)	1.8° ± 0.7°	2.0°	1.2° ± 0.7°	1.4°

Comparisons between the four fixation models and the intact model

The percentage of ROM of the four fixation models with respect to the intact model was compared in terms of the degree of ROM in each direction of movement. The percentage of ROM of the S-I-C group was lowest in all directions of motion (flexion: 13.2%; extension: 13.5%; left bending: 35.0%; right bending: 33.9%; left rotation: 64.6%; right rotation: 65.6%), indicating the stability was the best. The percentage ROM of the S-L group was the highest in all directions of motion (flexion: 15.6%; extension: 15.4%; left bending: 39.7%; right bending: 37.8%; left rotation: 75.3%; right rotation: 76.5%), indicating the worst stability. The S-I group ranked second, and the S-L-C group ranked third with respect to stability (Fig. 6).

Stress distribution of the pedicle instrumentation system

von Mises stress distribution analysis showed that high stresses were mainly concentrated on the screws during flexion and extension. High stress in lateral bending was mainly concentrated on the longitudinal connecting rod. High stress was also concentrated at the junction of the transverse connecting rod and the longitudinal connecting rod under a rotation load (Fig. 7).

Maximum von Mises stress on the root of the pedicle screw

von Mises stresses of the pedicle screw neck of the S-L group were 30.9 MPa in flexion, 31.7 MPa in extension, 200.7 MPa in left lateral bending, 202.3 MPa in right lateral bending, 261.9 MPa in left rotation, and 265.3 MPa in right rotation. Stresses in the S-I group were 24.7 MPa in flexion, 25.7 MPa in extension, 141.8 MPa in left lateral bending, 144.3 MPa in right bending, 192.9 MPa in left rotation, and 191.2 MPa in right rotation. Stresses in the S-L-C group were 25.9 MPa in flexion, 26.1 MPa in extension, 156.5 MPa in left lateral bending, 258.4 MPa in right lateral bending, 200.4 MPa in left rotation, and 201.6 in right rotation. Stresses in the S-I-C group were 23.5 MPa in flexion, 24.6 MPa in extension, 128.6 MPa in left lateral bending, 130.2 MPa in right lateral bending, 162.3 MPa in left rotation, and 162.3 MPa in right rotation (Table 4).

Table 3 Range of motion of four fixations with different loading

Loading mode	S-L	S-I	S-L-C	S-I-C
Flexion	1.03°	0.95°	0.98°	0.87°
Extension	1.05°	0.98°	1.00°	0.92°
Left bending	2.92°	2.67°	2.75°	2.57°
Right bending	2.80°	2.54°	2.61°	2.51°
Left rotation	2.60°	2.32°	2.46°	2.23°
Right rotation	2.60°	2.32°	2.46°	2.23°

Discussion

Surgical management of a thoracolumbar burst fracture varies according to many factors. Fracture morphology, neurologic status, and surgeon preference all play major roles in deciding the surgical approach. An anterior approach to the fracture site can directly decompress the neural elements, and the reconstruction ca be performed by simultaneous iliac bone graft and plating. Hitchon et al. [15] and Sasso et al. [16] reported that the anterior approach was superior to the posterior approach in its ability to maintain the kyphotic correction at final

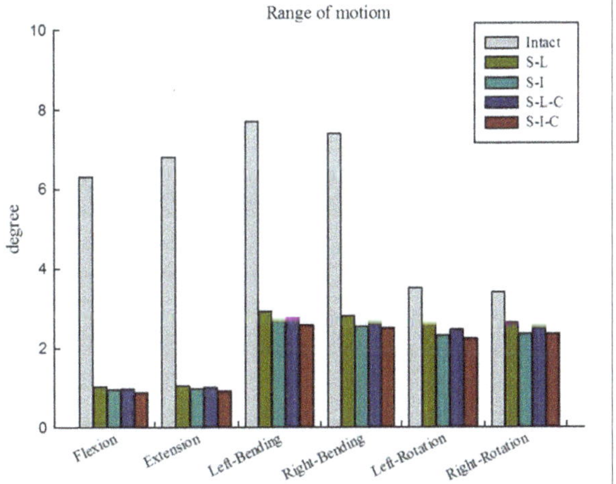

Fig. 6 Range of motion (ROM). Compared to the intact normal spine model, the four fixation models showed a decreased ROM in all directions. S-I-C fixation had the lowest ROM

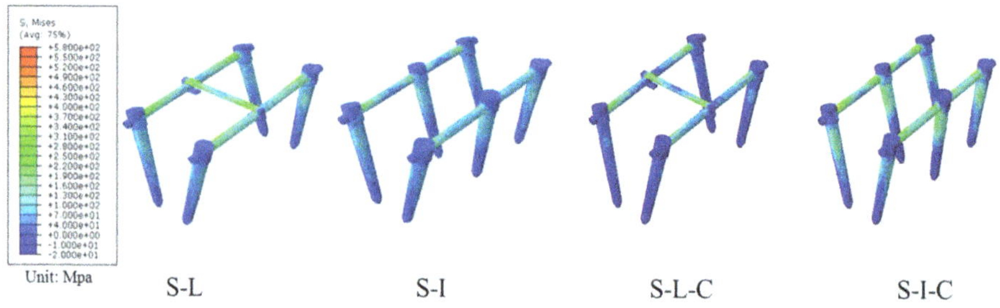

Fig. 7 Stress nephogram of the pedicle screws and rods with rotation stress

follow-up, but both approaches achieved similar in clinical results. A major disadvantage of anterior surgery is potential donor site morbidity from harvesting iliac tricortical bone graft. In addition, the cost of the anterior approach is generally greater than that of the posterior approach. We usually use a posterior approach for the repair of thoracolumbar burst fractures, which is one of the reasons that led to the current study.

Traditional one-above and one-below short-segment posterior instrumentation has the potential for early implant failure and re-kyphosis due to lack of anterior support of the defect inside the injured vertebra. Several techniques, such as reinforcement with additional screws at the fractured level, or augmentation with any kind of bone cement to fill the defect of the fractured vertebra, have been proposed to improve the stability of the posterior instrumentation construct, and thus prevent implant failure and enhance fracture union [17–20]. However, no studies examined reinforcement of a fractured vertebra with a combination of bone cement with two additional fracture-level screws. Several biomechanical studies have suggested that reinforcement with fracture-level screws could improve the biomechanical stability of the construct [21–23]. Clinical studies have also suggested that reinforcement with additional screws at the fractured level can provide better kyphotic correction, more effectively restore fractured vertebra height, and allow earlier ambulation for patients with thoracolumbar burst fractures [24, 25]. On the contrary, authors have also claimed that a fractured vertebra augmented by absorbable bone cement followed by a posterior short-segment construct can provide satisfactory clinical results, with a low implant failure rate of 0% to 5% [19, 20]. Xu et al. [26] designed a FE model of a thoracolumbar burst fracture, and demonstrated that vertebroplasty inside the fractured vertebra can significantly reduce the stresses of the pedicle instrumentations and spine to prevent kyphotic correction loss and implant failure. In a clinical study, Liao et al. [27] showed that two screws placed inside the fractured vertebra with short-segment instrumentation was associated with shorter surgical time and less implant failure as compared to augmentation with injectable calcium sulphate/phosphate cement following posterior short-segment instrumentation.

Table 4 Maximum von Mises stress on the root of the pedicle screw

Loading mode	S-L	S-I	S-L-C	S-I-C
Flexion	30.9 MPa	24.7 MPa	25.9 MPa	23.5 MPa
Extension	31.7 MPa	25.7 MPa	26.1 MPa	24.6 MPa
Left bending	200.7 MPa	141.8 MPa	156.5 MPa	128.6 MPa
Right bending	202.3 MPa	144.3 MPa	258.4 MPa	103.2 MPa
Left rotation	261.9 MPa	192.9 MPa	200.4 MPa	162.3 MPa
Right rotation	265.3 MPa	191.2 MPa	201.6 MPa	162.3 MPa

In the current study, the four fixation models all demonstrated decreased ROM in all directions as compared with the intact spine model. ROM in flexion, extension, axial rotation, and lateral bending was the smallest in the S-I-C fixation model, followed by the S-I and S-L-C fixation models; the greatest ROM was seen in the S-L fixation model. The S-I-C and the S-I fixation model both contained six screws in the construct; the S-L-C and the S-L fixation only had four screws in the construct. Reinforcement with two additional screws at the fractured level can enhance biomechanical stability; and these results were similar to a previous FE study by Li et al. [28]. Two additional screws inside the fractured vertebra was also stronger than when bone cement was used inside the fractured level (S-I fixation model versus S-L-C fixation model). This result was similar to the clinical results demonstrated by Liao et al. [27].

The pedicle screw is considered to be the weakest point of the posterior fixation, and implant failure is usually caused by screw loosening or screw root breakage [29]. It has also been shown that the pedicle screws still continue to bear most of the load after fusion [30, 31]. To prevent early screw breakage, and to prolong the life of the screw, it is necessary to prevent the load on the screw from reaching the fatigue load. For this reason, we evaluated the maximum von Mises stress on the root of the pedicle screws in the four fixation models. A lower stress distribution around the root of the pedicle screw means the less chance of pedicle screw breakage. The maximum von Mises stress of the pedicle screws in the S-L group was higher than that in the other three fixation groups. In the S-I-C group, the maximum von Mises stress of the pedicle screw in all directions was the lowest. These results indicate that using two additional screws inside the fractured vertebra can reduce the stress on the pedicle screw root. Further augmentation with bone cement at the fractured level can further reduce the stress around the pedicle screw root, and further decrease the probability of screw failure. In addition, we found the pedicle screw root under lateral bending and axial rotation load sustained higher von Mises stresses, as finding similar to that of Xu et al. [32].

Injectable bone substitutes such as calcium sulfate, calcium phosphate cement, and hydroxyapatite cement are widely used for filling bone defects. These bone substitutes not only have osteoconductive ability to promote bone union, but also provide initial mechanical support. Evaniew et al. [33] used calcium sulfate/phosphate cement to manage patients with bone defects after curettage of primary tumor. Orsini et al. [34] demonstrated that calcium sulfate cement could promote new bone formation in a rabbit model of bone defects. Furthermore, Xu et al. [26] used a FE model to show that cement augmentation of a fractured vertebra could decrease the von Mises stress on the rods by 50% and on the screws by 40%. In the current study, however, the initial stability provided by bone cement inside the fractured vertebra did not achieve the stability provided by two additional screws. Nevertheless, an advantage of bone cements is that they can stimulate bone healing inside the vertebra, which screws cannot provide. Therefore, a combination of bone cement and two additional screws inside the fractured vertebra along with short-segment instrumentation may be an ideal surgical method for thoracolumbar burst fractures because provides greater initial stability, and also stimulates bone growth.

There are limitations of this study that should be considered. First, the FE spine models were reconstructed from data of a single patient, and thus is not representative of various ages or different sexes. Second, most cases of thoracolumbar burst fractures are associated with injury to the upper endplate and/or adjacent intervertebral disc. This was not addressed in the current models. Removal of the upper end-plate of the vertebrae in the FE model may better reflect the real injury pattern of a burst fracture. However, the main purpose of this study was to compare different fixation techniques, not different injuries. Third, because the current FE study only provided comparison data for the stability of different fixation methods, and the material representations of the biological structures were assumed to be linearly elastic, biomechanical studies of cadavers are necessary to validate the results for clinical practice. If the results are validated in cadaver studies, clinical cohort studies would be warranted.

Conclusion

Additional bilateral pedicle screws combined with cement augmentation vertebroplasty at the level of the fractured vertebra results in a stiffer construct and lower von Mises stress on the pedicle screws as compared with other types of posterior short-segment fixations. Four-screws plus a link resulted in the highest stress on the screws, suggesting this method would be associated with a higher incidence of implant failure and re-kyphosis. The S-I-C fixation was the strongest posterior short-segment fixation method for thoracolumbar burst fractures.

Abbreviation

FE: Finite element; ROM: Range of motion

Acknowledgements

None.

Funding

This study was funded by the Chang Gung Memorial Hospital Research Fund. The grant number is CRRPG3E0151.

Author contributions

JCL provided the concept of the study and wrote the manuscript. WPC designed the study and took responsibility for revising the manuscript. HW designed the study and performed the anaalyses. All authors read and approved the final manuscript.

Competing interest

The authors declare that they have no competing interests.

Consent for publication

"Not applicable"

Author details

[1]Department of Orthopedic Surgery, Bone and Joint Research Center, Chang Gung Memorial Hospital, Chang Gung University, Taoyuan, Taiwan. [2]Department of Mechanical Engineering, National Taipei University of Technology, 1, Sec. 3, Chung-Hsiao E. Rd, Taipei 10608, Taiwan.

Reference

1. Benson DR, Burkus JK, Montesano PX, Sutherland TB, McLain RF. Unstable thoracolumbar and lumbar burst fractures treated with the AO fixateur interne. J Spinal Disord. 1992;5:335–43.
2. Crawford NR, Dickman CA. Construction of local vertebral coordinate systems using a digitizing probe. Tech Note Spine. 1997;22:559–63.
3. Limb D, Shaw DL, Dickson RA. Neurological injury in thoracolumbar burst fractures. J Bone Joint Surg Br. 1995;77:774–7.

4. Kaneda K, Taneichi H, Abumi K, Hashimoto T, Satoh S, Fujiya M. Anterior decompression and stabilization with the Kaneda device for thoracolumbar burst fractures associated with neurological deficits. J Bone Joint Surg Am. 1997;79:69–83.
5. Steffee AD, Biscup RS, Sitkowski DJ. Segmental spine plates with pedicle screw fixation. A new internal fixation device for disorders of the lumbar and thoracolumbar spine. Clin Orthop Relat Res. 1986;203:45–53.
6. Müller U, Berlemann U, Sledge J, Schwarzenbach O. Treatment of thoracolumbar burst fractures without neurologic deficit by indirect reduction and posterior instrumentation: bisegmental stabilization with monosegmental fusion. Eur Spine J. 1999;8:284–9.
7. Liao JC, Fan KF, Keorochana G, Chen WJ, Chen LH. Transpedicular grafting after short-segment pedicle instrumentation for thoracolumbar burst fracture: calcium sulfate cement versus autogenous iliac bone graft. Spine. 2010;35:1482–8.
8. Korovessis P, Hadjipavlou A, Repantis T. Minimal invasive short posterior instrumentation plus balloon kyphoplasty with calcium phosphate for burst and severe compression lumbar fractures. Spine. 2008;33:658–67.
9. Norton RP, Milne EL, Kaimrajh DN, Eismont FJ, Latta LL, Williams SK. Biomechanical analysis of four- versus six-screw constructs for short-segment pedicle screw and rod instrumentation of unstable thoracolumbar fractures. Spine J. 2014;14:1734–9. See comment in PubMed Commons below
10. Chosa E, Goto K, Totoribe K, Tajima N. Analysis of the effect of lumbar spine fusion on the superior adjacent intervertebral disk in the presence of disk degeneration, using the three-dimensional finite element method. J Spinal Disord Tech. 2004;17:134–9.
11. Park WM, Park YS, Kim K, Kim YH. Biomechanical comparison of instrumentation techniques in treatment of thoracolumbar burst fractures: a finite element analysis. J Orthop Sci. 2009;14:443–9.
12. Qiu TX, Tan KW, Lee VS, Teo EC. Investigation of thoracolumbar T12-L1 burst fracture mechanism using finite element method. Med Eng Phys. 2006;28: 656–64.
13. Qiu TX, Teo EC, Zhang QH. Effect of bilateral facetectomy of thoracolumbar spine T11-L1 on spinal stability. Med Biol Eng Comput. 2006;44:363–70.
14. Panjabi MM, Oxland TR, Lin RM, McGowen TW. Thoracolumbar burst fracture. A biomechanical investigation of its multidirectional flexibility. Spine. 1994;19:578–85.
15. Hitchon PW, Torner J, Eichholz KM, Beeler SN. Comparison of anterolateral and posterior approaches in the management of thoracolumbar burst fractures. J Neurosurg Spine. 2006;5:117–25.
16. Sasso RC, Renkens K, Hanson D, Reilly T, McGuire RA Jr, Best NM. Unstable thoracolumbar burst fractures: anterior-only versus short-segment posterior fixation. J Spinal Disord Tech. 2006;19:242–8.
17. Guven O, Kocaoglu B, Bezer M, Aydin N, Nalbantoglu U. The use of screw at the fracture level in the treatment of thoracolumbar burst fractures. J Spinal Disord Tech. 2009;22:417–21.
18. Farrokhi MR, Razmkon A, Maghami Z, Nikoo Z. Inclusion of the fracture level in short segment fixation of thoracolumbar fractures. Eur Spine J. 2010;19:1651–6.
19. Marco RA, Meyer BC, Kushwaha VP. Thoracolumbar burst fractures treated with posterior decompression and pedicle screw instrumentation supplemented with balloon-assisted vertebroplasty and calcium phosphate reconstruction. Surgical technique. J Bone Joint Surg Am. 2010;92(Suppl 1 Pt 1):67–76.
20. Shen YX, Zhang P, Zhao JG, Xu W, Fan ZH, Lu ZF, et al. Pedicle screw instrumentation plus augmentation vertebroplasty using calcium sulfate for thoracolumbar burst fractures without neurologic deficits. Orthop Surg. 2011;3:1–6.
21. Anekstein Y, Brosh T, Mirovsky Y. Intermediate screws in short segment pedicular fixation for thoracic and lumbar fractures: a biomechanical study. J Spinal Disord Tech. 2007;20:72-77.
22. Baaj AA, Reyes PM, Yaqoobi AS, Uribe JS, Vale FL, Theodore N, et al. Biomechanical advantage of the index-level pedicle screw in unstable thoracolumbar junction fractures. J Neurosurg Spine. 2011;14:192–7.
23. Wang H, Li C, Liu T, Zhao WD, Zhou Y. Biomechanical efficacy of monoaxial or polyaxial pedicle screw and additional screw insertion at the level of fracture, in lumbar burst fracture: an experimental study. Indian J Orthop. 2012;46:395–401.
24. Mahar A, Kim C, Wedemeyer M, Mitsunaga L, Odell T, Johnson B, et al. Short-segment fixation of lumbar burst fractures using pedicle fixation at the level of the fracture. Spine. 2007;32:1503–7.
25. Tian JW, Wang L, Xia T, Liu CY, Zhao QH, Dong SH. Posterior short-segmental fixation combined with intermediate screws vs conventional intersegmental fixation for monosegmental thoracolumbar fractures. Orthopedics. 2011;34:e389–96.
26. Xu G, Fu X, Du C, Ma J, Li Z, Ma X. Biomechanical effects of vertebroplasty on thoracolumbar burst fracture with transpedicular fixation: a finite element model analysis. Orthop Traumatol Surg Res. 2014;100:379–83.
27. Liao JC, Fan KF. Posterior short-segment fixation in thoracolumbar unstable burst fractures - Transpedicular grafting or six-screw construct? Clin Neurol Neurosurg. 2016;153:56–63.
28. Li C, Zhou Y, Wang H, Liu J, Xiang L. Treatment of unstable thoracolumbar fractures through short segment pedicle screw fixation techniques using pedicle fixation at the level of the fracture: a finite element analysis. PLoS One. 2014;9:e99156.
29. Moran JM, Berg WS, Berry JL, Geiger JM, Steffee AD. Transpedicular screw fixation. J Orthop Res. 1989;7:107–14.
30. Chen CS, Cheng CK, Liu CL. A biomechanical comparison of posterolateral fusion and posterior fusion in the lumbar spine. J Spinal Disord Tech. 2002; 15:53–63.
31. Suda K, Ito M, Abumi K, Haba H, Taneichi H, Kaneda K. Radiological risk factors of pseudoarthrosis and/or instrument breakage after PLF with the pedicle screw system in isthmic spondylolisthesis. J Spinal Disord Tech. 2006;19:541–6.
32. Xu G, Fu X, Du C, Ma J, Li Z, Tian P, et al. Biomechanical comparison of mono-segment transpedicular fixation with short-segment fixation for treatment of thoracolumbar fractures: a finite element analysis. Proc Inst Mech Eng H. 2014;228:1005–13.
33. Evaniew N, Tan V, Parasu N, Jurriaans E, Finlay K, Deheshi B, et al. Use of a calcium sulfate-calcium phosphate synthetic bone graft composite in the surgical management of primary bone tumors. Orthopedics. 2013;36:e216–22.
34. Orsini G, Ricci J, Scarano A, Pecora G, Petrone G, Iezzi G, et al. Bone-defect healing with calcium-sulfate particles and cement: an experimental study in rabbit. J Biomed Mater Res B Appl Biomater. 2004;68:199–208. See comment in PubMed Commons below

5

A cross-sectional study of the effects of load carriage on running characteristics and tibial mechanical stress: implications for stress-fracture injuries in women

Chun Xu[1], Amy Silder[2], Ju Zhang[3], Jaques Reifman[1*] and Ginu Unnikrishnan[1]

Abstract

Background: Load carriage is associated with musculoskeletal injuries, such as stress fractures, during military basic combat training. By investigating the influence of load carriage during exercises on the kinematics and kinetics of the body and on the biomechanical responses of bones, such as the tibia, we can quantify the role of load carriage on bone health.

Methods: We conducted a cross-sectional study using an integrated musculoskeletal-finite-element model to analyze how the amount of load carriage in women affected the kinematics and kinetics of the body, as well as the tibial mechanical stress during running. We also compared the biomechanics of walking (studied previously) and running under various load-carriage conditions.

Results: We observed substantial changes in both hip kinematics and kinetics during running when subjects carried a load. Relative to those observed during running without load, the joint reaction forces at the hip increased by an average of 49.1% body weight when subjects carried a load that was 30% of their body weight (ankle, 4.8%; knee, 20.6%). These results indicate that the hip extensor muscles in women are the main power generators when running with load carriage. When comparing running with walking, finite element analysis revealed that the peak tibial stress during running (tension, 90.6 MPa; compression, 136.2 MPa) was more than three times as great as that during walking (tension, 24.1 MPa; compression, 40.3 MPa), whereas the cumulative stress within one stride did not differ substantially between running (15.2 MPa · s) and walking (13.6 MPa · s).

Conclusions: Our findings highlight the critical role of hip extensor muscles and their potential injury in women when running with load carriage. More importantly, our results underscore the need to incorporate the cumulative effect of mechanical stress when evaluating injury risk under various exercise conditions. The results from our study help to elucidate the mechanisms of stress fracture in women.

Keywords: Stress fracture, Tibial mechanical stress, Finite element analysis, Running mechanics, Load carriage

* Correspondence: jaques.reifman.civ@mail.mil
[1]Department of Defense Biotechnology High Performance Computing Software Applications Institute, Telemedicine and Advanced Technology Research Center, United States Army Medical Research and Materiel Command, Fort Detrick, Maryland, USA
Full list of author information is available at the end of the article

Background

The frequent occurrence of stress-fracture injuries during basic combat training (BCT) remains a leading concern for the United States (US) military [1]. Epidemiological studies have shown that the most commonly injured sites for stress fractures include the tibia, femoral neck, tarsal navicular, metatarsals, and pelvis [2–4]. Stress fractures are caused by repeated application of sub-critical mechanical insults associated with common BCT exercises, including walking, running, and jumping [1, 5–7]. Furthermore, military personnel are often required to carry loads that reach a considerable percentage of their body weight, which have been shown to be associated with an increased risk of stress fracture [8, 9]. To understand the impact of load carriage and ultimately help reduce the risk of stress fracture, previous studies have examined systematic changes in metabolic parameters (e.g., energy cost) [10–12], ground reaction forces (GRFs) [13], joint kinematics [10, 14], and muscle activities [15] due to load carriage. However, the effects of load carriage on bone biomechanical responses (e.g., bone stress and strain), which play a crucial role in bone health, have been less extensively investigated.

The technical challenges and ethical restrictions associated with implanting strain gauges make it impractical to experimentally measure bone strains in healthy individuals [16]. Therefore, computational methods have been implemented in recent years to quantify mechanical bone stress and strain [17]. For example, our group has developed an integrated musculoskeletal-finite-element (FE) modeling framework and used it to quantify the impact of load carriage during walking in a woman [18] on a number of measures, including joint kinematics, joint kinetics (joint reaction forces or JRFs), and biomechanical responses of the tibia (i.e., spatiotemporal stress distribution, and its cumulative effect during one gait cycle).

Previous studies have shown that the muscles involved during walking and running are almost identical, and that switching from walking to running is associated with changes in both the timing and intensity of muscle activation [19]. However, our understanding of how the body adjusts its kinetics, kinematics, and biomechanics over a range of load carriages during running remains fragmentary. Here, we sought to answer the following research question: how do the joint angles, JRFs, and tibial mechanical stresses change in response to load carriage when women run at their preferred speeds? We hypothesized that: *1*) running with load carriage would increase both peak JRFs and the percentage of the tibial volume subjected to high stress and *2*) the changes in JRFs and tibial stress would not be proportional to the change in load carriage.

Methods

We performed musculoskeletal-FE analyses by using a recently reported method [18]. Figure 1 shows an overview of our integrated approach.

Experiments

Our musculoskeletal analyses were based on data obtained from motion-capture experiments described by Silder et al. [20]. Briefly, four female recreational runners [age, 29.8 yr (95% CI: 27.8, 31.7); mass, 60.0 kg (55.8, 64.3); height: 1.68 m (1.66, 1.71); body mass index (BMI): 21.2 kg/m^2 (19.8, 22.6)] ran on a force-sensing treadmill (Bertec Corporation, Columbus, OH, USA), at their preferred speeds without carrying any load (0% baseline model) or carrying a load of 20% or 30% of their body weight (BW) by using an adjustable weight vest. For each participant, 29 retroreflective markers were secured on specific anatomical locations, including the clavicle bone, arms, trunk, pelvis, thighs, shanks, and feet. All subjects were free of injury (current or past) and signed a written consent form approved by the Stanford University Institutional Review Board. The output from the motion-capture experiments included marker trajectories, GRFs, and electromyography (EMG) recordings.

Musculoskeletal analysis

We used the AnyBody Modeling System™ (AnyBody Technology, Aalborg, Denmark) to perform musculoskeletal analyses based on the motion-capture data. We first filtered the marker trajectories and GRF recordings with a low-pass fourth-order Butterworth filter (cutoff frequency, 8 Hz). In the absence of subject-specific anatomical and musculoskeletal parameters, we used the anthropometric data to scale a previously validated whole-body musculoskeletal model [21]. The lower extremities of the musculoskeletal model consisted of seven rigid bodies, including the pelvis, thigh, shank, and foot, as well as 55 Hill-type muscles per leg [22]. We modeled the hip joints as spherical joints (enabling flexion/extension, internal/external rotation, and abduction/adduction movements), and the knee and ankle joints as revolute joints (allowing flexion/extension rotation). A revolute joint connected the patella to the femur, which allowed a small degree of rotation but no translation. A patellar tendon connected the patella segment to the tibia.

One common challenge associated with musculoskeletal modeling based on motion-capture experiments is determining the length of each body segment [23]. This is because the joints are located deep below the skin and the tissues, making it difficult to measure their true positions without advanced imaging techniques. Therefore, we first obtained the joint positions and orientations by using a least-squares parameter identification algorithm

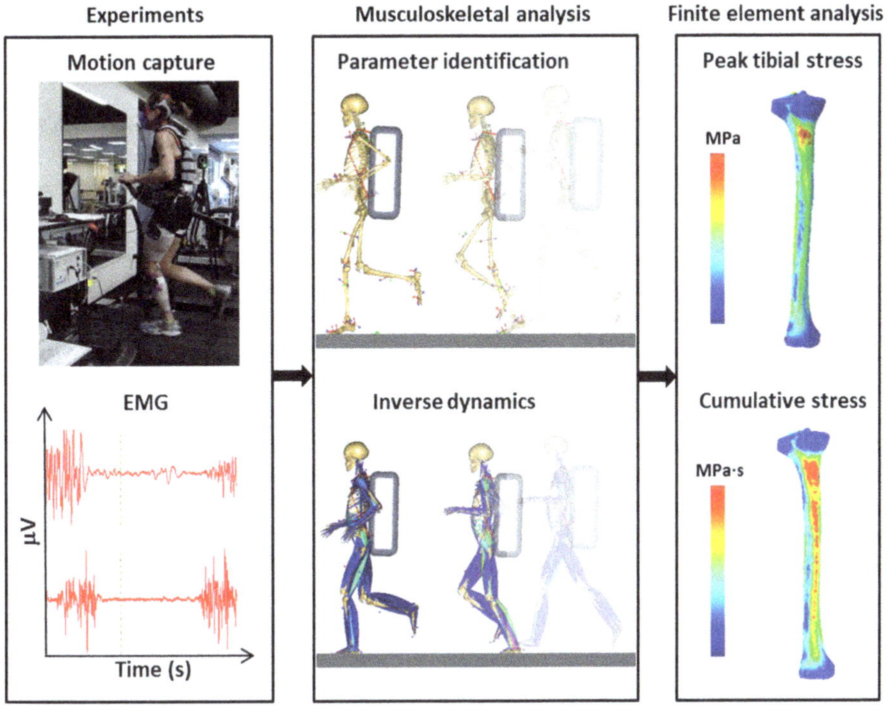

Fig. 1 Flowchart of the integrated musculoskeletal-finite-element modeling method. EMG: electromyography

that minimizes the errors between markers defined in the model and those tracked in the experiment [23]. We used an inverse dynamics approach to compute muscle activities and JRFs over one running cycle, where muscle activity was defined as the muscle force divided by muscle strength [21]. We performed whole-body musculoskeletal analysis for running without a load (0%), or with a load of 20% or 30% BW for all four subjects. We normalized the moments and JRFs for each participant by the body mass to enable consistent comparisons.

FE analysis

Details of the FE analysis method have been reported previously [18]. Briefly, we first generated a tetrahedral FE mesh from computed tomography images of a sex-, age-, and BMI-matched subject from the Victorian Institute of Forensic Medicine (Melbourne, Victoria, Australia) database. Subsequently, we used a mesh-morphing and material-property-mapping algorithm to derive heterogeneous bone material properties for each tibia model of interest [24, 25]. This procedure produced an average of 147,357 unique linear elastic and isotropic material properties for the tibia model. Finally, we exported the material property definitions into an ABAQUS input file for structural analysis (ABAQUS 6.12, Dassault Systèmes, Vélizy-Villacoublay, France).

We used the muscle forces and bone forces/moments obtained from the musculoskeletal analysis to specify the loading conditions for the FE analysis. Specifically, we first identified muscle/ligament insertion points from the musculoskeletal model to construct FE constraint nodes, which were then coupled to the outer surface of the tibial FE meshes. Through this procedure, we specified an average of 171 couplings between the muscle/ligament nodes and the tibial FE meshes. We defined the joint contact forces in a similar manner. Finally, we performed mesh convergence studies, using the FE loading conditions defined for the baseline model. We determined 3.5 mm as an adequate edge-length for our 10-node quadratic tetrahedral mesh.

From the FE analyses, we determined the spatiotemporal tibial stress distribution, and then evaluated the per-cycle cumulative effects of tibial stress (MPa · s) by integrating the FE-predicted nodal stress values over time [26]. In the absence of any experimentally measured threshold above which the tibial mechanical stress becomes harmful, we first determined three stress thresholds from the baseline model that divided the tibia into four zones of equal volume (i.e., 25% of the total volume). Then, we calculated the changes in volumetric fraction at load carriage conditions of 20% and 30% BW according to the determined stress thresholds. Lastly, we quantified the changes in the volumetric fraction of cumulative stress due to load carriage in a similar manner.

Results

Muscle activities

To ensure the validity of the musculoskeletal model—that it correctly predicted the muscle activation needed to produce the measured whole-body kinematics—we compared the time courses of the predicted muscle forces and EMG recordings under baseline conditions [27]. We observed good agreement between the predicted and measured muscle activity profiles under the baseline condition after taking into account the electromechanical delay, which represents the time lag between the onset of muscle activation (measured by EMG) and muscle force generation (predicted by the model) [28] (Fig. 2: red, model predictions; green, EMG measurements). Specifically, the model correctly predicted activation of the ankle plantarflexor muscles (soleus and gastrocnemius) during mid-stance and of the ankle dorsiflexor muscles (tibialis anterior) during the late-swing and early-stance phases. Consistent with the EMG recordings, the model predicted medial hamstring activation in the latter half of the swing phase. The model also predicted peak biceps femoris activation during the early stance phase, while the EMG recordings from this muscle peaked earlier (albeit at a lower level), at the end of the swing phase of the previous stride. The model predicted the onset of knee extensor (vastus lateralis, vastus medialis, and rectus femoris) activity at mid-stance to absorb the shock. In addition, the model predicted low muscle activity in the vastus lateralis throughout the swing phase, although two of four subjects' EMG recordings showed muscle activities only during the late-swing phase. This indicates considerable inter-subject variability in the EMG recordings.

Kinematics and kinetics

All participants adopted a rear-foot-strike running style except one subject, who was a forefoot-strike runner. Their running speeds were 3.4, 3.0, 3.5, and 3.6 m/s. Figures 3, 4 and 5 depict the means and SDs of the kinematic (Fig. 3) and kinetic (Figs. 4 and 5) parameters at each joint during running with and without load carriage; their peak values are summarized in Table 1. Consistent with the results of a previous study [20], load carriage increased the stance time and magnitude of the GRFs. Specifically, Table 1 shows

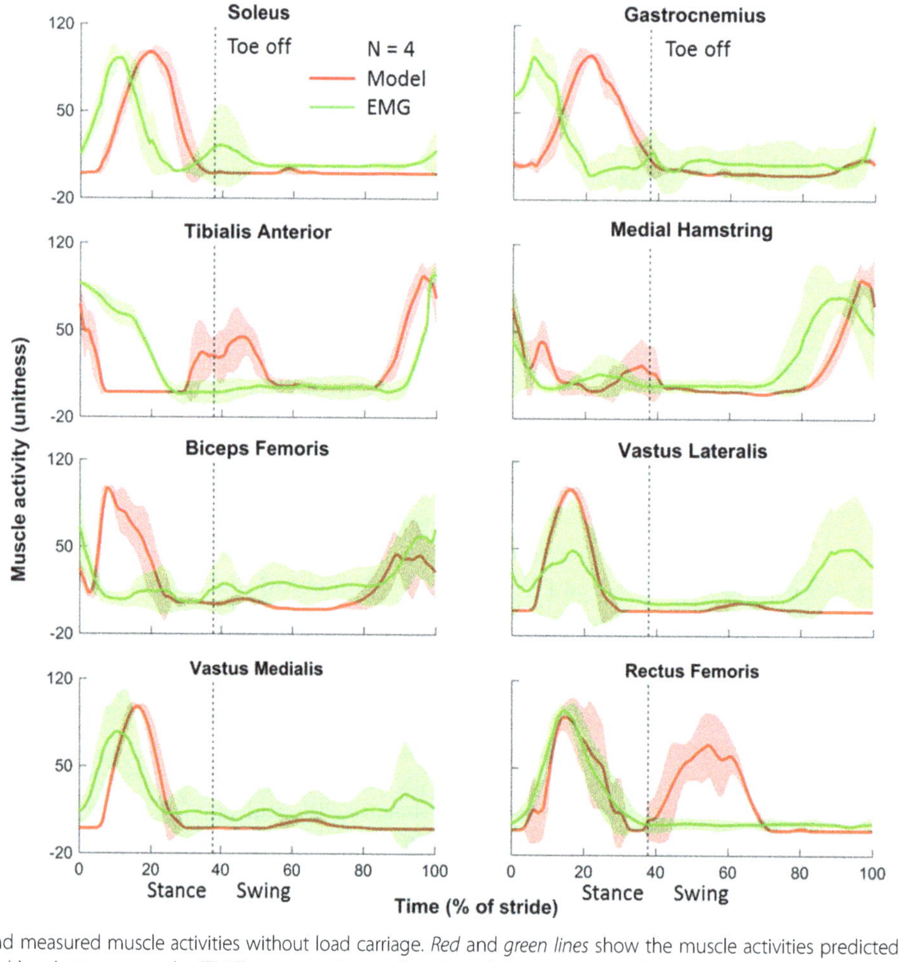

Fig. 2 Predicted and measured muscle activities without load carriage. *Red* and *green lines* show the muscle activities predicted by the model and those measured by electromyography (EMG), respectively, as a function of the percentage of stride. We normalized the magnitudes by the maximal values for each curve. The solid lines represent the group averages of simulated and measured muscle activities ($N = 4$). The shaded areas represent the group-averaged EMG linear envelopes (mean ± one standard deviation). The vertical dashed line, which represents the toe-off point for each condition, separates the stance phase (before toe off) from the swing phase (after toe off)

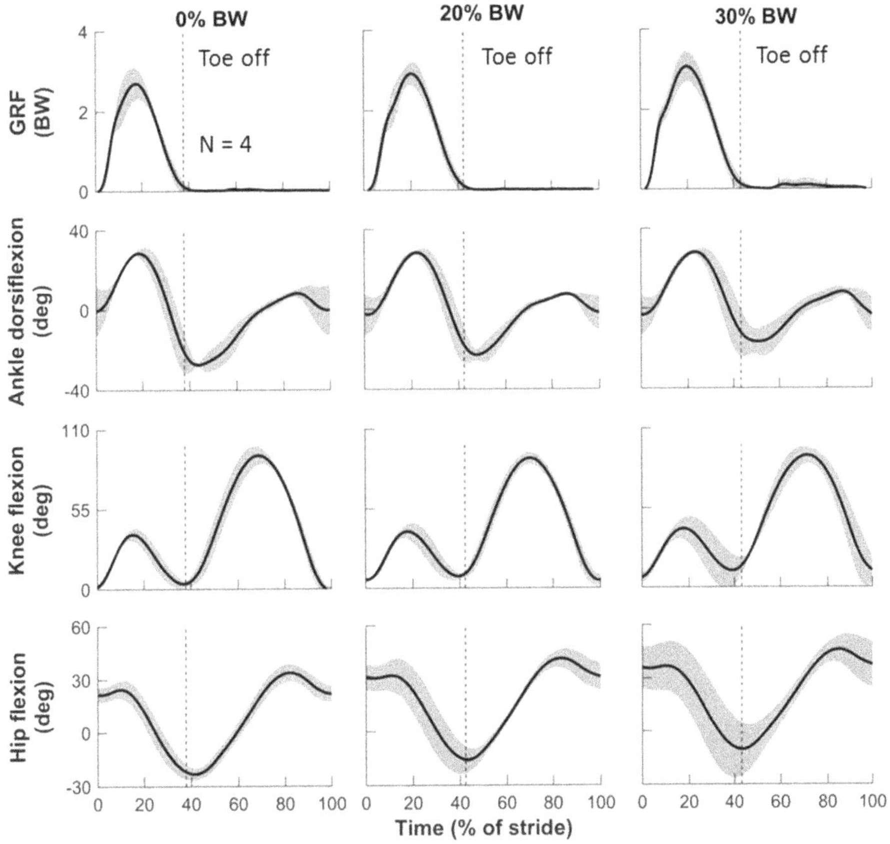

Fig. 3 Joint kinematics at different loads during one gait cycle in the sagittal plane. Solid lines represent means of four subjects. Shaded areas represent one standard deviation above and below the means. For convenience, the first row shows ground reaction force (GRF). Each graph begins and ends at initial contact. The vertical dashed line, which represents the toe-off point for each condition, separates the stance phase (before toe off) from the swing phase (after toe off). Positive angles represent flexion, and negative values represent extension. BW: body weight; deg: degree

that carrying a 30% BW load increased the stance from 37.8% (SD = 1.1) in the baseline condition to 43.2% (SD =1.8) of a gait cycle (i.e., an average increase of 14.3%). The peak vertical GRF increased from 2.7 BW (SD = 0.4) in the baseline condition to 3.1 BW (SD = 0.4) for 30% BW load carriage (i.e., an average increase of 14.8%; Fig. 3, Table 1).

When running with a 30% BW load carriage, the peak ankle dorsiflexion and plantarflexion decreased from 28.5 deg (SD = 2.2) and 27.4 deg (SD = 1.1) in the baseline condition to 27.9 deg (SD = 1.5) and 17.9 deg (SD = 6.7) after toe off, respectively (i.e., an average decrease of 2.1% and 34.7%, respectively; Fig. 3, Table 1). The peak ankle plantarflexion moment increased from 3.4 N · m/kg (SD = 0.3) in the baseline condition to 3.7 N · m/kg (SD = 0.3) (i.e., an average increase of 8.8%; Fig. 4, Table 1). The peak ankle JRFs increased from 12.6 BW (SD = 0.8) in the baseline condition to 13.2 BW (SD = 1.6) (i.e., an average increase of 4.8%; Fig. 5, Table 1).

The knee was flexed throughout the entire running gait, with one flexion peak occurring near mid-stance and the other near mid-swing. During the absorption phase of the stance, the knee flexed to approximately 45 deg. This was followed by the maximal knee flexion during the swing phase, which reached approximately 90 deg (Fig. 3). We did not observe systematic changes in knee angles or knee moments as the load increased (Figs. 3 and 4, Table 1). When running without a load, the knee, among the lower-extremity structures examined, was exposed to the greatest JRFs, which reached as much as 14.1 BW (SD = 2.3) [ankle, 12.6 BW (SD = 0.8); hip, 10.8 BW (SD = 1.4)]. Running with a 30% BW load increased the knee JRFs to 17.0 BW (SD = 3.0), corresponding to a 20.6% increase in average peak knee JRFs (Fig. 5, Table 1).

Carrying a 30% BW load while running limited hip extension but increased hip flexion. The peak hip extension at toe off decreased from 23.2 deg (SD = 3.5) in the baseline condition to 10.5 deg (SD = 14.8) (i.e., an average decrease of 54.7%; Fig. 3, Table 1). All subjects leaned forward to compensate for the reduced hip extension, as evidenced by the increased peak hip flexion before the terminal swing phase from 33.8 deg (SD = 5.1) in the baseline condition to 45.8 deg (SD = 7.9) with a 30% BW load (i.e., an average increase of 35.5%; Fig. 3, Table 1). We did not observe

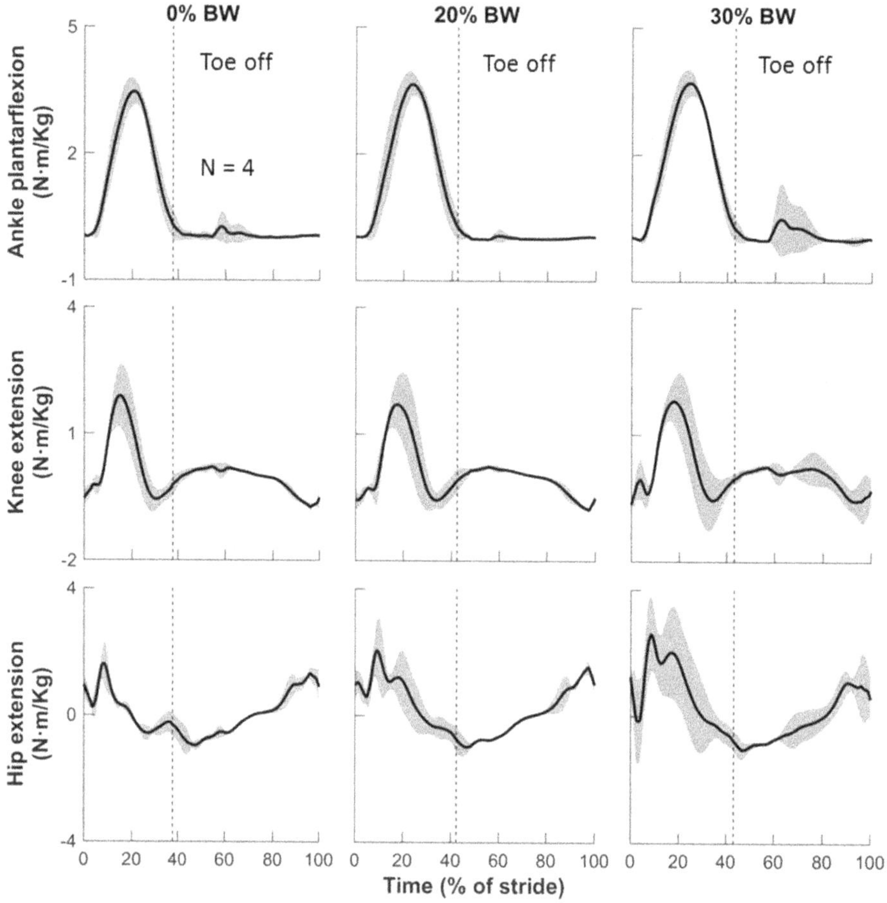

Fig. 4 Joint moments at different loads during one gait cycle in the sagittal plane. Solid lines represent means of four subjects. Shaded areas represent one standard deviation above and below the means. Each graph begins and ends at initial contact. The vertical dashed line, which represents the toe-off point for each condition, separates the stance phase (before toe off) from the swing phase (after toe off). Results are normalized by body mass (in kg). Positive angles and moments represent extension, and negative values represent flexion. BW: body weight

systematic changes in hip adduction and external rotation in response to load carriage. The mean peak hip flexion and extension moment increased from 1.0 N · m/kg (SD = 0.1) and 1.6 N · m/kg (SD = 0.7) in the baseline condition to 1.1 N · m/kg (SD = 0.3) and 2.6 N · m/kg (SD = 1.2), respectively (i.e., an average increase of 10.0% and 62.5%, respectively; Fig. 4, Table 1). The mean peak hip JRFs increased from 10.8 BW (SD = 1.4) to 16.1 BW (SD = 3.2) (i.e., an average increase of 49.1%; Fig. 5, Table 1).

Tibial stress and cumulative stress

Figure 6 shows von Mises stress distributions in the tibia of one subject when running without a load, with a 20% BW load, and with a 30% BW load. For all subjects, the load-related changes in von Mises stress (Fig. 6a) were less pronounced than those in cumulative stress (Fig. 6b). The observed high-stress regions were mainly on the medial-posterior side of the upper diaphysis, corresponding to the location where the semitendinosus muscle of the hamstring inserted, and the posterior side of the mid-diaphysis, corresponding to the location of the superficial posterior muscle compartment, including the gastrocnemius and soleus muscles. Similar to our previous findings of load carriage during walking, the anterior crest of the tibia was exposed to tension, and the posterior aspect subjected to compression [18]. However, the peak values of tibial von Mises stress appeared to be unaffected by load carriage (Table 2).

In the baseline model, we identified pseudo-thresholds in the peak von Mises stress distributions [1.3 MPa (SD = 0.0), 4.6 MPa (SD = 0.2), and 17.8 MPa (SD = 1.4)] and cumulative stress distributions [0.2 MPa · s (SD = 0.0), 0.7 MPa · s (SD = 0.1), and 2.4 MPa · s (SD = 0.1)] for the three load conditions. Histograms of the tibial stress distribution indicated that the average percentage of the tibia exposed to stresses between 4.7 MPa and 17.8 MPa increased from 25.0% at baseline to 25.8% or 29.4% when carrying a 20% or 30% BW load, respectively, while the fraction of the tibia subjected to stresses greater than 17.8 MPa

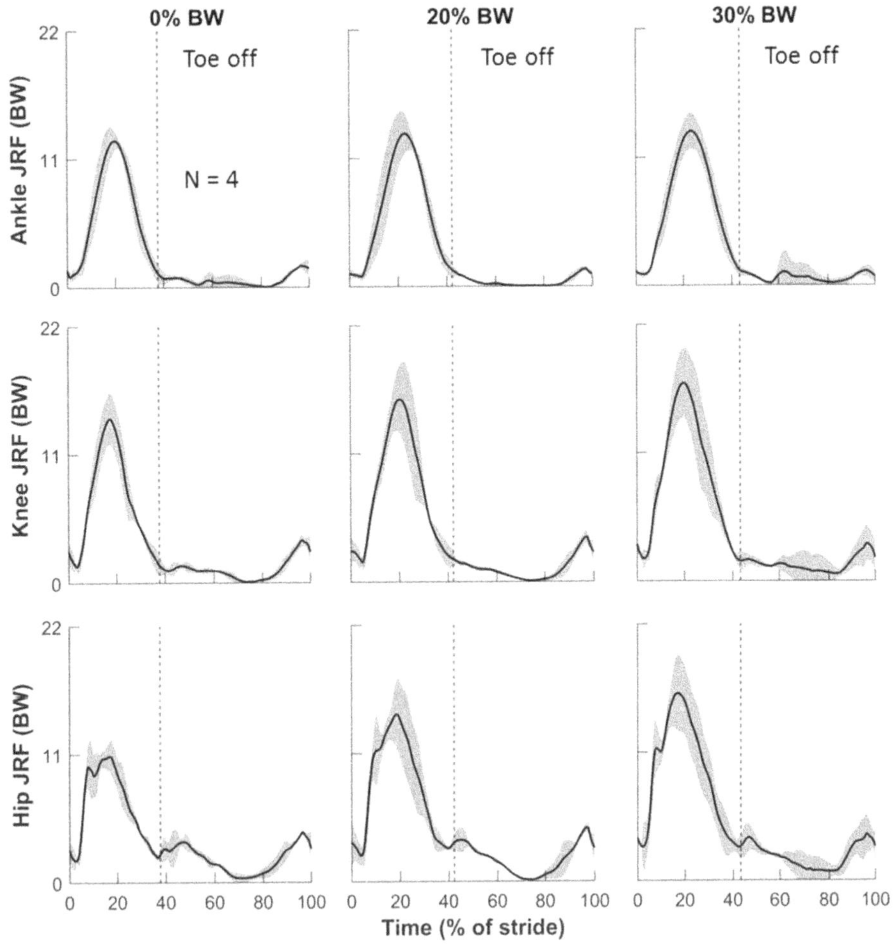

Fig. 5 Joint reaction forces (JRFs) at different loads during one gait cycle. Solid lines represent means of four subjects. Shaded areas represent one standard deviation above and below the means. Each graph begins and ends at initial contact. The vertical dashed line, which represents the toe-off point for each condition, separates the stance phase (before toe off) from the swing phase (after toe off). Results are shown as normalized dimensionless quantities. BW: body weight

increased from 25.0% at baseline to 27.2% or 25.7% when carrying a 20% or 30% BW load, respectively (Fig. 7a). The average percentage of the tibia exposed to cumulative stresses between 0.7 MPa · s and 2.4 MPa · s increased from 25.0% at baseline to 26.9% or 28.9% when carrying a 20% or 30% BW load, respectively, while the fraction of the tibia subjected to cumulative stresses greater than 2.4 MPa · s increased from 25.0% at baseline to 26.1% or 27.8% when the subject carried a load of 20% or 30% of BW, respectively (Fig. 7b). Consequently, the tibial volume subjected to "high" stress (>4.7 MPa) increased from 50.0% in the baseline running condition to 53.0% (= 25.8% + 27.2%) and 55.1% (= 29.4% + 25.7%) when carrying 20% and 30% BW loads, respectively (Fig. 7a). Likewise, the tibial volume subjected to "high" cumulative stress (> 0.7 MPa · s) increased from 50.0% in the baseline running condition to 53.0% (= 26.9% + 26.1%) and 56.7% (= 28.9% + 27.8%) when carrying 20% and 30% BW loads, respectively (Fig. 7b).

Discussion

We performed integrated musculoskeletal-FE simulations to emulate the effects of load carriage on joint kinematics, joint kinetics, tibial mechanical stress, and cumulative tibial stress per gait cycle in four women running at their preferred speeds. We chose the tibia as the bone of interest because it is the most frequently injured site in athletes [29–31] and military recruits [32]. We chose female subjects because of the growing number of women serving in the Army [33]. As are their male counterparts, women are required to wear body armor and carry heavy loads averaging 45.5 kg [34]. Consequently, they are at a higher risk for developing stress-fracture injuries than are men [33].

In support of our first hypothesis, both the peak JRFs and the percentage of the tibial volume subjected to high stresses and cumulative stresses per cycle increased with an increase in load carriage. It is noteworthy that the fraction of tibial volume subjected to pre-defined stress

Table 1 Mean and standard deviation of peak joint angles, joint moments, and joint reaction forces while running without a load (0%) or with an additional load of 20% or 30% of body weight (BW) ($N = 4$)

	Load carriage (% BW)		
	0	20	30
Stance duration (%)	37.8 (1.1)	42.3 (2.5)	43.2 (1.8)
Ground reaction force (BW)	2.7 (0.4)	2.9 (0.3)	3.1 (0.4)
Peak joint angles (degree)			
Ankle			
Dorsiflexion	28.5 (2.2)	28.2 (1.7)	27.9 (1.5)
Plantarflexion	27.4 (1.1)	22.9 (3.0)	17.9 (6.7)
Knee			
Flexion during stance phase	37.7 (4.5)	39.1 (5.2)	40.6 (7.9)
Flexion during swing phase	92.0 (6.3)	89.5 (4.3)	90.7 (5.9)
Hip			
Flexion	33.8 (5.1)	41.3 (5.5)	45.8 (7.9)
Extension	23.2 (3.5)	15.8 (7.3)	10.5 (14.8)
Adduction	5.3 (2.0)	5.8 (0.9)	5.0 (1.9)
External rotation	6.4 (2.4)	6.3 (3.5)	7.9 (2.7)
Peak joint moments (N · m/kg)			
Ankle			
Plantarflexion	3.4 (0.3)	3.6 (0.3)	3.7 (0.3)
Knee			
Flexion	0.7 (0.1)	0.8 (0.1)	0.7 (0.1)
Extension	1.9 (0.7)	1.7 (0.7)	1.8 (0.5)
Hip			
Flexion	1.0 (0.1)	1.0 (0.2)	1.1 (0.3)
Extension	1.6 (0.7)	2.1 (0.9)	2.6 (1.2)
Peak joint reaction forces (BW)			
Ankle	12.6 (0.8)	13.1 (1.7)	13.2 (1.6)
Knee	14.1 (2.3)	15.6 (2.9)	17.0 (3.0)
Hip	10.8 (1.4)	14.4 (3.0)	16.1 (3.2)

thresholds changed in response to load carriage in a non-monotonic manner. Specifically, carrying a 30% BW load increased the average peak JRFs of the ankle, knee, and hip by 4.8%, 20.6%, and 49.1%, respectively, when compared with the baseline condition (Table 1). The tibial volume subjected to stresses between 4.7 MPa and 17.8 MPa increased from 25.0% for the baseline condition to 25.8% for a 20% BW and 29.4% for a 30% BW load carriage, whereas that subjected to stresses greater than17.8 MPa increased from 25.0% for the baseline condition to 27.2% for 20% BW but only to 25.7% for 30% BW load carriage. This might be the result of the quadratic muscle-recruitment criterion adopted in the model, because such a mechanism, which tends to recruit more muscles during high-intensity tasks, distributes the load among several muscles spanning the joint to prevent a few muscles from being overloaded and consequently undergoing muscle fatigue [21]. Overall, the percentage changes in the JRFs, tibial peak stress, and cumulative stress were disproportional to that of the load carriage, consistent with our second hypothesis.

Our results showed that both the kinematics and kinetics of the hip changed substantially during running with load carriage. When compared with the baseline condition, carrying a 30% BW load decreased the mean peak hip extension at toe off by 54.7% and increased the mean peak hip flexion and extension moments by 10.0% and 62.5%, respectively, in addition to increasing the mean peak hip JRFs (49.1%, Table 1). These results highlight the importance of hip muscles in high-intensity physical activity (e.g., running with load carriage), and are supported by previous studies linking them with sports injuries. For example, in collegiate female athletes with patellofemoral injury, hip abductors and external rotators are significantly weaker in the injured leg than in the unaffected leg [35]. Furthermore, if the hip extensors do not generate enough power, either other muscles in the lower extremities will compensate for the reduced force, or movement patterns will change, which in turn may result in increased energy costs and early muscle fatigue [36]. Such changes may be related to a number of biomechanical alterations that potentially increase the risk of impact-related injuries in the lower extremities (e.g., Achilles tendinosis, patellofemoral dysfunction, and tibial stress fracture) [37]. Preparatory strength and endurance training exercises before military BCT, such as squats, incline sit-ups, leg raises, and interval training, which are designed to strengthen hip flexor muscles and pelvic-stabilizing muscles (gluteus medius), are effective in assisting prospective Service members to endure BCT without injuries [38].

Consistent with telemeterized bilateral joint-replacement studies [39, 40], our findings suggest that, for the subject who completed both walking [18] and running experiments, the peak running JRFs were more than two times greater than the peak walking JRFs, with the contribution from the hip muscles increasing during running with load carriage. Specifically, when running without a load, the knee experienced the highest JRF (15.8 BW vs. ankle, 11.3 BW; hip, 12.2 BW) for the subject who completed both walking and running experiments. In contrast, when walking without a load, her ankles were exposed to the highest JRF (4.7 BW vs. knee, 4.4 BW; hip, 4.3 BW). Carrying a 30% BW load increased her JRFs at the hip by 35.2% (ankle, 6.2%; knee, 20.1%) during running, as compared to an increase of 26.2% in her knee JRFs (ankle, 16.4%; hip, 19.0%) during walking [18]. Although this subject ran substantially slower than the others, her running speed (3.0 m/s) was still well above the preferred transition speed

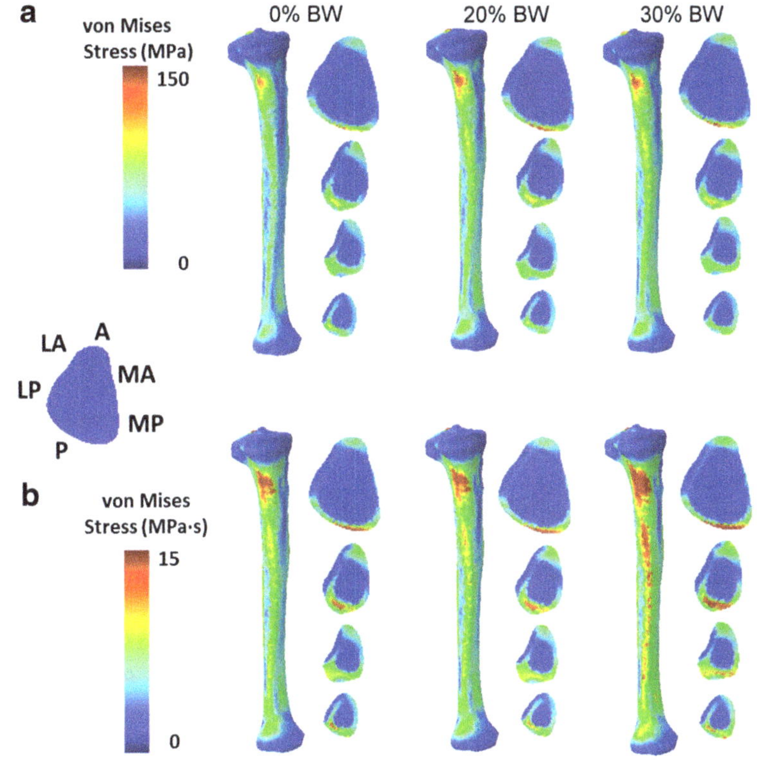

Fig. 6 Spatiotemporal distribution of tibial stresses. Top and bottom panels show tibial von Mises stresses (**a**) and cumulative tibial stresses (**b**), respectively, during one gait cycle without a load (0% baseline, left), with a 20% body weight (BW) load (center), and a 30% BW load (right). We divided the cross section of the left tibia into six sectors. A: Anterior; MA: Medial Anterior; MP: Medial Posterior; P: Posterior; LP: Lateral Posterior; LA: Lateral Anterior. To emphasize the high-stress region on the medial-posterior side, the anterior-posterior (A-P) axis of the 3-D tibia is set oblique relative to the page. Tibial cross sections are arranged with A-P axis running vertically along the page

between walking and running for nonrunners [2.01 (SD = 0.07) m/s] and runners [2.06 (SD = 0.07) m/s] [41]. Moreover, we observed the same trend in all running participants: the JRF at the knee was greater than that at the ankle or hip under the baseline running condition, whereas the hip JRF was more sensitive and increased markedly as the load carriage increased. The relatively small increase in the peak ankle JRFs in response to load carriage during running reflects the lower degree of the plantarflexor involvement in forward movements when running than when walking [18]. Likewise, the increase in hip JRFs associated with load carriage during running suggests that compared with walking, running requires a relatively greater contribution from the hip extensors to meet the increased mechanical and energetic demands of the leg [42].

Table 2 Mean and standard deviation of model-predicted peak tibial von Mises stresses during running without a load (0%), or with an additional load of 20% or 30% of body weight (BW) ($N = 4$)

Load carriage (% BW)	Tension (MPa)	Compression (MPa)
0	101.2 (10.7)	146.3 (8.9)
20	103.7 (17.7)	145.3 (10.1)
30	102.3 (26.0)	147.1 (19.9)

For the subject who completed both walking [18] and running experiments, the tibial stress during running was substantially different from that during walking. For the baseline condition, the peak running tibial stress (tension, 90.6 MPa; compression, 136.2 MPa) was more than three times greater than the peak walking tibial stress (tension, 24.1 MPa; compression, 40.3 MPa). Surprisingly, the cumulative stress per cycle for walking (13.6 MPa · s) was 88% of that for running (15.2 MPa · s). A one-time elevation of the peak JRF or tibial stress does not necessarily increase the risk of stress fracture, because elevated mechanical loading is only one factor that contributes to stress-fracture injuries. The total cumulative stress, which is affected by the duration of the stance (i.e., of foot-ground contact time) and is much shorter in running than in walking [43], plays a major role in the biomechanical and biological responses of bone, as do the total time and frequency of training [1].

During BCT, military recruits on average run 36 min and march 129 min a day, depending on their company and initial fitness level [44, 45]. Assuming that a BCT recruit adopts a common step frequency of 60 steps/min

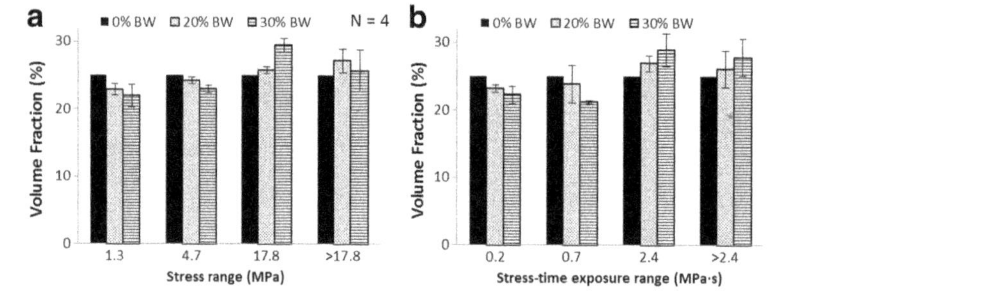

Fig. 7 Histograms of tibial volume fractions subjected to different stress levels. Left and right panels show the tibial volume fractions subjected to different levels of stress (**a**) and cumulative stress (**b**), respectively, as a function of carried load. BW: body weight

for walking and a recommended step frequency of 180 steps/min for running [46], the peak cumulative tibial stress to complete a 36-min running distance reaches 98,496 MPa · s [15.2 (cumulative stress per running cycle) × 180 × 36], and that to complete a 129-min walking distance reaches 105,264 MPa · s [13.6 (cumulative stress per walking cycle) × 60 × 129]. When carrying a 30% BW load under these conditions, the daily cumulative stress due to 36 min of running is 83.3% of that due to 129 min of walking. In other words, the biomechanical impact on the tibia resulting of marching for 129 min is equivalent to that of running for 43 min when the individual carries a 30% BW load. The relatively shorter duration of ground contact in running presumably offsets the effect of the high tibial stress per stride. This is an important finding because, while Service members are not encouraged to run while carrying heavy loads during military training, they are required to complete long-distance tactical foot marches carrying mission-essential equipment (up to 25 kg or 45% BW), which, in essence, leads to the same cumulative stress as a short run with load. If the cumulative effect of internal forces and bone stresses increases the risk of stress-fracture injury, our results suggest that BCT recruits could be more prone to injury when marching an excessive distance than when running a short distance.

One major limitation of the present study stems from the simplifications and assumptions made to construct the model. For example, the knee joint in the current model does not include medial and lateral compartments of joint loads, nor does it fully incorporate complex three-dimensional motions, including translations and rotations. In the absence of medical images necessary for reconstructing subject-specific tibial geometrical structures for FE analyses, we used anthropometric measurements to scale a 50th percentile European female generic musculoskeletal model. Similarly, given that all participants were young and healthy (i.e., ~30 years old), we used tibial material properties mapped from a BMI-matched subject of the same sex for the FE analysis. This approach, along with the use of assumptions regarding material properties (e.g., linear elasticity and isotropy) may affect tibial stress/strain predictions. Furthermore, we chose an effort-based cost function to solve the muscle redundancy problem in the musculoskeletal model. Although this commonly used method predicted patterns of muscle activation qualitatively similar to those of the EMG recordings, it is not suitable for predicting subject-specific muscle activities. This is evident from the discrepancy between the predictions and EMG recordings in the tibialis anterior activation at toe off and rectus femoris activation during early swing (Fig. 2). Lastly, although we quantified the biomechanical alterations during running with load carriage, we only assessed acute effects and did not test for a cause-and-effect relationship between load carriage and stress fracture. Therefore, until more research is conducted in this area, we believe it is premature to identify a correlation between our results and clinically observed injury sites.

Conclusion

Our study shows how the kinetics and kinematics of the body, as well as bone mechanical stress, adjust over a range of load carriages during running. Our findings highlight the critical role of the hip extensor muscles and their potential injury in women when running with load carriage. More importantly, our results underscore the need to incorporate the cumulative effect of mechanical stress when evaluating injury risk under various exercise conditions. These analyses provide insights into the biomechanical alterations of bone that cannot be captured through traditional force platform measurements. Such findings should serve as a foundation for identifying the mechanical determinants for optimizing military training.

Abbreviations

BCT: basic combat training; BMI: body mass index; BW: body weight; EMG: electromyography; FE: finite element; GRF: ground reaction force; JRF: joint reaction forces; SD: standard deviation; US: United States

Acknowledgements

We thank Dr. Tatsuya Oyama for editorial assistance. We also acknowledge the high-performance computing resources made available by the US Department of Defense High Performance Computing Modernization Program at the Air Force Research Laboratory.

Funding
This research was sponsored by the US Army Network Science Initiative and a grant from the Defense Health Program managed by the Military Operational Medicine Research Program, US Army Medical Research and Materiel Command, Fort Detrick, Maryland.

Authors' contributions
CX, GU, and JR designed the study. CX developed the computational model, performed simulations, analyzed the results, and drafted the manuscript. GU and JR contributed to data evaluation and manuscript preparation. AS performed data collection and provided feedback on data interpretation. JZ contributed in the mapping of bone material properties. All authors edited the manuscript and reviewed the final version.

Competing interests
The authors declare no competing interests. The opinions and assertions contained herein are the private views of the authors and are not to be construed as official or as reflecting the views of the US Army or of the US Department of Defense. This paper has been approved for public release with unlimited distribution.

Consent for publication
The authors obtained a written consent to publish the identifiable image in Fig. 1.

Author details
[1]Department of Defense Biotechnology High Performance Computing Software Applications Institute, Telemedicine and Advanced Technology Research Center, United States Army Medical Research and Materiel Command, Fort Detrick, Maryland, USA. [2]Department of Bioengineering, Stanford University, Stanford, California, USA. [3]Auckland Bioengineering Institute, University of Auckland, Auckland, New Zealand.

References
1. Jones BH, Hansen BC. An armed forces epidemiological board evaluation of injuries in the military. Am J Prev Med. 2000;18(3 Suppl):14–25.
2. Boden BP, Osbahr DC. High-risk stress fractures: evaluation and treatment. J Am Acad Orthop Surg. 2000;8(6):344–53.
3. Brukner P, Bradshaw C, Khan KM, White S, Crossley K. Stress fractures: a review of 180 cases. Clin J Sport Med. 1996;6(2):85–9.
4. Fredericson M, Bergman AG, Hoffman KL, Dillingham MS. Tibial stress reaction in runners. Correlation of clinical symptoms and scintigraphy with a new magnetic resonance imaging grading system. Am J Sports Med. 1995;23(4):472–81.
5. Knapik J, Montain SJ, McGraw S, Grier T, Ely M, Jones BH. Stress fracture risk factors in basic combat training. Int J Sports Med. 2012;33(11):940–6. doi:10.1055/s-0032-1311583.
6. Jones BH, Perrotta DM, Canham-Chervak ML, Nee MA, Brundage JF. Injuries in the military: a review and commentary focused on prevention. Am J Prev Med. 2000;18(3 Suppl):71–84.
7. Knapik JJ, Darakjy S, Hauret KG, Canada S, Marin R, Jones BH. Ambulatory physical activity during United States Army basic combat training. Int J Sports Med. 2007;28(2):106–15. doi:10.1055/s-2006-924147.
8. Seay JF, Fellin RE, Sauer SG, Frykman PN, Bensel CK. Lower extremity biomechanical changes associated with symmetrical torso loading during simulated marching. Mil Med. 2014;179(1):85–91. doi:10.7205/MILMED-D-13-00090.
9. Silder A, Delp SL, Besier T. Men and women adopt similar walking mechanics and muscle activation patterns during load carriage. J Biomech. 2013;46(14):2522–8. doi:10.1016/j.jbiomech.2013.06.020.
10. Quesada PM, Mengelkoch LJ, Hale RC, Simon SR. Biomechanical and metabolic effects of varying backpack loading on simulated marching. Ergonomics. 2000;43(3):293–309. doi:10.1080/001401300184413.
11. Pedersen AV, Stokke R, Mamen A. Effects of extra load position on energy expenditure in treadmill running. Eur J Appl Physiol. 2007;102(1):27–31. doi:10.1007/s00421-007-0553-1.
12. Ricciardi R, Deuster PA, Talbot LA. Metabolic demands of body armor on physical performance in simulated conditions. Mil Med. 2008;173(9):817–24.
13. Birrell SA, Hooper RH, Haslam RA. The effect of military load carriage on ground reaction forces. Gait Posture. 2007;26(4):611–4. doi:10.1016/j.gaitpost.2006.12.008.
14. Liew BX, Morris S, Netto K. Joint power and kinematics coordination in load carriage running: Implications for performance and injury. Gait Posture. 2016;47:74–9. doi:10.1016/j.gaitpost.2016.04.014.
15. Neumann DA, Hase AD. An electromyographic analysis of the hip abductors during load carriage: implications for hip joint protection. J Orthop Sports Phys Ther. 1994;19(5):296–304. doi:10.2519/jospt.1994.19.5.296.
16. Milgrom C, Finestone A, Simkin A, Ekenman I, Mendelson S, Millgram M, et al. In-vivo strain measurements to evaluate the strengthening potential of exercises on the tibial bone. J Bone Joint Surg Br. 2000;82(4):591–4.
17. Bhatia VA, Edwards WB, Troy KL. Predicting surface strains at the human distal radius during an in vivo loading task–finite element model validation and application. J Biomech. 2014;47(11):2759–65. doi:10.1016/j.jbiomech.2014.04.050.
18. Xu C, Silder A, Zhang J, Hughes J, Unnikrishnan G, Reifman J, et al. An integrated musculoskeletal-finite-element model to evaluate effects of load carriage on the tibia during walking. J Biomech Eng. 2016;138(10). doi:10.1115/1.4034216.
19. Cappellini G, Ivanenko YP, Poppele RE, Lacquaniti F. Motor patterns in human walking and running. J Neurophysiol. 2006;95(6):3426–37. doi:10.1152/jn.00081.2006.
20. Silder A, Besier T, Delp SL. Running with a load increases leg stiffness. J Biomech. 2015;48(6):1003–8. doi:10.1016/j.jbiomech.2015.01.051.
21. Damsgaard M, Rasmussen J, Christensen ST, Surma E, Zee M. Analysis of musculoskeletal systems in the AnyBody Modeling System. Simul Model Pract Theory. 2006;14:1100–11.
22. Klein Horsman MD, Koopman HF, van der Helm FC, Prose LP, Veeger HE. Morphological muscle and joint parameters for musculoskeletal modelling of the lower extremity. Clin Biomech (Bristol, Avon). 2007;22(2):239–47. doi:10.1016/j.clinbiomech.2006.10.003.
23. Andersen MS, Damsgaard M, MacWilliams B, Rasmussen J. A computationally efficient optimisation-based method for parameter identification of kinematically determinate and over-determinate biomechanical systems. Comput Methods Biomech Biomed Eng. 2010;13(2):171–83. doi:10.1080/10255840903067080.
24. Zhang J, Sorby H, Clement J, Thomas CDL, Hunter P, Nielsen P, et al., editors. The MAP Client: User-Friendly Musculoskeletal Modelling Workflows. 6th International Symposium, ISBMS 2014; 2014; Strasbourg, France.
25. Fernandez JW, Mithraratne P, Thrupp SF, Tawhai MH, Hunter PJ. Anatomically based geometric modelling of the musculo-skeletal system and other organs. Biomech Model Mechan. 2004;2(3):139–55. doi:10.1007/s10237-003-0036-1.
26. Maxian TA, Brown TD, Weinstein SL. Chronic stress tolerance levels for human articular cartilage: Two nonuniform contact models applied to long-term follow-up of CDH. J Biomech. 1995;28(2):159–66.
27. Erdemir A, McLean S, Herzog W, van den Bogert AJ. Model-based estimation of muscle forces exerted during movements. Clin Biomech (Bristol, Avon). 2007;22(2):131–54. doi:10.1016/j.clinbiomech.2006.09.005.
28. Cavanagh PR, Komi PV. Electromechanical delay in human skeletal muscle under concentric and eccentric contractions. Eur J Appl Physiol. 1979;42(3):159–63.
29. Estrada K, Styrkarsdottir U, Evangelou E, Hsu YH, Duncan EL, Ntzani EE, et al. Genome-wide meta-analysis identifies 56 bone mineral density loci and reveals 14 loci associated with risk of fracture. Nat Genet. 2012;44(5):491–501. doi:10.1038/ng.2249.
30. Sanderlin BW, Raspa RF. Common stress fractures. Am Fam Physician. 2003;68(8):1527–32.
31. Bennell KL, Malcolm SA, Thomas SA, Wark JD, Brukner PD. The incidence and distribution of stress fractures in competitive track and field athletes. A twelve-month prospective study. Am J Sports Med. 1996;24(2):211–7.
32. Milgrom C, Giladi M, Stein M, Kashtan H, Margulies JY, Chisin R, et al. Stress fractures in military recruits. A prospective study showing an unusually high incidence. J Bone Joint Surg Br. 1985;67(5):732–5.
33. Shaffer RA, Rauh MJ, Brodine SK, Trone DW, Macera CA. Predictors of stress fracture susceptibility in young female recruits. Am J Sports Med. 2006;34(1):108–15. doi:10.1177/0363546505278703.
34. Seay JF. Biomechanics of load carriage–historical perspectives and recent insights. J Strength Cond Res. 2015;29 Suppl 11:S129–33. doi:10.1519/JSC.0000000000001031.
35. Cichanowski HR, Schmitt JS, Johnson RJ, Niemuth PE. Hip strength in collegiate female athletes with patellofemoral pain. Med Sci Sports Exerc. 2007;39(8):1227–32. doi:10.1249/mss.0b013e3180601109.

36. Wang H, Frame J, Ozimek E, Leib D, Dugan EL. The effects of load carriage and muscle fatigue on lower-extremity joint mechanics. Res Q Exerc Sport. 2013;84(3):305–12. doi:10.1080/02701367.2013.814097.
37. Santamaria LJ, Webster KE. The effect of fatigue on lower-limb biomechanics during single-limb landings: a systematic review. J Orthop Sports Phys Ther. 2010;40(8):464–73. doi:10.2519/jospt.2010.3295.
38. Henning P, Khamoui AV, Brown LE. Preparatory strength and endurance training for U.S. Army Basic Combat Training. Strength Cond J. 2011;33(5): 48–57. doi:10.1519/SSC.0b013e31822fdb2e.
39. Bergmann G, Graichen F, Rohlmann A. Hip joint loading during walking and running, measured in two patients. J Biomech. 1993;26(8):969–90.
40. Pandy MG, Andriacchi TP. Muscle and joint function in human locomotion. Annu Rev Biomed Eng. 2010;12:401–33. doi:10.1146/annurev-bioeng-070909-105259.
41. Rotstein A, Inbar O, Berginsky T, Meckel Y. Preferred transition speed between walking and running: effects of training status. Med Sci Sports Exerc. 2005;37(11):1864–70.
42. Sasaki K, Neptune RR. Differences in muscle function during walking and running at the same speed. J Biomech. 2006;39(11):2005–13. doi:10.1016/j.jbiomech.2005.06.019.
43. Miller RH, Edwards WB, Brandon SC, Morton AM, Deluzio KJ. Why don't most runners get knee osteoarthritis? A case for per-unit-distance loads. Med Sci Sports Exerc. 2014;46(3):572–9. doi:10.1249/MSS.0000000000000135.
44. Redmond JE, Cohen BS, Simpson K, Spiering BA, Sharp MA. Measuring physical activity during US Army Basic Combat Training: a comparison of 3 methods. US Army Med Dep J. 2013:48–54.
45. Simpson K, Redmond JE, Cohen BS, Hendrickson NR, Spiering BA, Steelman R, et al. Quantification of physical activity performed during US Army Basic Combat Training. US Army Med Dep J. 2013:55–65.
46. Perl DP, Daoud AI, Lieberman DE. Effects of footwear and strike type on running economy. Med Sci Sports Exerc. 2012;44(7):1335–43. doi:10.1249/MSS.0b013e318247989e.

6

Concomitant glenohumeral injuries in Neer type II distal clavicle fractures

Tobias Helfen[1*], Georg Siebenbürger[1], Florian Haasters[2], Wolfgang Böcker[1] and Ben Ockert[1]

Abstract

Background: To identify the prevalence of concomitant glenohumeral injuries in surgically treated Neer type II distal clavicle fractures and relate its clinical importance.

Methods: Between 11/2011 and 11/2015 41 patients, suffering from a displaced and unstable distal clavicle fracture were included. 20 patients (group 1) received surgical treatment by means of plate osteosynthesis in combination with an arthroscopically assisted coraco-clavicular ligament augmentation. In group 2 ($n = 21$ patients) the fracture was treated by hooked plating solely, and diagnostic arthroscopy was conducted during hardware retrieval after the fracture had healed. All arthroscopies were performed in a standardized fashion, images were blinded retrospectively, and evaluated by two independent investigators.

Results: In total, concomitant glenohumeral pathologies were found in 26.8% of cases (41 patients, mean age 43.6 ± 16. 6 years). In Group 1 ($n = 20$, arthroscopically assisted fracture treatment) the prevalence was 25%, in Group 2 ($n = 21$, diagnostic arthroscopy during implant removal) 28.5% ($p = 0.75$). Concomitant glenohumeral injuries included Labrum- and SLAP-tears, partial and full thickness rotator cuff tears as well as lesions to the biceps pulley system. Concomitant injuries were addressed in 2 patients of group 1 (10%, 2× labrum repair) and in 3 patients of group 2 (14.3%, of Group 2 (2× arthroscopic cuff repair of full thickness tear, 1× subpectoral biceps tenodesis in an type IV SLAP lesion, $p = 0.68$).

Conclusion: The present study could clarify the acute and for the first time mid-term implication and clinical relevance of concomitant glenohumeral injuries. They have been observed in averaged 27% of Neer type II distal clavicle fractures at these two times. However, the findings of this study show that not all concomitant lesions remain symptomatic. While lesions are still present after fracture healing, it's treatment may be depicted upon symptoms at the time of implant removal. In turn, early diagnosis and treatment of concomitant injuries seems reasonable, as untreated injuries can remain symptomatic for more than 6 months after the fracture and recovery may be delayed.

Keywords: Distal clavicle fracture, Concomitant injuries, Arthroscopic treatment, Osteosynthesis

Background

Fractures of the distal clavicle account for approximately 17% of all clavicle fractures [1]. For stable and non-displaced fractures conservative treatment leads to satisfactory outcome, however in unstable fractures surgical treatment is recommended [2]. Surgical treatment consists of closed or open reduction followed by fracture fixation, nevertheless, numerous surgical techniques have been described including k-wire, plating, hookplating or suture fixation.

* Correspondence: tobias.helfen@med.uni-muenchen.de
[1]Department General, Trauma and Reconstructive Surgery, Ludwig Maximilians University, Munich University Hospital, Nußbaumstr. 20, 80336 Munich, Germany

Recently, arthroscopic assisted treatment of displaced distal clavicle fractures has been reported with the advantage of a minimal invasive approach, early recovery and good functional outcome. However, as arthroscopic assisted treatment is increasingly performed concomitant intraarticular glenohumeral pathologies are observed with distal clavicle fractures [3]. Most commonly, injuries involve the superior labrum anterior-posterior complex (SLAP), the biceps pulley or the rotator cuff and account for approximately 25–46% of cases.

Associated glenohumeral injuries have been described in acute distal clavicle fracture, as well as in dislocation of the acromioclavicular joint, however, the implication and clinical relevance in the treatment of distal clavicle fractures is yet unknown [4–6]. Purpose of this retrospective study was to evaluate the prevalence of concomitant injuries in surgically treated displaced distal clavicle fractures. Furthermore, glenohumeral lesions should be evaluated for clinical relevance. We hypothesised that the prevalence of concomitant injuries is similar when assessed during diagnostic arthroscopy of successfully healed distal clavicle fractures and would represent a pathology with clinical implication.

Methods

This retrospective study was conducted by approval of the local ethical board. Between November 2011 and November 2015, patients ≥18 years of age with a displaced fracture of the distal clavicle were included and surgically treated. Patients with a history of shoulder surgery or symptoms of glenohumeral pathology (instability, rotator-cuff tear, biceps tendon pathology) prior to the fracture event were excluded.

Fracture displacement was identified on standard radiographs in anterior-posterior as well as in Rockwood's view and were classified as described by Neer [2]. Patients were excluded if the fracture was non displaced or other than a Neer II type. All remaining patients were subsequent divided according to the received treatment in 2 groups.

In group 1 ($n = 20$) patients received surgical treatment by means of locked plating and arthroscopically assisted coracoclavicular fixation (Clavicle Fracture System, Arthrex®, Naples, USA). Arthroscopically assisted coracoclavicular fixation consisted of a thorough diagnostic arthroscopy through a standard posterior portal including 8 steps of imaging: After entrance into the glenohumeral joint by use of blunt trocar, the first view was the triangle formed by the long biceps tendon, the humeral head and the subscapularis tendon. 2nd view was onto the biceps origin and the superior labrum anterior-posterior (SLAP) complex. The biceps origin was manipulated using a probe in order to detect a SLAP lesion. 3rd and 4th views included the medial and lateral Pulley system, the superior glenohumeral ligament (SGHL) and the encircled long biceps tendon. Hereafter the articular surface of the glenoid and humerus and the medial gleno-humeral ligament (MGHL) were examined (5th view). The 6th view was on the supraspinatus tendon and the footprint in abduction and external rotation, while the 7th view was used to exclude infraspinatus tendon tears and avulsion of the teres minor or a posterior avulsion of the glenohumeral ligament (reversed HAGL). Finally, the 8th view was to assess the axillary recess for the presence of loose bodies, lesions to the inferior gleno-humeral ligament (IGHL) and HAGL lesions. Cartilage injury of the glenoid or the humeral head was evaluated for in all of 8 standard views. Subacromial arthroscopy was not performed in patients of group 1.

Patients of group 2 ($n = 21$) received open reduction and locking plate osteosynthesis with 3.5 mm Clavicle Hook Plate (LCP, DePuy Synthes®, Zuchwil, Switzerland). All patients of group 2 underwent diagnostic arthroscopy at the time of implant removal, which was then performed in the identical manner as described above. In addition, a subacromial arthroscopy was conducted prior to implant removal.

Patients of both groups were clinically and radiographically followed for 12 months. Functional outcome has been recorded and is presented by the Constant Score (CS), the Oxford Shoulder Score (OSS) and the abduction. Arthroscopic images were blinded retrospectively in order to eliminate interpretational bias by the surgeon or the physical examination. All images were evaluated independently by two investigators. Full thickness rotator cuff tears were classified according to Bateman [7], partial supraspinatus tendon lesions were classified in accordance to Ellman [8], subscapularis tendon lesions were further classified as described by Fox and Romeo [9]. Injuries of the superior labrum in relation to the biceps tendon anchor were classified according to Snyder et al. [6] and Maffet et al. [10] Lesions of the pulley system were classified as described by Habermeyer et al. [11]

Data was enrolled through Microsoft Excel 2010 (Microsoft, Redmond, WA), followed by a statistical analysis using IBM SPSS Statistics, version 25 (SPSS, Chicago, IL). Data are given in terms of the arithmetic mean and standard deviation. The study of Pauly et al. was used to estimate the power and sample Size [12]. The authors reported the prevalence of concomitant intra-articular pathologies following high-grade dislocation of the acromioclavicular (AC) joint with 15%. Based on these findings, a sample size of 35 is needed with a 95.0% confidence interval and a normal approximation of 0.150. Frequencies were calculated for ordinal data, and the χ^2 test was applied for group comparison. Rational data were described by mean and standard deviation. To compare the groups, analysis of variance and post hoc tests were used for parametric data, and the Mann-Whitney *U* test was used for nonparametric data. $P \leq .05$ was considered significant for differences in group comparison.

Results

Of 41 patients (mean age: 43.6 ± 16.6 years) with a Neer type II displaced fracture of the distal clavicle, concomitant glenohumeral pathologies were found in 11 patients (27%).

In Group 1 ($n = 20$, mean age: 53 ± 17.5 years, fracture pattern: Neer IIa $n = 3$, Neer IIb = 17) concomitant glenohumeral pathologies were detected in 5 patients (25%) during primary arthroscopically assisted treatment (Table 1). In

Table 1 Distribution and significance of concomitant injuries

Concomitant injury	Group 1[n]	Group 2[n]	*p*-value
SLAP-lesion	0 (0%)	1 (4.7%)	*1*
SSP-transmural tear	1 (5%)	2 (9.5%)	*1*
SSP-partial rupture	2 (10%)	3 (14.3%)	*1*
SSC partial rupture	0 (0%)	1 (4.7%)	*1*
Pulley lesion	0 (0%)	1 (4.7%)	*1*
Labrum lesion	2 (10%)	0 (0%)	*0.23*
Bursitis glenohumeral	0 (0%)	2 (9.5%)	*0.48*

Group 2 ($n = 21$, mean age: 39.7 ± 14.6, $p = 0.01$, fracture pattern: Neer IIa $n = 1$, Neer IIb = 20) glenohumeral pathologies were found in 6 patients (28.5%) during diagnostic arthroscopy at the time of hardware removal 6.7 ± 3.5 months following primary non-arthroscopic treatment. Concomitant glenohumeral injuries included SLAP-lesions, SSP transmural and partial lesions, SSC partial lesions as well as Pulley and Bankart lesions. (Table 1). Distribution of classification of the injuries is shown in Table 2.

A distinct treatment, other than debridement, was performed in 2 patients (10%, 2 x labrum refixation) of Group 1 and in 3 patients of group 2 (14.3%, 2× arthroscopic cuff repair, 1 x subpectoral biceps tenodesis in SLAP type IV). A characteristic example for the findings is shown in Fig. 1. Of group 2, 5 patients (23.8%) patients presented with ongoing clinical symptoms related to the glenohumeral finding. 1 patient (4.8%) showed a positive Jobe's Test (full thickness rotator cuff tear and 1 patient had a positive O'Brien's Test (SLAP type IV lesion). The last case is exemplary presented in Fig. 2. Three patients of group 2 (14.3%) complained of persisting subacromial impingement symptoms until hook plate removal, without glenohumeral finding.

Results of the CS and the OSS as well as the degrees of abduction are shown in Tables 3 and 4. Functional outcome parameters were mainly superior in group 1. Significance was given only in the overall abduction values regardless of concomitant injuries. In the subgroup of existing concomitant injuries of group 2 implant removal and late arthroscopy benefits the patients' functional outcome of all measured functional outcome parameters.

Table 2 Distribution of degrees of injuries according to their individual classification

Injury classification	Group 1	Group 2
SLAP-lesion *(Snyder)*	–	N = 1 *(VI)*
SSP transmural tear *(Bateman)*	N = 1 *(II)*[a]	N – 1 *(III)*
		N = 1 *(VI)*
SSP-partial rupture *(Ellman)*	N = 2 *(I)*[a]	N = 2 *(I)*a
		N = 1 *(II)*a
SSC partial rupture *(Fox/Romeo)*	–	N = 1 *(Ib)*a
Pulley lesion *(Habermayer)*	–	N = 1 *(II)*a
Labrum lesions	N = 2	–

[a]only arthroscopic debridement

Discussion

Fractures to the distal third of the clavicle represent 10–30% of all clavicle fractures and can be treated conservatively with satisfying outcome in the majority of cases. However, symptomatic non-union under conservative treatment exists and therefore, distal clavicle fractures with instability should be treated operatively, with respect to patient's age and functional demands. Over the last decades, surgical treatment of distal clavicle fractures developed from open reduction and fixation by k-wires, conventional plates or hook-plating to minimal invasive approaches and arthroscopically assisted fracture management. Arthroscopically assisted fracture fixation may be beneficial in terms of minimally invasive approach as well as assessment and treatment of associated glenohumeral lesions. While impaired functional outcome and prolonged pain was historically contributed to fracture non-union, several authors noted that other reasons for a limited shoulder function may be present [13]. In this context, due to an increase of arthroscopic assisted fracture treatment, concomitant glenohumeral lesions were observed more frequently and proclaimed as potentially causing shoulder dysfunction [14].

Beirer et al. detected concomitant intra-articular glenohumeral injuries in 13 of 28 patients (46.4%) with initially suspected isolated lateral clavicle fracture. Surgical treatment was performed in 8 of 28 cases (28.6%) of which superior-labrum-anterior-posterior (SLAP) lesions, injuries to the pulley-complex as well as rotator cuff tears were regarded as relevant injuries. The authors concluded that subsequent surgical treatment of these formerly missed but therapy-relevant injuries may increase functional outcome and reduce complication rate. However, several arthroscopic and imaging studies have shown that there are glenohumeral pathologies in otherwise asymptomatic patients. Tempelhof et al. showed a prevalence of rotator cuff tears in 13% of patients aged 50 to 59 years with an overall rate of 23% of all patients with asymptomatic shoulders [15].

In the present study glenohumeral injuries, concomitant to a displaced fracture of the distal clavicle were found in 27% of cases. This result supports the data of existing studies reporting of acute determined concomitant glenohumeral injuries in 25–46% of patients with distal clavicle fractures [3]. For the first time, our study showed that glenohumeral pathologies are not only observed during primary arthroscopic fracture treatment, but are also present more than 6 months thereafter. No study exists to show late arthroscopy findings in distal clavicle fractures. With the particular collective of

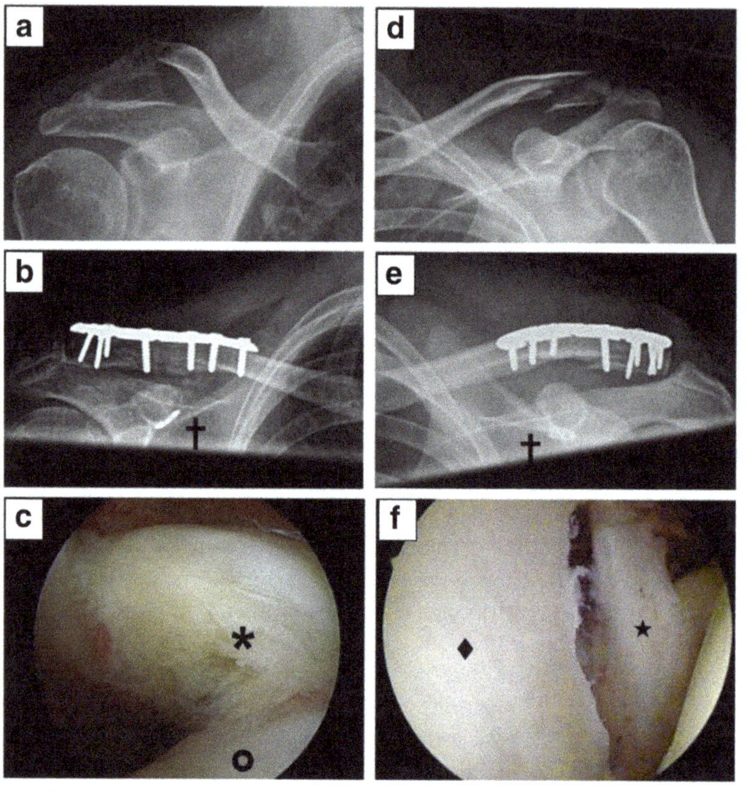

Fig. 1 Findings of Group 1 (initial arthroscopy). **a-c** 53 years old female with Neer type IIb fracture treated by plate osteosynthesis with coraco-clavicular augmentation [†]. **a** Preoperative x-ray. **b** Postoperative x-ray. **c** SSC Lesion (Fox/Romeo Ib) [*] humeral head in front [O]. **d-e** 32 years old male with Neer type IIb fracture treated by plate osteosynthesis with coraco-clavicular augmentation [†]. **d** Preoperative x-ray. **e** Postoperative x-ray. **f** anterior Bankart Lesion [★], glenoid in the front[♦]

patients undergone late arthroscopy we could examine this issue.

Some concomitant injuries could potentially heal others are clinically irrelevant. In some cases this turns out only in the further course of healing. In 21 patients (group 2) of our study the fracture was treated non-arthroscopically, but diagnostic arthroscopy was conducted 6.7 ± 3.5 months thereafter and glenohumeral lesions were found in 6 patients (28.5%). Interestingly, this result was similar to patients of group 1 (25%) which shows that lesions may not dissolve over time. In contrast, not all patients that suffered from a glenohumeral lesion were symptomatic at that time. However, 2 patients were symptomatic and diagnostic arthroscopy revealed a full thickness rotator cuff tear. While both patients were asymptomatic before the fracture event there is little to judge, whether this cuff tear was a result of the trauma, or not. Nevertheless, Tempelhof et al. proclaim that there are certain parameters that may convent an asymptomatic rotator cuff tear into a symptomatic tear, however, for a fracture of the distal clavicle this remains speculative [16]. Symptoms may have been misinterpreted as unspecific subacromial impingement caused by the implant itself. One may argue that symptoms may have resolved with hardware removal alone.

There are several limitations of this study: First, the number of patients is low and the results may be biased due to a retrospective design. Secondly, patients were excluded if the fracture was not classified as Neer type II. Thus, this study does not evaluate the total amount of concomitant glenohumeral lesions in distal clavicle fractures. In fact, there may have be a selection bias because of the indication for an arthroscopically assisted approach with coracoclavicular ligament augmentation. However, we suggest that a Neer type IIb fracture represents a distal clavicle fracture with extensive tissue damage, to be distinguished from the more mild type I injuries, according to Neer himself [16]. During the period of study both implant types have been applied. In the early phase hook plate system dominated, later subsequently locked plating and arthroscopically assisted coracoclavicular fixation has become the method of choice. The study period implies a development process of the implants. For this reason we were unable to randomize and thus study is retrospective. Our preliminary and already published work regarding the used implants has demonstrated a tendency better functional outcome after the arthroscopically assisted osteosynthesis [17]. Therefore this treatment has become to our method of choice. The tendency of better functional outcome was further strengthened by this study.

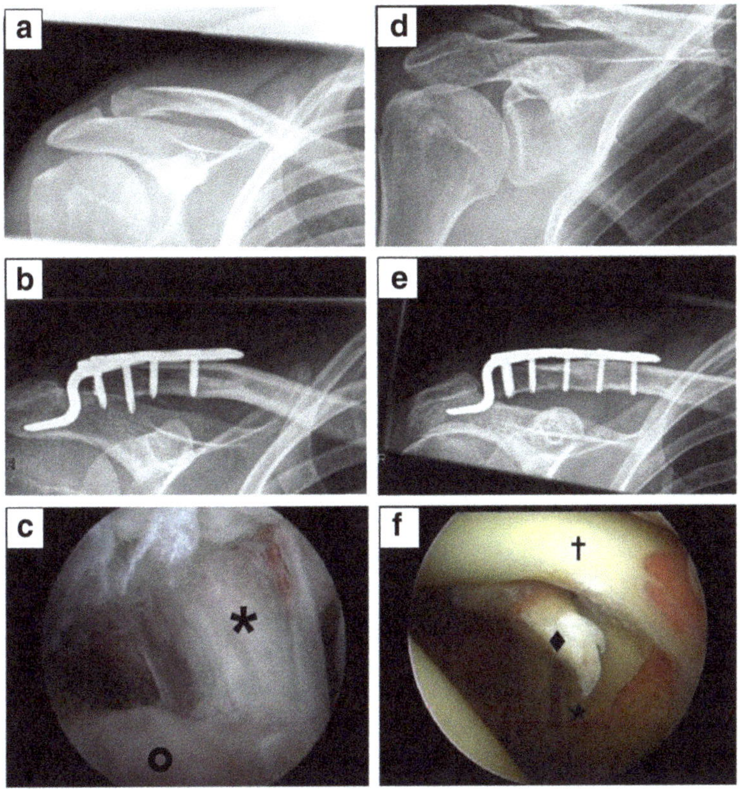

Fig. 2 Findings of Group 2 (late arthroscopy). **a-c** 40 years old male with Neer type IIb fracture treated by hook-plate osteosynthesis. **a** Preoperative x-ray. **b** Postoperative x-ray. **c** SSP transmural Lesion (Bateman III) [✱], footprint area in front [O]. **d-e** 24 years old male with Neer type IIb fracture treated by hook-plate osteosynthesis. **d** Preoperative x-ray. **e** Postoperative x-ray. **f** SLAP Lesion (Snyder IV) [♦], long biceps tendon[†], glenoid [★]

There is no recommendation such fractures to be referred only by arthroscopic experienced surgeons. However the awareness in case of persistent complaints either to perform an arthroscopically assisted implant removal or at least MRI-Imaging after implant removal is necessary. This treatment phase is not that critical of the time; priming of arthroscopically assisted implant removal should be possible.

Table 3 Functional outcome

	Group 1	Group 2	*[p]*
CS total	92.2 ± 5.6	90.6 ± 8.9	*0.49*
CS (-CI)	93.6 ± 4.9	90.9 ± 9.7	*0.33*
CS (+CI)	87 ± 1.9	88.8 ± 1.9	*0.43*
OSS total	46.9 ± 2.4	45.6 ± 4.9	*0.28*
OSS (-CI)	45.5 ± 5.6	47.4 ± 2	*0.23*
OSS (+CI)	44.8 ± 3.3	43.3 ± 6.7	*0.69*
CS (late)	-	90.8 ± 1.9	
OSS (late)	-	45.3 ± 4.6	

CS Constant Score, *(-CI)* without concomitant injuries, *(+CI)* with concomitant injuries, *OSS* Oxford Shoulder Score, *(late)* after late arthroscopy and surgical intervention

Conclusion

Concomitant intra-articular glenohumeral injuries in type Neer II distal clavicle fractures are not only observed during fracture treatment, but also 7 months thereafter in more than a quarter of cases. As glenohumeral lesions may not dissolve over time, diagnostic arthroscopy is recommended in cases were hardware removal is indicated and the patient is symptomatic. In turn, early diagnosis and treatment of relevant concomitant intra-articular glenohumeral injuries is reasonable, as delayed diagnosis and treatments might delay recovery. Whether or not glenohumeral pathologies concomitant to a distal clavicle fracture are of traumatic origin, however, remains uncertain.

Table 4 Range of Motion (Abduction)

	Group 1	Group 2	*[p]*
Abduction [°]	179 ± 3	172 ± 13	*0.02*
Abd [°] (-CI)	180 ± 2	174 ± 13	*0.06*
Abd [°] (+CI)	177 ± 4	163 ± 17	*0.15*
Abd [°] (late)	-	169 ± 9	

(-CI) without concomitant injuries, *(+CI)* with concomitant injuries, *(late)* after late arthroscopy and surgical intervention

Abbreviations

AC: Acromioclavicular; CS: Constant score; HAGL: Posterior avulsion of the glenohumeral ligament; IGHL: Inferior gleno-humeral ligament; LCP: Locking compression plate; LMU: Ludwig Maximilians University; MGHL: Medial gleno-humeral ligament; MRI: Magnetic Resonance Imaging; OSS: Oxford shoulder score; SGHL: Superior glenohumeral ligament; SLAP: Superior labrum anterior-posterior complex

Acknowledgements

Not applicable

Funding

Study was not funded.

Authors' contributions

TH: planning study, writing and ethic's approval; GS patients examination and scheduling; FH surgeon and statistics; WB surgron, consultation, proofreading; BO surgeon, idea to study, writing esp. discussion. All authors have read and approved the manuscript.

Consent for publication

Not applicable

Competing interests

The authors declare that they have no competing interests.

Author details

[1]Department General, Trauma and Reconstructive Surgery, Ludwig Maximilians University, Munich University Hospital, Nußbaumstr. 20, 80336 Munich, Germany. [2]Department Knee, Hip and Shoulder Surgery, Schön Klinik Munich-Harlaching, Harlachinger Str. 51, 54817 Munich, Germany.

References

1. Postacchini F, Gumina S, De Santis P, Albo F. Epidemiology of clavicle fractures. J Shoulder Elbow Surg. 2002;11(5):452–6.
2. Neer CS 2nd. Fractures of the distal third of the clavicle. Clin Orthop Relat Res. 1968;58:43–50.
3. Beirer M, Zyskowski M, Cronlein M, Pforringer D, Schmitt-Sody M, Sandmann G, Huber-Wagner S, Biberthaler P, Kirchhoff C. Concomitant intra-articular glenohumeral injuries in displaced fractures of the lateral clavicle. Knee Surg Sports Traumatol Arthrosc. 2015;5(10):3237–41.
4. Biz C, Berizzi A, Cappellari A, Crimì A, Tamburin S, Iacobellis C. The treatment of acute Rockwood type III acromio-clavicular joint dislocations by two different surgical techniques. Acta Biomed. 2015;86(3):251–9.
5. Tischer T, Salzmann GM, El-Azab H, Vogt S, Imhoff AB. Incidence of associated injuries with acute acromioclavicular joint dislocations types III through V. Am J Sports Med. 2009;37(1):136–9.
6. Snyder SJ, Karzel RP, Del Pizzo W, Ferkel RD, Friedman MJ. SLAP lesions of the shoulder. Arthroscopy. 1990;6(4):274–9.
7. Bayne O. BJL-trosrof-trctlBJ. In: Welsh R, editor. Surgery of the shoulder. Philadelphia: CV Mosby. 1994; p. 167–71.
8. Ellman H. Diagnosis and treatment of incomplete rotator cuff tears. Clin Orthop Relat Res. 1990;254:64–74.
9. Fox JANMA, Romeo AA. Arthroscopic subscapularis repair. Tech Should Elbow Surg. 2003;4:154–68.
10. Maffet MW, Gartsman GM, Moseley B. Superior labrum-biceps tendon complex lesions of the shoulder. Am J Sports Med. 1995;23(1):93–8.
11. Habermeyer P, Magosch P, Pritsch M, Scheibel MT, Lichtenberg S. Anterosuperior impingement of the shoulder as a result of pulley lesions: a prospective arthroscopic study. J Shoulder Elbow Surg. 2004;13(1):5–12.
12. Pauly S, Gerhardt C, Haas NP, Scheibel M. Prevalence of concomitant intraarticular lesions in patients treated operatively for high-grade acromioclavicular joint separations. Knee Surg Sports Traumatol Arthrosc. 2009;17(5):513–7.
13. O'Donnell TM, McKenna JV, Kenny P, Keogh P, O'Flanagan SJ. Concomitant injuries to the ipsilateral shoulder in patients with a fracture of the diaphysis of the humerus. J Bone Joint Surg B. 2008;90(1):61–5.
14. Gartsman GM, Roddey TS, Hammerman SM. Arthroscopic treatment of anterior-inferior glenohumeral instability. Two to five-year follow-up. J Bone Joint Surg Am. 2000;82-A(7):991–1003.
15. Tempelhof S, Rupp S, Seil R. Age-related prevalence of rotator cuff tears in asymptomatic shoulders. J Shoulder Elbow Surg. 1999;8(4):296–9.
16. Neer CS 2nd. Fracture of the distal clavicle with detachment of the coracoclavicular ligaments in adults. J Trauma. 1963;3:99–110.
17. Helfen T, Siebenburger G, Ockert B, Haasters F. Therapy of acute acromioclavicular joint instability. Meta-analysis of arthroscopic/minimally invasive versus open procedures. Unfallchirurg. 2015;118(5):415–26.

7

Association of vertebral compression fractures with physical performance measures among community-dwelling Japanese women aged 40 years and older

Kazuhiko Arima[1*], Yasuyo Abe[1], Takayuki Nishimura[1], Takuhiro Okabe[1,2], Yoshihito Tomita[1,2], Satoshi Mizukami[1,2], Mitsuo Kanagae[1,2] and Kiyoshi Aoyagi[1]

Abstract

Background: Numerous reported studies have shown that vertebral compression fractures are associated with impaired function or disability; however, few examined their association with objective measures of physical performance or functioning.

Methods: We examined the association of vertebral compression fractures with physical performance measures in 556 Japanese women aged 40–89 years. Lateral spine radiographs were obtained and radiographic vertebral compression fractures were assessed by quantitative morphometry, defined as vertebral heights more than 3 SD below the normal mean. Measures of physical performance included walking speed, chair stand time and functional reach. Adjusted means of performance-based measures according to the number and severity of vertebral compression fractures were calculated using general linear modeling methods.

Results: After adjusting for age, body mass index, back pain, number of painful joints, number of comorbidities and regular physical activities, the walking speed of women with two or more compression fractures (1.17 m/s) was significantly slower than that of women without compression fracture (1.24 m/s) ($p = 0.03$). Compared with women without compression fracture, chair stand time was longer in women with two or more compression fractures ($p = 0.01$), and functional reach was shorter ($p = 0.01$). No significant differences were observed in walking speed, chair stand time, or functional reach between women with one compression fracture and those without compression fracture.

Conclusions: Having multiple vertebral compression fractures affects physical performance in community-dwelling Japanese women. Poor physical functioning may lead to functional dependence, accelerated bone loss, and increased risk for falls, injuries, and fractures. Preventing vertebral compression fracture is considered important for preserving the independence of older adults.

Keywords: Vertebral compression fractures, Physical performance, Walking speed, Chair stand time, Functional reach test

* Correspondence: kzarima-ngs@umin.ac.jp
[1]Department of Public Health, Nagasaki University Graduate School of Biomedical Sciences, 1-12-4 Sakamoto, Nagasaki 852-8523, Japan
Full list of author information is available at the end of the article

Background

Osteoporosis has been characterized as a skeletal disorder of reduced bone strength that leads to an increased risk for fracture [1]. The estimated number of patients with lumbar spine (L2-L4) and femoral neck osteoporosis in Japan was approximately 6.4 and 11 million, respectively [2]. Vertebral compression fracture is the most prevalent manifestation of osteoporosis [3]. Vertebral fractures were reported to occur in approximately 20% of postmenopausal women in population-based studies [4–6], but two-thirds of vertebral fractures do not come to clinical attention [7, 8], because symptoms are absent or missed [9, 10]. In Japan, medical and care expenditures on spine fracture were estimated at 9,895 hundred million yen [11],

Physical performance measures have been applied in geriatric studies. Poor physical performance measures are associated with medical problems [12], disability in activities of daily living (ADL) [13, 14], and increased risk of falls [15–17]. Thus, physical performance measures capture information about these physical factors above. In addition, the elderly with poor physical performance have an increased risk of hip and non-spine fractures and lower bone mineral density [18–20].

Numerous studies showed that vertebral compression fractures are associated with back pain, impaired function or disability [21–29], most of which used subjective measures, not objective ones. A few published studies examined the association of the number of vertebral compression fractures with objective measures of physical performance and functioning [23, 25, 26, 30]. We examined the association of the number and severity of vertebral compression fractures with objective measures of physical performance among community-dwelling Japanese women.

Methods

Study design and participants

The subjects were Japanese women aged 40–89 years who participated in the Hizen-Oshima Study. Details of the Hizen-Oshima Study have been published previously [27, 31]. We recruited community-dwelling women aged 40 years and older in Oshima, Nagasaki prefecture, Japan. The women were identified by the municipal electoral list and were invited to participate through a single mailing. The town of Oshima has a population of approximately 5800; all women aged 40 and older (n >2000) were invited to participate. The examinations were performed at the Oshima Health Center between 1998 and 1999. A total of 586 women participated in the study. The mean age of participants (63.9 years) was significantly higher than that of non-participants (61.1 years). All participants were noninstitutionalized and living independently. All subjects gave written informed consent before enrolling. Recently, Cawthon et al. [30] reported that poorer physical performance was associated with an increased risk of incident radiographic vertebral fracture in men. We analyzed our baseline data of women in order to reinforce this evidence.

Spine radiographs and vertebral compression fractures

Lateral radiographs were obtained with the subject lying in a lateral decubitus position with knees bent. All radiographs were obtained using a tube-to-film distance of 105 cm, with the tube positioned approximately over T-8 for thoracic films and L-2 for lumbar films. The anterior, medial, and posterior heights of each vertebral body (T-4 to L-4) were measured on the lateral films with the aid of a microcomputer-linked caliper. Vertebral heights were measured on the thoracic film for thoracic vertebrae, and on the lumbar film for lumbar vertebrae. The points indicating the border of the vertebral centrum were chosen based on the procedure described by Gallagher et al. [32] and Spencer et al. [33]. Radiographic images were evaluated by one orthopedic surgical specialist (KA). A vertebral compression fracture was defined as a vertebra with at least one dimension (anterior, medial, or posterior height) more than 3 standard deviations (SDs) below the vertebra-specific population mean on the radiographs [34]. For example, the means and SDs of the anterior, medial, or posterior heights of subjects' T4 vertebrae were calculated. ([Mean anterior height of T4] - [3 × SD of anterior height of T4]; [mean medial height of T4] - [3 × SD of medial height of T4]; and [mean posterior height of T4 - [3 × SD of posterior height of T4]) were calculated. Each calculated value was compared with the actual anterior, medial, or posterior height. If at least one dimension (actual anterior, medial, or posterior height) was less than the calculated value, it was regarded as a T4 vertebral compression fracture. Furthermore, based on the extent of vertebral height reduction, mild compression fracture was recorded as 3–4 SDs, and severe compression fracture as >4 SDs below the normal mean value. Mild vertebral compression fracture was defined as at least one mild compression fracture without severe compression fractures (at least one mild but no severe compression fracture). Severe vertebral compression fracture was defined as one or more severe compression fractures (at least one severe compression fracture).

Measurements

All participants were asked if they experienced back pain on most days during the previous month, and if they had any comorbidity, including cancer, heart disease, kidney disease, liver disease, diabetes mellitus, history of gastrectomy, thyroid disease, collagen disease, lung disease, stroke, or Parkinson's disease. Information on regular physical activity was collected; participants were asked whether they do any physical activity (e.g., walking, jogging, or bicycling) long enough to work up a sweat at least once a week. Information on the number of painful non-spine joints was based on the subject's response to the following question: "Which of your joints have ever been painful on most days during the previous month?" Specific response categories (shoulders, elbows, wrists, hands and fingers, hips, knees, ankles, and feet) for both sides of the body were provided on an illustration of the skeleton.

Measures of physical performance included walking speed (assessment of balance and lower extremity strength) [35], chair stand time (assessment of lower extremity strength) [36] and functional reach (assessment of balance and posture) [37], according to the previous report [19]. These performances are reported to be associated with balance, posture or lower limb strength [35–39]. Women who had difficulty performing the test safely, such as needing a walking aid, recent lower limb fracture or operation or neurological comorbidity, were not examined. Trained physical therapists conducted the performance tests. Walking speed was calculated as the time required for subjects to walk a 6-m course bounded by two lines at their usual pace (average of two trials). Chair stand time was measured as the time it took (average of two trials) to stand up from a standard chair five times; the subjects were asked not to use their arms for assistance. Functional reach was calculated as the difference between two measurements (average of three trials), as follows: the subjects first stood comfortably upright, facing forward, hand in a fist, with their arm extended next to a yardstick mounted on a wall. They then reached forward as far as possible without stepping or losing their balance. Height and weight were measured in light clothing and without shoes. Body mass index (BMI) was calculated as weight (kg)/height (m)^2.

Statistical analysis

Women with missing values for any variables were excluded from analysis, leaving 556 women for data analysis. Analysis of variance (ANOVA) and multiple comparisons using the Tukey method for continuous variables and Fisher's exact test for categorical variables were used to determine the significance of differences among groups according to the number of vertebral compression fractures (no, one, and two or more). Age-specific means of physical performance measures were performed using ANOVA. Adjusted means of performance-based measures according to the number of vertebral compression fractures (no, one, and two or more) and the severity of vertebral compression fracture (no, at least one mild but no severe, and at least one severe) were calculated using general linear modeling methods (analysis of covariance). Age, BMI, back pain, number of non-spine painful joints, the number of comorbidities and regular physical activity was included simultaneously in the model as covariates. We examined the independent association of each variable above with physical performance measures. All statistical analyses were performed using SAS version 9.2 software (SAS Institute, Cary, NC, USA).

Results

Characteristics of subjects are shown in Table 1. The mean age of subjects was 64.4 years old. Mean walking speed was 1.24 m/s, mean chair stand time was 9.4 s, and mean functional reach was 25.6 cm. A total of 30% of the subjects had back pain, and 52% engaged in regular physical activity; 14.2% (79) had one or more vertebral compression fractures; 6.9% (38) had one compression fracture; and 7.4% (41) had two or more compression fractures. Women with vertebral compression fractures were significantly older, shorter and lighter than those without vertebral compression fracture. Women with vertebral compression fractures had significantly poorer physical performance (slower walking speed, longer chair stand time and shorter functional reach) and more prevalent back pain compared with those without vertebral compression fracture.

Table 2 shows mean and standard deviation (SD) of vertebral height, and %height reduction values [(mean-vertebral height)/mean] corresponding to mild (mean-3SD) and severe (mean-4SD) vertebral fracture cutoffs for each vertebral dimension. Percent height reduction values corresponding to mild vertebral fracture cutoffs were between 20.3 and 38.3%, and those corresponding to severe vertebral fracture cutoffs were between 27.0 and 51.0%.

Physical performance decreased with age (Table 3); walking speed and functional reach decreased, and chair stand time increased (longer time required to complete the test represents a decline in function).

Table 4 shows the adjusted means of physical performance measurements according to the number of vertebral compression fractures. After adjusting for age, BMI, back pain, number of non-spine painful joints, the number of comorbidities and regular physical activity, the walking speed of women with two or more compression fractures (1.17 m/s) was significantly slower than that of women without compression fracture (1.24 m/s) ($p = 0.03$). Compared with women without compression fracture, chair stand time was longer in women with two or more compression fractures (10.4 s vs. 9.3 s) ($p = 0.01$), and functional reach was shorter (23.2 cm vs. 25.9 cm) ($p = 0.01$). No significant

Table 1 Basic characteristics of subjects according to compression fracture status ($n = 556$)

Variable	Total ($n = 556$)	No compression fracture ($n = 477$)	One compression fracture ($n = 38$)	Two or more compression fractures ($n = 41$)
	Mean (SD, 95% CI)			
Age (years)	64.4 (9.5, 63.6–65.2)	63.1 (9.3, 62.3–64.0)	69.5 (6.9, 67.2–71.8) [a]	73.6 (7.1, 71.3–75.8) [a]
Height (cm)	149.7 (6.1, 149.2–150.2)	150.5 (5.7, 150.0–151.0)	146.2 (5.5, 144.4–148.0) [a]	143.6 (6.6, 141.6–145.7) [a]
Weight (kg)	52.4 (8.7, 51.7–53.1)	53.1 (8.7, 52.3–53.9)	49.7 (7.6, 47.2–52.2) [a]	46.8 (7.4, 44.5–49.2) [a]
Body mass index (kg/m^2)	23.3 (3.4, 23.1–23.6)	23.4 (3.5, 23.1–23.7)	23.2 (3.5, 22.1–24.4)	22.6 (2.7, 21.8–23.5)
Walking speed (m/s)	1.24 (0.25, 1.22–1.26)	1.26 (0.24, 1.24–1.28)	1.17 (0.28, 1.08–1.26)	1.05 (0.24, 0.97–1.13) [a]
Chair stand time (s)	9.4 (3.1, 9.1–9.6)	9.1 (2.8, 8.8–9.3)	10.3 (2.9, 9.4–11.3) [a]	11.8 (4.4, 10.4–13.2) [a]
Functional reach (cm)	25.6 (7.2, 25.0–26.2)	26.3 (7.0, 25.7–27.0)	22.7 (6.8, 20.5–25.0) [a]	19.7 (6.8, 17.6–21.9) [a]
	Number (%)			
Back pain	164 (29.5)	128 (26.8)	18 (47.4) [b]	18 (43.9) [b]
Regular physical activity	288 (51.8)	248 (52.0)	23 (60.5)	17 (41.5)
Postmenopausal women	510 (91.7)	431 (90.4)	38 (100.0) [b]	41 (100.0) [b]
	Median (1st, 3rd quartile)			
No. of non-spine painful joints	0 (0, 2)	0 (0, 2)	0.5 (0, 2)	0 (0, 2)
No. of comorbidity	0 (0, 1)	0 (0, 1)	0 (0, 1)	0 (0, 1)

[a] $P < 0.05$ compared with no compression fracture (ANOVA & Tukey method)
[b] $P < 0.05$ compared with no compression fracture (Fisher's exact test)

differences were observed in walking speed, chair stand time, or functional reach between subjects with one compression fracture and those without compression fracture. In a multivariate model, slower walking speed was associated with older age, number of non-spine painful joints, number of comorbidities and lack of regular physical activity. Longer chair stand time was associated with older age, number of non-spine painful joints and lack of regular physical activity. Shorter functional reach was associated with older age. Additionally, we did the same analysis including upper or lower extremity joint pain instead of non-spinal painful joints. Slower walking speed was independently associated with number of upper and lower extremity joint pain, and chair stand time with lower extremity joint pain.

We also compared multivariate-adjusted means of physical performance measures according to severity of vertebral compression fracture. Women with severe vertebral compression fractures (at least one severe compression fracture) had significantly slower walking speed ($p = 0.03$) and longer chair stand time ($p = 0.01$) compared with women without compression fracture (data not shown). No significant differences were observed in walking speed and chair stand time between women with mild compression fracture (at least one mild but no severe compression fracture) and those without. Functional reach tended to be shorter in those with mild compression fracture ($p = 0.06$) and severe compression fracture ($p = 0.08$) than in those with no compression fracture. Women with severe vertebral compression fractures tended to have multiple vertebral compression fractures; median number (range) of vertebral compression fractures was 1 (1–3) in women with mild vertebral compression fracture and 2 (1–12) in those with severe vertebral compression fracture.

We examined multivariate-adjusted means of physical performance measures according to location of vertebral compression fracture (thoracic vs. lumbar). Longer chair stand time was associated with one thoracic compression fracture. Shorter functional reach was associated with two or more thoracic compression fracture.

Discussion

We showed that two or more vertebral compression fractures were associated with poor physical performance in walking speed, chair stand time, and functional reach. Huang et al. [25] reported that the number of recent vertebral fractures was associated with reduced functional reach and walking speed. Pluijm et al. [26] reported that the number of vertebral deformities was significantly associated with poor performance (cardigan test, walking test and chair stand test). These findings suggest that vertebral compression fracture affects various physical performance measures.

Previous studies have shown the relationship between vertebral compression fractures and impaired function (difficulty with activities of daily living [ADL]) or disability [21–29]. Poor physical performance test results (decreased functional reach and walking speed, and increased chair stand time) are reported to be predictors

Table 2 Mean and standard deviation (SD) of vertebral height (mm) and % reduction values [(mean-vertebral height)/mean]

	mean	SD	Mild % reduction: 100*[1 - (mean-3SD)/mean] (%)	Severe % reduction: 100*[1 - (mean-4SD)/mean] (%)
T4A	18.75	1.40	22.4	29.8
T5A	19.10	1.50	23.6	31.5
T6A	19.13	1.87	29.3	39.1
T7A	19.43	1.90	29.4	39.2
T8A	19.98	2.19	33.0	43.9
T9A	20.80	2.11	30.5	40.7
T10A	21.67	1.81	25.1	33.4
T11A	22.30	2.10	28.3	37.7
T12A	23.90	3.05	38.3	51.0
L1A	26.19	3.07	35.2	46.9
L2A	27.66	2.95	32.0	42.7
L3A	28.77	2.49	26.0	34.6
L4A	28.32	2.48	26.2	35.0
T4M	18.87	1.44	22.9	30.5
T5M	19.33	1.44	22.4	29.8
T6M	19.63	1.66	25.4	33.8
T7M	19.88	1.83	27.6	36.8
T8M	20.19	2.02	30.1	40.1
T9M	20.81	1.93	27.9	37.2
T10M	21.70	1.83	25.3	33.8
T11M	22.90	1.92	25.1	33.4
T12M	24.61	3.00	36.6	48.7
L1M	26.52	3.29	37.2	49.7
L2M	27.35	2.96	32.5	43.3
L3M	27.94	2.53	27.2	36.3
L4M	27.57	2.80	30.5	40.6
T4P	20.57	1.68	24.6	32.8
T5P	21.26	1.60	22.6	30.1
T6P	21.83	1.57	21.6	28.8
T7P	22.21	1.68	22.7	30.2
T8P	22.25	1.70	22.9	30.5
T9P	22.37	1.69	22.7	30.2
T10P	23.44	1.68	21.5	28.6
T11P	25.19	1.95	23.2	31.0
T12P	27.67	2.18	23.7	31.6
L1P	29.72	2.19	22.1	29.4
L2P	30.09	2.03	20.3	27.0
L3P	29.70	2.02	20.4	27.2
L4P	27.95	2.22	23.9	31.8

of impaired function or disability [13, 40, 41]. Vertebral compression fractures are likely to cause functional limitations, such as difficulty with ADL and physical performance.

Abnormal trunk posture resulting from vertebral compression fractures has been reported to be associated with functional disabilities [42, 43]. Antonelli-Incalzi et al. [44] showed that longer occiput-wall

Table 3 Means (SD) of physical performance measures by age group

Age group (years)	40–49 (n = 41)	50–59 (n = 118)	60–69 (n = 211)	70–79 (n = 161)	80- (n = 25)	P for trend
Walking speed (m/s)	1.44 (0.20)	1.34 (0.19)	1.29 (0.22)	1.10 (0.22)	0.93 (0.24)	<0.0001
Chair stand time (s)	6.7 (1.2)	8.1 (1.7)	9.1 (2.3)	10.7 (3.1)	13.4 (6.2)	<0.0001
Functional reach (cm)	33.0 (5.9)	29.8 (6.1)	25.0 (6.3)	22.6 (6.4)	18.2 (6.4)	<0.0001

distance, which indirectly evaluates thoracic kyphosis due to vertebral compression fractures [45], was associated with slower walking speed, reduced balance, and longer chair stand time in elderly women. Hirose et al. [46] showed that abnormal posture of the trunk (thoracic and lumbar kyphosis) was associated with slower walking speed and shorter functional reach among the community-dwelling elderly population. In our study,

Table 4 Multivariate-adjusted mean (standard error) of walking speed, chair stand time and functional reach according to number of vertebral compression fractures

	Vertebral compression fracture	Adjusted mean (SE)	P value
Walking speed (m/s)	No	1.24 (0.01)	
	One	1.23 (0.03)	0.68
	Two or more	1.17 (0.03)	0.03 [a]
Adjusted factors		Estimate (SE)	
Age (year)	+1 year	−0.012 (0.001)	<0.001
BMI	+1 kg/m^2	−0.003 (0.003)	0.22
Back pain	1, yes; 0, no	−0.023 (0.020)	0.24
No. of non-spine painful joints	+1	−0.018 (0.004)	<0.001
No. of comorbidity	+1	−0.039 (0.014)	0.005
Regular physical activity	1, yes; 0, no	0.041 (0.017)	0.02
Chair stand time (s)	No	9.3 (0.1)	
	One	9.6 (0.4)	0.41
	Two or more	10.4 (0.4)	0.01 [a]
Adjusted factors			
Age (year)	+1 year	0.14 (0.13)	<0.001
BMI	+1 kg/m^2	−0.004 (0.03)	0.91
Back pain	1, yes; 0, no	0.04 (0.25)	0.87
No. of non-spine painful joints	+1	0.16 (0.05)	0.003
No. of comorbidity	+1	0.25 (0.18)	0.16
Regular physical activity	1, yes; 0, no	−0.70 (0.22)	0.002
Functional reach (cm)	No	25.9 (0.3)	
	One	24.7 (1.0)	0.28
	Two or more	23.2 (1.0)	0.01 [a]
Adjusted factors			
Age (year)	+1 year	−0.37 (0.03)	<0.001
BMI	+1 kg/m^2	−0.12 (0.08)	0.12
Back pain	1, yes; 0, no	−0.85 (0.60)	0.16
No. of non-spine painful joints	+1	0.08 (0.13)	0.52
No. of comorbidity	+1	−0.04 (0.42)	0.92
Regular physical activity	1, yes; 0, no	0.17 (0.53)	0.75

BMI Body mass index

[a] compared with women without compression fracture

longer chair stand time was associated with one thoracic compression fracture, and shorter functional reach was associated with two or more thoracic compression fracture.

We previously reported that spinal posture in forward inclination was associated with impaired physical performance in 6-m walking time, chair stand time, and functional reach [39]. Lyles et al. [23] postulated that osteoporotic compression fractures affect the alignment of the entire trunk, leading to a reduction in motion and strength. The shift forward in the center of gravity that occurs with progressive kyphosis from vertebral compression fracture could make trunk movements in a forward direction more unsteady and limited.

Some vertebral compression fractures are associated with increased risk of back pain [22, 25, 47]. In situations in which both vertebral compression fracture and back pain are present, functional losses could occur from the symptoms caused by the compression fracture and/or from the alteration in trunk alignment [29]. In this study, having vertebral compression fractures was significantly associated with poor physical performance independent of back pain and other covariates. These results possibly mean vertebral compression fractures affect physical performances via abnormal trunk posture.

Comorbidities are associated with decreased physical function, and the more the number of comorbidities is, the poorer the physical function is [48]. Thus, we included the number of comorbidities in the model as a covariate.

Our definition of vertebral compression fracture used the vertebral height and its SD, according to Ross et al. [34]; they reported that the cutoff of 3 SD rarely misclassified normal vertebrae as fractured (specificity = 99.9%). However, this cutoff correctly identified about 70% of the incident fractures. A less stringent criterion (2 SD below the mean: specificity = 97.7%) identified about 85–90% of true fractures. Thus, our results may have underestimated the prevalence of compression fractures, which may contribute to Type II error of the association.

The study has several limitations. First, because this was a cross-sectional design, a causal relationship was not necessarily shown by our results. Longitudinal studies are required to clarify the relationships between vertebral compression fracture and physical performance. Second, the subjects were community-dwelling women who voluntarily participated; women with poorer physical performance might not have participated in the present study, which might have affected the results. Third, there are no results of the Timed Up & Go Test of physical performance in our analysis. Fourth, the present study included only Japanese women; therefore, it may be not possible to extrapolate the results to men or people of other ethnicities. Nevertheless, the present data clearly showed an association of vertebral compression fracture with deterioration of physical performance, independent of age and other covariates.

Conclusion

Our results suggest that multiple vertebral compression fractures affect physical performance (slower walking speed, lower chair stand time and shorter functional reach) in community-dwelling Japanese women, independent of age and other covariates. Because poor physical functioning may lead to functional dependence, accelerated bone loss, and increased risk for falls, injuries (e.g., sprain, abrasion, laceration or dislocation after falling), and fractures [25], preventing vertebral compression fracture is important for the preservation of older adults' independence.

Abbreviations

ADL: Activities of daily living; BMI: Body mass index

Acknowledgements

None.

Funding

Not applicable.

Authors' contributions

Making substantial contributions to conception and design: KA, YA, TN, TO, YT and KA. Acquisition of data: KA, YA, TN, TO, YT, SM, MK. Analysis and interpretation of data: KA, YA, TN and KA. Drafting the manuscript: KA, YA, TN, YT and KA. All authors read and approved the final manuscript.

Competing interests

The authors declare that they have no competing interest.

Consent for publication

Not applicable.

Author details

[1]Department of Public Health, Nagasaki University Graduate School of Biomedical Sciences, 1-12-4 Sakamoto, Nagasaki 852-8523, Japan.
[2]Department of Rehabilitation, Nishi-Isahaya Hospital, Isahaya, Japan.

References

1. Nih Consensus Development Panel on Osteoporosis Prevention D. Therapy: Osteoporosis prevention, diagnosis, and therapy. JAMA. 2001;285(6):785–95.
2. Yoshimura N, Muraki S, Oka H, Mabuchi A, En-Yo Y, Yoshida M, Saika A, Yoshida H, Suzuki T, Yamamoto S, et al. Prevalence of knee osteoarthritis, lumbar spondylosis, and osteoporosis in Japanese men and women: the

research on osteoarthritis/osteoporosis against disability study. J Bone Miner Metab. 2009;27(5):620–8.

3. Ross PD. Clinical consequences of vertebral fractures. Am J Med. 1997; 103(2A):30S–42. discussion 42S-43S.
4. Eastell R, Cedel SL, Wahner HW, Riggs BL, Melton 3rd LJ. Classification of vertebral fractures. J Bone Miner Res. 1991;6(3):207–15.
5. Sadat-Ali M, Gullenpet AH, Al-Mulhim F, Al Turki H, Al-Shammary H, Al-Elq A, Al-Othman A. Osteoporosis-related vertebral fractures in postmenopausal women: prevalence in a Saudi Arabian sample. East Mediterr Health J. 2009; 15(6):1420–5.
6. Clark P, Cons-Molina F, Deleze M, Ragi S, Haddock L, Zanchetta JR, Jaller JJ, Palermo L, Talavera JO, Messina DO, et al. The prevalence of radiographic vertebral fractures in Latin American countries: the Latin American Vertebral Osteoporosis Study (LAVOS). Osteoporos Int. 2009;20(2):275–82.
7. Spector TD, McCloskey EV, Doyle DV, Kanis JA. Prevalence of vertebral fracture in women and the relationship with bone density and symptoms: the Chingford Study. J Bone Miner Res. 1993;8(7):817–22.
8. O'Neill TW, Felsenberg D, Varlow J, Cooper C, Kanis JA, Silman AJ. The prevalence of vertebral deformity in european men and women: the European Vertebral Osteoporosis Study. J Bone Miner Res. 1996;11(7):1010–8.
9. Fechtenbaum J, Cropet C, Kolta S, Verdoncq B, Orcel P, Roux C. Reporting of vertebral fractures on spine X-rays. Osteoporos Int. 2005;16(12):1823–6.
10. McKiernan FE. The broadening spectrum of osteoporotic vertebral fracture. Skeletal Radiol. 2009;38(4):303–8.
11. Harada A, World Health O. Absolute risk for fracture and WHO guideline. Economic analysis of pharmacotherapy for osteoporosis. Clin Calcium. 2007; 17(7):1029–34.
12. Perkowski LC, Stroup-Benham CA, Markides KS, Lichtenstein MJ, Angel RJ, Guralnik JM, Goodwin JS. Lower-extremity functioning in older Mexican Americans and its association with medical problems. J Am Geriatr Soc. 1998;46(4):411–8.
13. Ensrud KE, Nevitt MC, Yunis C, Cauley JA, Seeley DG, Fox KM, Cummings SR. Correlates of impaired function in older women. J Am Geriatr Soc. 1994; 42(5):481–9.
14. Kim MJ, Yabushita N, Kim MK, Matsuo T, Okuno J, Tanaka K. Alternative items for identifying hierarchical levels of physical disability by using physical performance tests in women aged 75 years and older. Geriatr Gerontol Int. 2010;10(4):302–10.
15. Morita M, Takamura N, Kusano Y, Abe Y, Moji K, Takemoto T, Aoyagi K. Relationship between falls and physical performance measures among community-dwelling elderly women in Japan. Aging Clin Exp Res. 2005; 17(3):211–6.
16. Nevitt MC, Cummings SR, Kidd S, Black D. Risk factors for recurrent nonsyncopal falls. A prospective study. JAMA. 1989;261(18):2663–8.
17. Davis JW, Ross PD, Nevitt MC, Wasnich RD. Risk factors for falls and for serious injuries on falling among older Japanese women in Hawaii. J Am Geriatr Soc. 1999;47(7):792–8.
18. Cummings SR, Nevitt MC, Browner WS, Stone K, Fox KM, Ensrud KE, Cauley J, Black D, Vogt TM. Risk factors for hip fracture in white women. Study of Osteoporotic Fractures Research Group. N Engl J Med. 1995;332(12):767–73.
19. Aoyagi K, Ross PD, Hayashi T, Okano K, Moji K, Sasayama H, Yahata Y, Takemoto T. Calcaneus bone mineral density is lower among men and women with lower physical performance. Calcif Tissue Int. 2000;67(2):106–10.
20. Cawthon PM, Fullman RL, Marshall L, Mackey DC, Fink HA, Cauley JA, Cummings SR, Orwoll ES, Ensrud KE. Osteoporotic Fractures in Men Research G: Physical performance and risk of hip fractures in older men. J Bone Miner Res. 2008;23(7):1037–44.
21. Ross PD, Ettinger B, Davis JW, Melton 3rd LJ, Wasnich RD. Evaluation of adverse health outcomes associated with vertebral fractures. Osteoporos Int. 1991;1(3):134–40.
22. Ettinger B, Black DM, Nevitt MC, Rundle AC, Cauley JA, Cummings SR, Genant HK. Contribution of vertebral deformities to chronic back pain and disability. The Study of Osteoporotic Fractures Research Group. J Bone Miner Res. 1992;7(4):449–56.
23. Lyles KW, Gold DT, Shipp KM, Pieper CF, Martinez S, Mulhausen PL. Association of osteoporotic vertebral compression fractures with impaired functional status. Am J Med. 1993;94(6):595–601.
24. Ross PD, Davis JW, Epstein RS, Wasnich RD. Pain and disability associated with new vertebral fractures and other spinal conditions. J Clin Epidemiol. 1994;47(3):231–9.
25. Huang C, Ross PD, Wasnich RD. Vertebral fracture and other predictors of physical impairment and health care utilization. Arch Intern Med. 1996; 156(21):2469–75.
26. Pluijm SM, Tromp AM, Smit JH, Deeg DJ, Lips P. Consequences of vertebral deformities in older men and women. J Bone Miner Res. 2000;15(8):1564–72.
27. Jinbayashi H, Aoyagi K, Ross PD, Ito M, Shindo H, Takemoto T. Prevalence of vertebral deformity and its associations with physical impairment among Japanese women: The Hizen-Oshima Study. Osteoporos Int. 2002;13(9):723–30.
28. O'Neill TW, Cockerill W, Matthis C, Raspe HH, Lunt M, Cooper C, Banzer D, Cannata JB, Naves M, Felsch B, et al. Back pain, disability, and radiographic vertebral fracture in European women: a prospective study. Osteoporos Int. 2004;15(9):760–5.
29. Edmond SL, Kiel DP, Samelson EJ, Kelly-Hayes M, Felson DT. Vertebral deformity, back symptoms, and functional limitations among older women: the Framingham Study. Osteoporos Int. 2005;16(9):1086–95.
30. Cawthon PM, Blackwell TL, Marshall LM, Fink HA, Kado DM, Ensrud KE, Cauley JA, Black D, Orwoll ES, Cummings SR, et al. Physical performance and radiographic and clinical vertebral fractures in older men. J Bone Miner Res. 2014;29(9):2101–8.
31. Yoshida S, Aoyagi K, Felson DT, Aliabadi P, Shindo H, Takemoto T. Comparison of the prevalence of radiographic osteoarthritis of the knee and hand between Japan and the United States. J Rheumatol. 2002;29(7):1454–8.
32. Gallagher JC, Hedlund LR, Stoner S, Meeger C. Vertebral morphometry: normative data. Bone Miner. 1988;4(2):189–96.
33. Spencer NESP, Cummings SR, Genant HK. Placement of points for digitizing spine films. J Bone Miner Res (abstract). 1990;5 Suppl 2:247.
34. Ross PD, Davis JW, Epstein RS, Wasnich RD. Ability of vertebral dimensions from a single radiograph to identify fractures. Calcif Tissue Int. 1992;51(2):95–9.
35. Imms FJ, Edholm OG. Studies of gait and mobility in the elderly. Age Ageing. 1981;10(3):147–56.
36. Csuka M, McCarty DJ. Simple method for measurement of lower extremity muscle strength. Am J Med. 1985;78(1):77–81.
37. Duncan PW, Weiner DK, Chandler J, Studenski S. Functional reach: a new clinical measure of balance. J Gerontol. 1990;45(6):M192–7.
38. Davis JW, Ross PD, Preston SD, Nevitt MC, Wasnich RD. Strength, physical activity, and body mass index: relationship to performance-based measures and activities of daily living among older Japanese women in Hawaii. J Am Geriatr Soc. 1998;46(3):274–9.
39. Abe Y, Aoyagi K, Tsurumoto T, Chen CY, Kanagae M, Mizukami S, Ye Z, Kusano Y. Association of spinal inclination with physical performance measures among community-dwelling Japanese women aged 40 years and older. Geriatr Gerontol Int. 2013;13(4):881–6.
40. Fried LP, Young Y, Rubin G, Bandeen-Roche K. Self-reported preclinical disability identifies older women with early declines in performance and early disease. J Clin Epidemiol. 2001;54(9):889–901.
41. Weiner DK, Duncan PW, Chandler J, Studenski SA. Functional reach: a marker of physical frailty. J Am Geriatr Soc. 1992;40(3):203–7.
42. Kado DM, Huang MH, Barrett-Connor E, Greendale GA. Hyperkyphotic posture and poor physical functional ability in older community-dwelling men and women: the Rancho Bernardo study. J Gerontol A Biol Sci Med Sci. 2005;60(5):633–7.
43. Takahashi T, Ishida K, Hirose D, Nagano Y, Okumiya K, Nishinaga M, Matsubayashi K, Doi Y, Tani T, Yamamoto H. Trunk deformity is associated with a reduction in outdoor activities of daily living and life satisfaction in community-dwelling older people. Osteoporos Int. 2005;16(3):273–9.
44. Antonelli-Incalzi R, Pedone C, Cesari M, Di Iorio A, Bandinelli S, Ferrucci L. Relationship between the occiput-wall distance and physical performance in the elderly: a cross sectional study. Aging Clin Exp Res. 2007;19(3):207–12.
45. Green AD, Colon-Emeric CS, Bastian L, Drake MT, Lyles KW. Does this woman have osteoporosis? JAMA. 2004;292(23):2890–900.
46. Hirose D, Ishida K, Nagano Y, Takahashi T, Yamamoto H. Posture of the trunk in the sagittal plane is associated with gait in community-dwelling elderly population. Clin Biomech (Bristol, Avon). 2004;19(1):57–63.
47. Kitahara H, Ye Z, Aoyagi K, Ross PD, Abe Y, Honda S, Kanagae M, Mizukami S, Kusano Y, Tomita M, et al. Associations of vertebral deformities and osteoarthritis with back pain among Japanese women: the Hizen-Oshima study. Osteoporos Int. 2013;24(3):907–15.
48. Groll DL, To T, Bombardier C, Wright JG. The development of a comorbidity index with physical function as the outcome. J Clin Epidemiol. 2005;58(6): 595–602.

8

Modified Essex-Lopresti procedure with percutaneous calcaneoplasty for comminuted intra-articular calcaneal fractures

Jen-Ta Shih, Chun-Lin Kuo, Tsu-Te Yeh, Hsain-Chung Shen, Ru-Yu Pan and Chia-Chun Wu*

Abstract

Background: The ideal treatment for comminuted intraarticular calcaneal fractures is still debated. Open reduction and internal fixation (ORIF) is the most popular surgical procedure; however, wound complications, implant choice, and infection remain major concerns. This study aimed to demonstrate the results of an innovative, minimally invasive surgical procedure, namely, a closed reduction technique using large-diameter Steinmann pins and percutaneous calcaneoplasty using injectable calcium sulfate cement (MIIG X3, Wright Medical Technology, Inc., Arlington, TN), in patients with comminuted calcaneal fractures.

Methods: From January 2012 to January 2014, 20 patients (three women, 17 men) with comminuted calcaneus fractures (Sanders classification type III and Essex-Lopresti classification joint-depression type fracture) were included. Plain films and CT scans were obtained preoperatively in all patients. The operation was performed within three days post-injury, and patients were not allowed to bear weight until three months postoperatively. During this period, the patients were educated on how to perform bed exercises for joints above the surgical site, including muscle strengthening and body conditioning. Early active range of motion exercises for the ankle and forefoot began 3 to 6 weeks postoperatively. All patients were followed up regularly. The results were assessed using the American Orthopaedic Foot and Ankle Society (AOFAS) ankle score and Böhler's angle of the calcaneus.

Results: After an average follow-up of two years, none of the patients required further surgery or experienced soft tissue complications. The clinical results were rated good to excellent on the AOFAS scale in 80% of the cases (16 of 20 patients), and most patients had pain relief and returned to their former daily activities at the same level as before the injury.

Conclusions: A modified Essex-Lopresti procedure with percutaneous calcaneoplasty appears to be a safe and effective procedure to treat comminuted calcaneal fractures with acceptable functional results. Long-term outcomes and additional cases using this technique are required to support our conclusion.

Keywords: Modified Essex-Lopresti, Minimally invasive, Calcaneoplasty, AOFAS ankle score, Calcaneal fractures

Background

Calcaneal fractures account for approximately 2% of all fractures, and displaced intra-articular fractures comprise 60% to 75% of these injuries [1]. These fractures increase the calcaneal width, involve the subtalar joint surface, and decrease Böhler's angle. Controversy still exists regarding their classification, treatment, and postoperative management, as well as the appropriate operative technique for this type of fracture; therefore, calcaneal fractures remain among the most challenging fractures for orthopaedic surgeons to treat. Closed reduction with percutaneous pinning, a minimally invasive technique, is believed to result in fewer soft tissue injuries and fewer wound complications [2]. Indications for this technique include the following: (a) Sanders 2C tongue-type fractures; (b)

* Correspondence: orthopedicsintsgh@gmail.com
Department of Orthopaedic Surgery, Tri-Service General Hospital, National Defense Medical Center, No. 325, Sec. 2, Chenggong Rd., Neihu Dist, Taipei City 11472, Taiwan, Republic of China

displaced calcaneal tuberosity fractures; (c) temporary stabilization of fractures with severe soft tissue compromise; and (d) fractures in patients with relative contraindications to open surgery. We have been using modified Essex-Lopresti reduction with percutaneous pinning and percutaneous calcaneoplasty with a minimally invasive injectable graft (MIIG) to augment treatment for comminuted calcaneal fractures since 2012 and herein describe our first 20 consecutive cases with an average follow-up of two years. The aim of the study was to demonstrate the clinical efficacy and safety of a minimally invasive surgical technique for comminuted calcaneal fractures that resolves the complications resulting from traditional ORIF.

Methods

The inclusion criteria were as follows: cases conforming to the diagnostic criteria for unilateral closed intra-articular calcaneal fractures and CT and X-ray examinations confirming a Sanders type III fracture and an Essex-Lopresti joint-depression type fracture (Fig. 1). Paediatric patients, patients with psychiatric disorders or accompanying severe trauma requiring another surgery, and patients with open fractures were excluded from the study. Informed consent was obtained from all eligible patients. Approval was obtained from the Institutional Review Board of Tri-Service General Hospital, National Defense Medical Center (approval number: 1–101–05-008). Chart data were analysed for patient demographics and surgical treatment details from the time of injury to the most recent follow-up. The American Orthopaedic Foot and Ankle Society (AOFAS) ankle/hindfoot score was utilized for clinical evaluation, with results graded as excellent (90), good (80), fair (70), and poor (< 70). Böhler's angle was calculated to assess bone reduction [3].

Operative technique

Patients were treated with minimally invasive manipulative reduction using large-diameter (3.2–4.0 mm) Steinmann pin fixation. The procedures were performed with patients in the lateral decubitus position under spinal anaesthesia. First, the heel was squeezed to reduce the calcaneal morphology, and the manipulation was performed continually during the operation. Guided by fluoroscopy, the first Steinmann pin was inserted from the superior external side of the calcaneal tuberosity and advanced to the forefoot without crossing the fracture line. With the forefoot plantarflexed, the Steinmann pin was pulled and poked toward the plantar foot, and reduction was performed to allow for calcaneal inversion and eversion as well as flexion and extension of the ankle. We utilized an iso-centric image intensifier intraoperatively to check lateral, Broden's and Harris axial views of the heel and thus confirmed that Böhler's angle was restored within the range of 20°–40°. The length and height of the calcaneus were restored as much as possible. The Steinmann pin was inserted into the tarsal bones after restoring the subtalar joint surface. A second Steinmann pin was inserted inferior to the first Steinmann pin and in the direction parallel to the inferior calcaneus for fracture fragment stabilization as well as fixation and support between the tarsal bones and the calcaneus. If necessary, a third Steinmann pin was inserted from the posterior of the calcaneus, traversing the fractured fragments of the subtalar joint and reaching the tarsal bones. We made a minimal incision through the modified sinus tarsi approach to elevate the articular surface, spread the fractured site, and remove blood clots with a suction tip under fluoroscopic guidance before the calcaneoplasty (Fig. 2). The augmentation was completed by the percutaneous injection of 10 ml of calcium sulfate cement (MIIG® X3, Wright Medical Technology, Inc., Arlington, TN) into the fractured site through a trocar. Cast immobilization was applied postoperatively, and protected weight-bearing ambulation was advised within 12 weeks. The pins were draped with antibiotic-coated dressings and were removed after 12 weeks in case of pin tract infection [4].

Results

We retrospectively reviewed 20 patients (three women and 17 men) with a mean age of 50 years (range, 31 to 66 years) who sustained comminuted intra-articular calcaneal fractures and were treated with closed reduction and percutaneous pinning combined with MIIG augmentation at our institution between January 2012 and January 2014. The injury mechanism was a fall from a height on hard ground in 13 cases and motor vehicle accidents in the remaining cases. Preoperatively, conventional X-ray and CT scan reconstructions were obtained

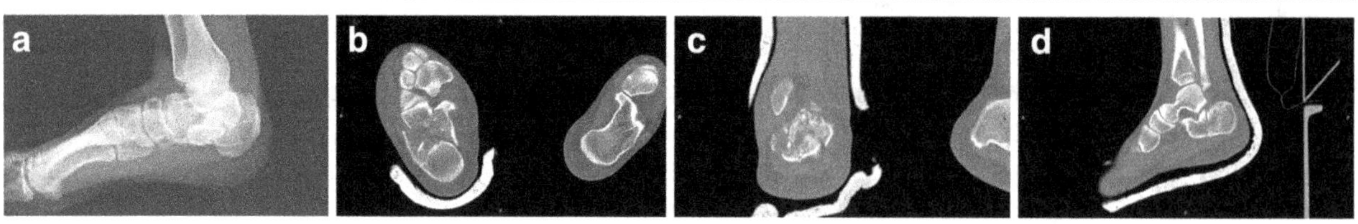

Fig. 1 Calcaneal fracture in a 61-year-old man. **a** Preoperative plain film demonstrating a nearly negative Böhler's angle, joint depression type; **b** CT scan demonstrating a Sanders type III fracture and increased calcaneal width in the axial plane, **c** coronal plane, and **d** sagittal plane

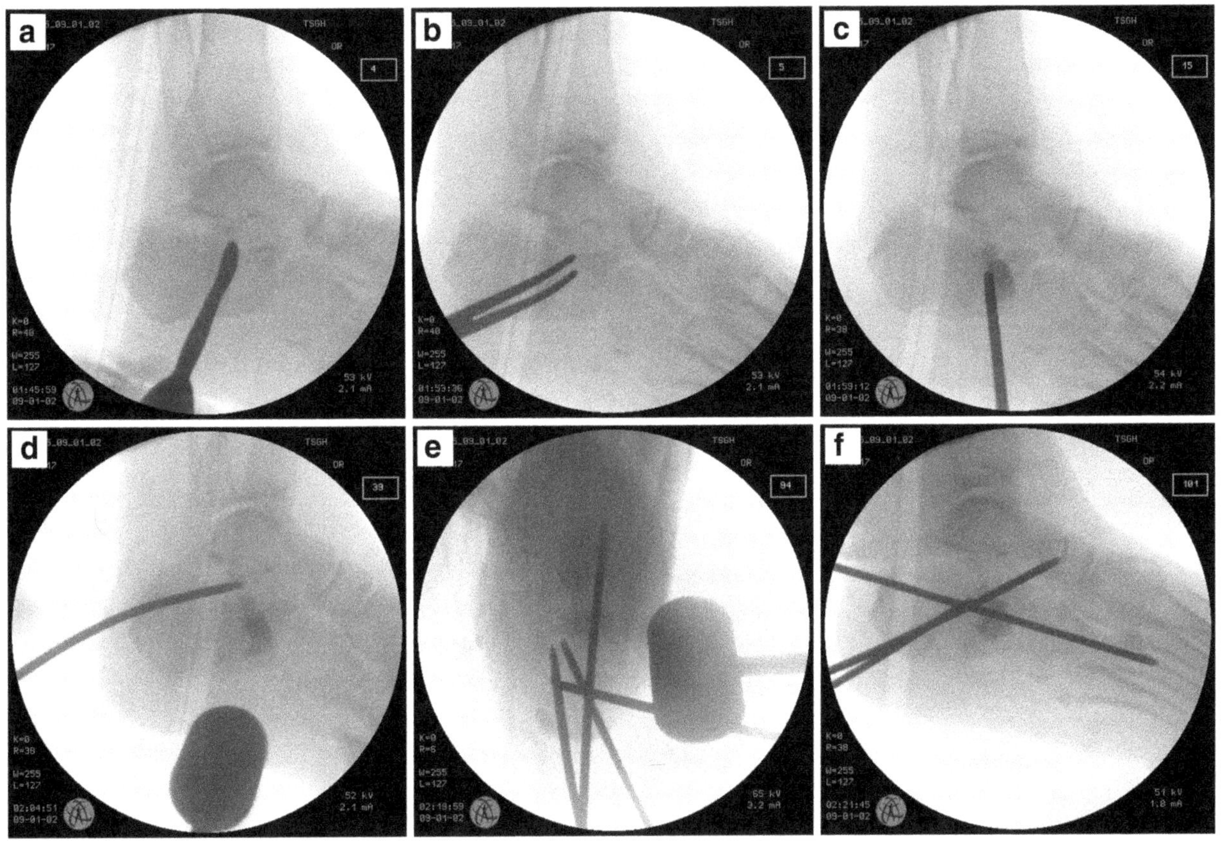

Fig. 2 Intraoperative images from an iso-centric image intensifier demonstrating reduction techniques and calcaneoplasty procedures. **a** A dull elevator was inserted through a small incision to elevate the articular surface; **b** a Kelly clamp was used to spread the fracture site; **c** MIIG was directly injected through a trocar to the fracture site; **d** a 3.2-mm Steinmann was applied as a joystick to perform the Essex-Lopresti manoeuvre; **e** Harris axial view demonstrating manipulation with a hammer and correction of the calcaneal axis using the distraction technique with Steinmann pins; and **f** fixation with Steinmann pins across joints to maintain the reduction

in all cases. Surgery was scheduled within three days because the success of manipulative reduction is correlated with early surgery and minimal soft tissue violation from the surgical technique. All cases progressed to bony union within 3 months. According to the AOFAS score, clinical results were excellent in 6 cases, good in 10 cases, and fair in 4 cases. The mean preoperative Böhler's angle was −1.8° (−16.1°–16.6°), while the mean postoperative value was 25.9° (20.8°–33.3°) (normal Böhler's angle is between 20° and 40°; Table 1). After an average follow-up of 2 years, the mean Böhler's angle of the injured calcaneus was 21.7° (17.4°–28.8°) (Fig. 3). Most patients returned to normal activities of daily living after 12 weeks or later. No wound complications or adverse reactions were observed.

Discussion

Most calcaneal fractures are high-energy injuries that are accompanied by various degrees of soft tissue damage. Open reduction using an extensile lateral approach has traditionally been used to treat displaced intra-articular calcaneal fractures, and the surgery is generally delayed until soft tissue swelling has subsided. The major complication associated with open reduction is wound complications, including plate exposure and skin edge necrosis. Despite the presence of advanced surgical techniques and more favourable designs and implant materials, the prevalence of wound complications remains high in open reduction [5]. Essex-Lopresti [6] described a percutaneous reduction manoeuvre several decades ago that was successfully performed by Tornetta [7] in 41 patients with tongue type IIC calcaneal fractures. The purpose of the manoeuvre is to disimpact the fracture by lifting one of the pins and simultaneously plantar flexing the foot. If reduction of the tongue fragment is successful, the second pin is advanced across the anterior process. Definitive fixation is achieved with a large cannulated lag screw that is inserted over the guide wire through small stab incisions placed around the guide pins. Currently, this minimally invasive surgical technique has become widely employed. The indications were limited to Sanders 2C tongue-type fractures, displaced calcaneal tuberosity fractures, and fractures in patients who are not amenable to open

Table 1 Patient data

Patient	Sex	Preop. BA	Postop. BA	Follow-up BA	Follow-up (months)	AOFAS score	Aetiology
1	M	−16.1	20.8	19.9	31	80	MVA
2	M	−11.8	22.3	18.7	33	81	Tumble
3	M	1.3	33.3	19.0	17	80	Tumble
4	F	−10	21.7	20.4	18	75	MVA
5	M	−2.5	26.6	21.4	31	87	MVA
6	M	0	22.5	21.2	26	90	Tumble
7	M	16.6	24.6	21.5	22	97	Tumble
8	M	−7.2	24.1	19.5	24	82	Tumble
9	M	13.8	25.8	21.9	15	93	Tumble
10	M	10.9	22.8	18.1	28	91	Tumble
11	F	9.0	31.1	24.5	16	78	MVA
12	M	−14.3	21.0	17.4	26	70	MVA
13	M	−15.9	30.1	24.0	22	86	Tumble
14	M	1.2	32.7	28.8	27	88	Tumble
15	M	3.2	28.9	26.4	21	86	Tumble
Patient	Sex	Preop. BA	Postop. BA	Follow-up BA	Follow-up (months)	AOFAS score	
16	M	−7.8	24.8	22.8	30	92	Tumble
17	M	−11.6	23.2	19.6	23	76	Tumble
18	M	−3.9	25.9	22.4	19	84	Tumble
19	F	1.7	24.8	18.2	26	82	MVA
20	M	7.5	30.6	28.5	22	94	MVA
Average		−1.8°	25.9°	21.7°	23.9	84.6	

BA Böhler's angle, *AOFAS* American Orthopaedic Foot and Ankle Society, *MVA* Motor vehicle accident

surgery. The minimally invasive reduction and fixation technique in the present study focused on treating complicated calcaneal fractures that are classified as Sanders type III joint depression fractures, which are considered to be one of the most challenging types of calcaneus fractures.

Calcaneal morphology is essential for hindfoot and ankle function, and fracture reduction helps to restore a congruent subtalar joint. Agren et al. [8] conducted a prospective, randomized, controlled multicentre trial to compare operative with nonoperative treatments of displaced intra-articular calcaneal fractures. Eighty-two patients were included. Operative treatment, despite increasing the risk of complications, appeared to have some benefits at eight to twelve years, including a trend towards increased patient-reported primary visual analogue scale (VAS) scores for pain and function and a reduced prevalence of posttraumatic arthritis evident on follow-up radiographs. Once poor calcaneal morphology and late post-traumatic arthritis develop, they may lead to persistent functional impairment requiring further treatment, such as subtalar arthrodesis [9]. The correlation between Böhler's angle and clinical outcomes in displaced intra-articular calcaneal fractures has been demonstrated [10]. In other words, restoration of hindfoot morphology

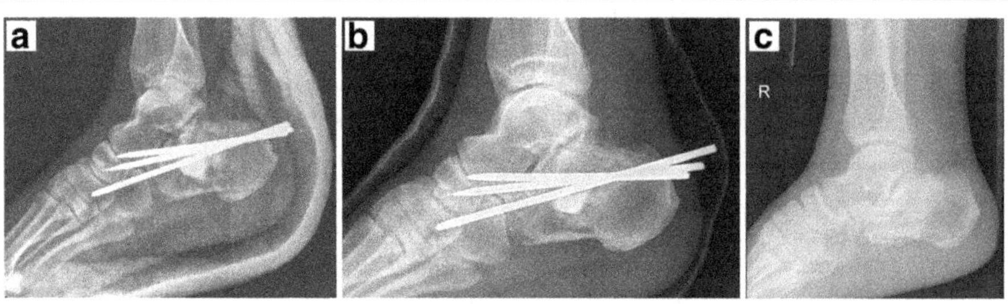

Fig. 3 Calcaneal fracture in a 61-year-old man (continued). **a** A postoperative plain film demonstrating restoration of Böhler's angle. **b** A postoperative plain film two months postoperatively. **c** A reduction of Böhler's angle was noted 20 months later

may be more important than the anatomical reduction of the posterior facet to achieve good clinical results in comminuted calcaneal fractures [11]. The surgical outcomes in our study demonstrated that minimally invasive manipulative reduction and percutaneous pinning can restore hindfoot morphology, with a mean increase in Böhler's angle of 27.7°. A mean loss of 4.2° at 2 years after the trauma was observed; however, the functional results remained satisfactory.

Traditionally, operative treatment for fractures should be performed within three weeks after the injury prior to early consolidation of the fracture; nevertheless, delaying definitive fixation of closed, intra-articular calcaneus fractures did not decrease wound complication rates when using the extensile lateral approach [12]. The time from injury to surgery in our study was three days or less. The benefits of our minimally invasive technique include the accessibility of manipulative reduction with early surgery and a low incidence of wound complications.

Stulik et al. [13] performed surgery within 48 h in 89% of the patients in their series and stated that earlier surgery facilitated reduction. However, the risk of deep infection and potential limb-threatening complications following open reduction and internal fixation of calcaneal fractures was significant [5]. deWall et al. [14] described a deep infection rate of 14.3% and a minor wound complication rate of 21.4% in 41 patients treated with open reduction via an extensile lateral approach, with no deep infections and a 6% minor wound complication rate in 79 patients who underwent percutaneous treatment. A relatively short operative time and less wound surface exposure may have contributed to these results.

Most injectable bone substitutes are calcium phosphate compounds, calcium sulfate compounds, or both. Following mixing, bone substitute pastes can be injected into a fracture space for augmentation as an alternative to a bone graft, and the mechanical strength of these pastes when compressed resembles that of cancellous bone [15]. Early clinical results have shown a reduced time to full weight-bearing when bone substitutes have been used for augmentation of calcaneal fractures [16]. Injectable calcium sulfate bone substitutes (MIIG® X3, Wright Medical Technology, Inc., Arlington, TN) were used for all patients in the present study. There was no increased risk of infection, and these substitutes provided more convenience during the operation. In fact, the use of autologous bone grafts has not been shown to have radiological or functional benefit [17]. Biggi et al. [18] described a percutaneous calcaneoplasty technique using balloon reduction and augmentation with injectable bone substitutes of calcium phosphate or cement, and this technique demonstrated good clinical results for treating calcaneal fractures without internal fixation.

Traditional extensile open surgery is technically demanding, and there is an extensive learning curve for surgeons who intend to achieve anatomic reduction and provide absolute stability for comminuted calcaneal fractures, as well as a prolonged operative time and extensive wound exposure. A minimally invasive technique achieves functional reduction, provides relative stability, minimizes soft tissue dissection, preserves the blood supply and, thus, may be more suitable given the characteristics of comminuted calcaneal fractures. It also offers an alternative approach in patients who have significant medical co-morbidities (smokers, diabetics, and patients with peripheral vascular disease or intolerance to prolonged surgery), in whom open reduction would be hazardous and non-operative treatment would be inadequate [19]. In fact, most surgeons learn the essentials of minimally invasive techniques earlier than previously thought [20]. Although this is a retrospective study with a limited number of cases and a two-year follow-up, the results are encouraging, suggesting that true minimally invasive percutaneous stabilization is an alternative for the surgical treatment of such challenging fractures.

Conclusion

To our knowledge, a minimally invasive technique combining a modified Essex-Lopresti manoeuvre and percutaneous calcaneoplasty with injectable bone substitutes of calcium sulfate has not been previously described in the literature. This technique can be performed in the presence of soft tissue swelling immediately following trauma, with a low incidence of wound infection/dehiscence. Although anatomic reduction of the articular surface cannot be achieved, this technique restores the calcaneal morphology by improving Böhler's angle and results in acceptable functional outcomes without major complications in patients with Sanders type III joint depression type calcaneal fractures. Further study of long-term outcomes and additional cases using this technique is required to support our conclusion.

Abbreviations

AOFAS: American Orthopaedic Foot and Ankle Society; MIIG: Minimally invasive injectable graft; ORIF: Open reduction and internal fixation

Acknowledgements

We would like to thank American Journal Experts (www.aje.com) for providing English language editing.

Funding

No funding was obtained for this study.

Authors' contributions

CW, TY, and CK conceptualized and designed the study. HS and RP acquired the data and assisted in drafting part of the manuscript and image management. JS interpreted the data and was a major contributor in drafting the manuscript. All authors read and approved the final manuscript.

Authors' information

CW is Associate Professor in Department of Orthopaedics at National Defense Medical Center in Taiwan. He fulfilled his fellowship in Georgetown University Hospital (Washington, DC), and specialized in bone and soft tissue reconstruction.

Consent for publication

Not applicable

Competing interests

The authors declare that they have no competing interests.

References

1. Mitchell MJ, McKinley JC, Robinson CM. The epidemiology of calcaneal fractures. Foot. 2009;19:197–200.
2. de Vroome SW, van der Linden FM. Cohort study on the percutaneous treatment of displaced intra-articular fractures of the calcaneus. Foot Ankle Int. 2014;35:156–62.
3. Su Y, Chen W, Zhang T, Wu X, Wu Z, Zhang Y. Bohler's angle's role in assessing the injury severity and functional outcome of internal fixation for displaced intra-articular calcaneal fractures: a retrospective study. BMC Surg. 2013;13:40.
4. Demcoe AR, Verhulsdonk M, Buckley RE. Complications when using threaded K-wire fixation for displaced intra-articular calcaneal fractures. Injury. 2009;40:1297–301.
5. Howard JL, Buckley R, McCormack R, Pate G, Leighton R, Petrie D, et al. Complications following management of displaced intra-articular calcaneal fractures: a prospective randomized trial comparing open reduction internal fixation with nonoperative management. J Orthop Trauma. 2003;17:241–9.
6. Essex-Lopresti P. The mechanism, reduction technique, and results in fractures of the OS calcis. Br J Surg. 1952;39:395–419.
7. Tornetta P 3rd. Percutaneous treatment of calcaneal fractures. Clin Orthop Relat Res. 2000;375:91–6.
8. Agren PH, Wretenberg P, Sayed-Noor AS. Operative versus nonoperative treatment of displaced intra-articular calcaneal fractures. J Bone Joint Surg Am. 2013;95:1351–7.
9. Radnay CS, Clare MP, Sanders RW. Subtalar fusion after displaced intra-articular calcaneal fractures: does initial operative treatment matter? J Bone Joint Surg Am. 2009;91:541–6.
10. Loucks C, Buckley R. Bohler's angle: correlation with outcome in displaced intra-articular calcaneal fractures. J Orthop Trauma. 1999;13:554–8.
11. van Hoeve S, Poeze M. Outcome of minimally invasive open and percutaneous techniques for repair of calcaneal fractures: a systematic review. J Foot Ankle Surg. 2016;55:1256–63.
12. Kwon JY, Guss D, Lin DE, Abousayed M, Jeng C, Kang S, et al. Effect of delay to definitive surgical fixation on wound complications in the treatment of closed, intra-articular calcaneus fractures. Foot Ankle Int. 2015;36:508–17.
13. Stulik J, Stehlik J, Rysavy M, Wozniak A. Minimally-invasive treatment of intra-articular fractures of the calcaneum. J Bone Joint Surg Br. 2006;88-B:1634–41.
14. deWall M, Henderson CE, McKinley TO, Phelps T, Dolan L, Marsh JL. Percutaneous reduction and fixation of displaced intra-articular calcaneus fractures. J Orthop Trauma. 2010;24:466–72.
15. Larsson S, Hannink G. Injectable bone-graft substitutes: current products, their characteristics and indications, and new developments. Injury. 2011;42:S30–4.
16. Larsson S, Bauer TW. Use of injectable calcium phosphate cement for fracture fixation: a review. Clin Orthop Relat Res. 2002;395:23–32.
17. Longino D, Buckley RE. Bone graft in the operative treatment of displaced intraarticular calcaneal fractures: is it helpful? J Orthop Trauma. 2001;15:280–6.
18. Biggi F, Di Fabio S, D'Antimo C, Isoni F, Salfi C, Trevisani S. Percutaneous calcaneoplasty in displaced intraarticular calcaneal fractures. J Orthop Traumatol. 2013;14:307–10.
19. Zhang T, Su Y, Chen W, Zhang Q, Wu Z, Zhang Y. Displaced intra-articular calcaneal fractures treated in a minimally invasive fashion: longitudinal approach versus sinus tarsi approach. J Bone Joint Surg Am. 2014;96:302–9.
20. Arastu M, Sheehan B, Buckley R. Minimally invasive reduction and fixation of displaced calcaneal fractures: surgical technique and radiographic analysis. Int Orthop. 2014;38:539–45.

9

Improving results in rat fracture models: enhancing the efficacy of biomechanical testing by a modification of the experimental setup

Peter Michael Prodinger[1*], Dominik Bürklein[2], Peter Foehr[3], Kilian Kreutzer[4], Hakan Pilge[5], Andreas Schmitt[6], Rüdiger v. Eisenhart-Rothe[1], Rainer Burgkart[1], Oliver Bissinger[7] and Thomas Tischer[8]

Abstract

Background: Animal fracture models, primarily performed in rats, are crucial to investigate normal and pathological bone healing. However, results of biomechanical testing representing a major outcome measure show high standard deviations often precluding statistical significance. Therefore, the aim of our study was a systematical examination of biomechanical characteristics of rat femurs during three-point bending. Furthermore, we tried to reduce variation of results by individually adapting the span of bearing and loading areas to the bone's length.

Methods: We examined 40 paired femurs of male Wistar-rats by DXA (BMD and BMC of the whole femur) and pQCT-scans at the levels of bearing and loading areas of the subsequent biomechanical three-point bending test. Individual adjustment of bearing and loading bars was done respecting the length of each specimen. Subgroups of light (< 400 g, $n = 22$) and heavy (> 400 g, $n = 18$) animals were formed and analysed separately. We furthermore compared the results of the individualised bending-setting to 20 femurs tested with a fix span of 15 mm.

Results: Femurs showed a length range of 34 to 46 mm. The failure loads ranged from 116 to 251 N (mean 175.4 ± 45.2 N; heavy animals mean 221 ± 18.9 N; light animals mean 138.1 ± 16.4 N) and stiffness ranged from 185 N/mm to 426 N/mm (mean 315.6 ± 63 N/mm; heavy animals mean 358.1 ± 34.64 N/mm; light animals mean 280.8 ± 59.85 N/mm). The correlation of densitometric techniques and failure loads was high (DXA $R^2 = 0.89$ and pQCT $R^2 = 0.88$). In comparison to femurs tested with a fix span, individual adaptation of biomechanical testing homogenized our data significantly. Most notably, the standard deviation of failure loads (221 ± 18.95 N individualized setting vs. 205.5 ± 30.36 N fixed) and stiffness (358.1 ± 34.64 N/mm individualized setting vs. 498.5 ± 104.8 N/mm fixed) was reduced by at least one third.

Conclusions: Total variation observed in any trait reflects biological and methodological variation. Precision of the method hence affects the statistical power of the study. By simply adapting the setting of the biomechanical testing, interindividual variation could be reduced, which improves the precision of the method significantly.

Keywords: Rat fracture studies, Three-point bending, Biomechanical testing, Animal model, pQCT

* Correspondence: peter.prodinger@tum.de
[1]Klinik für Orthopädie und Sportorthopädie, Klinikum rechts der Isar der Technischen Universität München, Ismaninger Straße 22, 81675 Munich, Germany
Full list of author information is available at the end of the article

Background

Preclinical research concerning normal and disturbed bone healing is usually done in small animal models [1–3]. Of those, rat fracture models are of paramount importance [4]. Still, a significant proportion (38%) of all published animal fracture studies used rats for their investigations [5]. Furthermore, they are useful to advance tissue-engineering methods and to characterize positive or negative effects of certain types of medication on bone healing that have been observed or suspected in the clinical use [6, 7].

Analysis of results is carried out by morphological and functional investigations. Regularly applied radiological procedures such as DXA, pQCT and Micro-CT provide detailed analyses of the bone microstructure [6, 8, 9]. In addition to bone density and mineral content, the raw data allows for a calculation and comparison of geometric parameters. Histological examinations enable cellular analyses and even dynamics in bone apposition can be visualized by fluorescence staining [10]. Of all the analytical methods mentioned – no matter how advanced and elaborated they might be - only functional trials using biomechanical testing provide answers to the most important question: the stability of bone [11].

Over the last few years, several experimental studies have been carried out on bone healing in animals under pharmacological influence [12–16]. While most of the studies showed significant differences in volume, formation and mineralization of the callus, these findings could often not be confirmed biomechanically. This led us to the question whether the apparent morphological variability is, in fact, irrelevant - or if the applied testing protocols are simply not good enough to measure small effects. In monitoring imaging technique developments over the past decades, the array of possibilities and their accuracy have expanded considerably [7, 17]. As a result, smaller effects could undoubtedly be verified through imaging. By contrast, biomechanical testing has not shown comparable progress.

Animal models often show a wide range of standard deviations in biomechanical testing protocols, leading to non-significant outcomes. Therefore, the aim of our study was to reduce variability and to obtain statistically sound results by doing a systematic examination of biomechanical characteristics of rat femora tested in an individualized setting. Furthermore, we think that there is a need for standardization of biomechanical testing procedures in small animal studies [18].

Methods

Animals

The study was performed in the animal facility of the Klinikum rechts der Isar, Technische Universität München and was evaluated and approved by the local authority (Regierung von Oberbayern, approval no. 55.2–1–54-2531-17-10) as required by German law.

As described previously [19], 20 male Wistar rats (individual testing setup) with a mean body weight of 476 ± 160 g (range between 240 and 720 g) and another 10 male Wistar rats (fixed testing setup) with a mean body weight of 634.5 ± 26.9 g (range between 585 and 679 g) were euthanised according to the recommendation of the European Union using a threefold overdose of Phenobarbital (90 mg/kg) i.v. Subsequently the extremities were dissected and both femurs ($n = 60$) harvested. Surrounding skin, muscle, and other soft tissues were removed. The bones were fixed and stored in 70% Methanol at 4 °C.

For further analysis, the individual testing setup group was divided into subgroups of animals below and above 400 g. Specimens below 400 g corresponded to young animals under 16 weeks, above 400 g to adults above 16 weeks of age.

High resolution dual energy X-ray absorptiometry (DXA)

The methodology of the radiological biomechanical analyses has been described before [19].

Bone mineral content (BMC) and lean mass was measured in all femurs of the individual testing group ($n = 40$) using a high resolution DXA scanner (pDEXA Sabre, Norland/Stratec, Stratec Medizintechnik, Pforzheim) [20]. The resolution was 100 μm × 100 μm (acquisition time: 5 mm/s, total time 40 min). By DXA the bone mass can be normalized to the surface area of the bones exposed to radiation (bone mineral density = BMD in in mg/cm^2), whereas analysis of the volumetric bone density (mg/cm^3) is not possible. This results in a higher BMD for bigger bones but not necessarily in discrepancies in volumetric density [21].

Immediately after DXA scanning, the length of the bones, as well as the anterior-posterior diameter at the middle of the diaphysis were assessed with a calliper.

Peripheral quantitative computed tomography (pQCT)

All femurs of the individualized bending setup ($n = 40$) were examined using a pQCT scanner (XCT Research SA+, Stratec Medizintechnik, Pforzheim). Before the measurement, excessive air was removed in a vacuum chamber (20 min). After a quick-view (Scout-View), transverse section images with a thickness of 500 μm and a spatial resolution within the image plane of 100 μm at the diaphysis and the distal and proximal metaphysis were acquired. Based on the scout-view, each bone's individual length was designated 100%. Measurement positions were defined at the distal femur metaphysis at 15, 17.5 and 20%, at the middle of the femur diaphysis at 40, 42.5 and 45% and proximal at 64, 66.5 and 69% of the femoral bone length [19]. The average value was calculated from the three cross section images at all sites. Positioning of bearing- and loading-bars during the subsequent three-point bending test corresponded to the pQCT transection positions.

Further analysis of the qualitative variables and evaluation of the cross-sections was done with the software provided by the manufacturer. We used peelmode 1 with a threshold of 600 mg/mm and peelmode 2 (40% surface with lowest density = trabecular compartment) to enable separate calculations of trabecular, cortical and subcortical bone properties [22].

The cortical mineral content, the cortical density and thickness of the cortical bone, the cortical bone cross section surface and its percentage of the whole cross section surface were assessed at the middle of the diaphysis. All parameters are supposed to indicate mechanical strength of the bone during bending. Furthermore, the area surface moment of inertia (IP), the moment of resistance, as well as minimal and maximum moment of inertia were determined.

Mechanical testing (Fig. 1)

After rehydration in saline solution, the bones were loaded until failure with a persistent test velocity of 5 mm/min (three-point setup, AP direction) using a Zwick material testing machine (Zwicki Line Z2.5, Zwick GmbH & Co, Ulm, Germany). Concerning the individualized setup group, the position of the supporting- and loading-bars corresponded to the pQCT assessment areas, with the force transmission at the evaluated middle position between the distal and proximal site. The distance between the bars was adapted relative for each bone, the bearing bars were adjusted between 15 and 20% distal and 64 to 69% of each femurs length proximal, the loading bar in the middle (40–45%, see Fig. 1). The tips of the bars were rounded with a diameter of 2.5 mm. A load-displacement diagram was recorded every 0.1 s during bending; thereby the failure load could be determined. We measured the reaction forces with a load cell for up to ±2.5 kN (Klasse 0.05, A.S.T. GmbH, Dresden, Germany). Stiffness was defined as linear regression of the force and displacement graph (testXpert V12, Zwick/Roell, Ulm, Germany).

The 20 femurs of the fixed setup group were tested biomechanically with a fix span of 15 mm between the supporting bars.

Statistical analysis

Acquired data was analysed using GraphPad Prism 5 (GraphPad Software, La Jolla, CA, USA). Descriptive statistics are given by mean ± standard deviation, as normal distribution could be assumed by the distribution of the single values. Percentage variation (CV%) was calculated as CV% = SD/Mean * 100. Group comparisons were performed by Student's t-test. *P*-values < 0.05 were declared as statistically significant different. The correlations were determined by the slope of linear regression graph (including the coefficient of determination R^2 and the 95% confidence intervals).

Results

Individualized bending setup

Femurs measured provided a length between 34 and 46 mm. Both femurs of one individual were very constant; especially in light animals, barely no side differences were evident. Subgroup analysis showed that the femoral length of light rats (< 400 g) was 35.5 ± 1.3 mm, heavy rat's (> 400 g) mean was 43.1 ± 1.6 mm.

The failure loads of all specimens ranged from 116 to 251 N (mean 175.4 ± 45.2 N), heavy animals had a mean of 221 ± 18.95 N; light animals showed a mean of 138.1 ± 16.38 N. The stiffness of all specimens showed a larger range of results than the failure loads

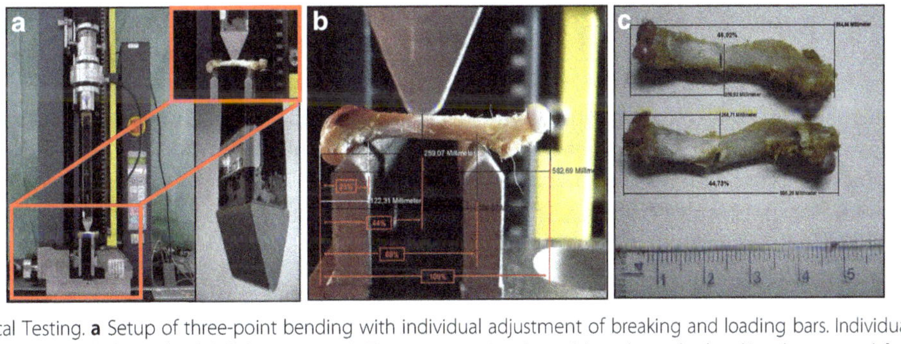

Fig. 1 Biomechanical Testing. **a** Setup of three-point bending with individual adjustment of breaking and loading bars. Individual adaption of the loading bars is facilitated by a helical wheel (left lower corner). The apparatus is relocatable to keep the breaking bar centred. **b** Individual adjustment of breaking and loading bars are identical to pQCT measurements. Every specimen was placed onto the flat area of the poplitheal plane (distal supporting bar), which is oriented in the frontal plane anatomically. Contact areas on the supporting bars were point-shaped proximally (just below the lesser trochanter) and either linear-shaped or two point-shaped (in case of prominent tails of the linea aspera) distally. This achieved a stable triangular-shaped bearing under loading, preventing rotational movements during the three-point bending test and standardizing the ap-orientation of the bone. **c** Rat femurs after mechanical testing, fracture occurred accurately at the predicted percentage

(Min 185 N/mm, Max 426 N/mm; Mean 315.6 ± 62.6 N/mm) (see Table 1).

Pairing of specimens (left vs. right) did not result in statistically significant differences altogether. However, we observed length differences of more than 1 mm in six of nine heavy animals (whereas in small animals both bones were almost equal). Furthermore, six of nine heavy rats showed a stronger right femur concerning the failure loads (which was not necessarily the longer bone, difference between the two groups still not statistically significant: $p = 0.072$), the left/right ratio in failure loads of small animals was almost balanced (5/6 in favor of right bones).

Interindividual variance (CV%) in failure load was 25.8% in all specimens and could be significantly reduced to under 9% if light animals were excluded, or 11.9% if heavy animals were excluded. The correlation of failure loads between the left and right side was higher in light animals ($R^2 = 0.86$), in heavy animals the coefficient of determination between the left and right side was only 0.4. Concerning the stiffness, a relatively weak correlation between both sides was observed either in light as in heavy specimens (see Fig. 2).

Over all, both densitometric techniques (DXA, pQCT) showed a high correlation between each other ($R^2 = 0.94$) (see Fig. 3a). The correlation of the densitometric techniques and the failure loads reached consistent and high values (DXA $R^2 = 0.89$ and pQCT $R^2 = 0.88$) (see Fig. 3b). The percentual deviation by the DXA for the BMD (left vs. right) was 0.6 ± 2,3% (BMC 1.5 ± 4.5%), by CT 2.5 ± 5.3% (n.s.).

Comparison individualized bending setup vs. fix span

In comparison to femurs tested with a fix span, individual adaptation of biomechanical testing improved the results significantly (see Table 2). Failure loads were higher using the individualized approach (mean 221 N adjusted setup vs. 205.5 N fixed span) and the standard deviation could be reduced by one-third (18.95 N adjusted setup vs. 30.36 N fixed). Concerning stiffness measurements, the changes caused by the treatment protocol appeared even bigger. By adapting the bars to the individual bones length, stiffness was reduced to a mean of 358.1 ± 34.6 N/mm, while femurs tested with a fix span showed a mean of 498.5 ± 104.8 N/mm. Besides reaching different absolute values, a diminution of the variation within the trait by individualized bending was feasible (see Fig. 4). Every single biomechanical and radiological measurement is depicted in the additional data sheet (Additional file 1).

Discussion

Accurate comparisons of biomechanical studies concerning bone strength are often impaired by lacking standardisation of the biomechanical testing protocols. Published techniques have included tensile testing, compressive loading, torsional testing, four-point bending and three-point bending tests [4, 23]. Of these, three-point bending is a simple, reproducible test, making it the preferred method of mechanical testing in small animal fracture models [4, 8, 24]. Usually, the three-point bending setup implies bearing bars with a fixed distance of 14 to 18 mm and a loading intender centred in between (regardless of individual bone length); force is applied perpendicularly to the bone with a constant speed of 2 to 5 mm/min [13, 25]. So even a simple procedure like three-point bending has experienced multiple modifications precluding comparability and integrity of data.

Preclinical animal models using rats have a high prognostic value concerning the efficacy and safety of drugs in humans [3, 6, 26]. Because the cellular phenotype of osteoblasts and osteoclasts is comparable, the effect of medication on bone and fracture healing in rats allows deductions about the human situation, designating these models ideal in exploring unknown or adverse effects on bone. However, the absence of the Haversian system and the presence of permanently open growth plates in rodents indicate fundamental discrepancies and prevents direct extrapolation of the results to humans [26]. Both, tibiae and femurs of rats are suitable for experimental studies. The tibia is surrounded by a thin soft tissue mantle allowing easy access to the bone and favouring this bone for closed fracture models without surgery [27]. Thus, the risk of generating concomitant fibular fractures is high and changes a stable into an unstable model, potentially implicating the need for secondary surgical stabilisation with a significant amount of complications [28]. The femur on the other hand is surrounded by a thick muscle layer impeding the generation of standardized fractures, but allowing the use of proper implants with

Table 1 Summary, biomechanical data, individualized-setting group

	Total $N = 40$	Light (< 400 g) $N = 22$	Heavy (> 400 g) $N = 18$	Light vs. Heavy
Lenght (mm)	38.9 (±4.1)	35.5 (±1.3)	43.1 (±1.6)	$p < 0.001$
Failure load (N)	175.4 (±45.2)	138.1 (±16.38)	221.0 (±18.95)	p < 0.001
Stiffness (N/mm)	315.6 (±63.0)	280.8 (±59.85)	358.1 (±34.64)	$p = 0.0003$

Means and standard deviations of length, failure load and stiffness. Total and subgroups of light and heavy animals separately

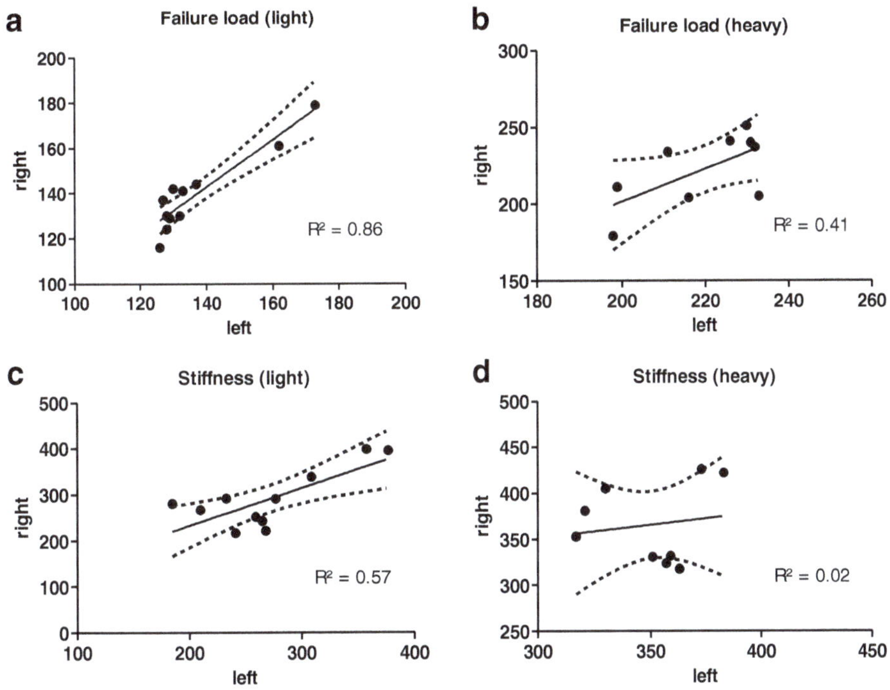

Fig. 2 Correlation graphs of failure loads and stiffness values, right versus left femur of each specimen (Bivariate Scattergrams with regression lines and 95% confidence bands). **a**, **b** Failure loads of the right versus the left femur. Light rats (> 400 g, **a**) show a strong correlation. In heavy animals (> 400 g, **b**) a wide range between both sides was evident. **c**, **d** Stiffness values of the right versus the left sides. In light and heavy animals, no correlations between both sides could be seen

acceptable complication rates. Furthermore, most, widely used fracture models are established regarding the femur offering the possibility for comparisons between different studies. To summarize, most authors would prefer the femur when fracture healing is the aim of the study [29].

Reviewing the recent literature, we surprisingly found that systematic tests/research on inter- and intra-individual differences of rat femurs are, for the most part, not available. Bones come in different shapes and sizes, and none have the geometry and gross morphology of an ideal mechanical test specimen. Hence, adapting the biomechanical testing setup to each bone individually seems a logical step to generate results that are more reliable. First and foremost the length of tested bones shows great impact on failure

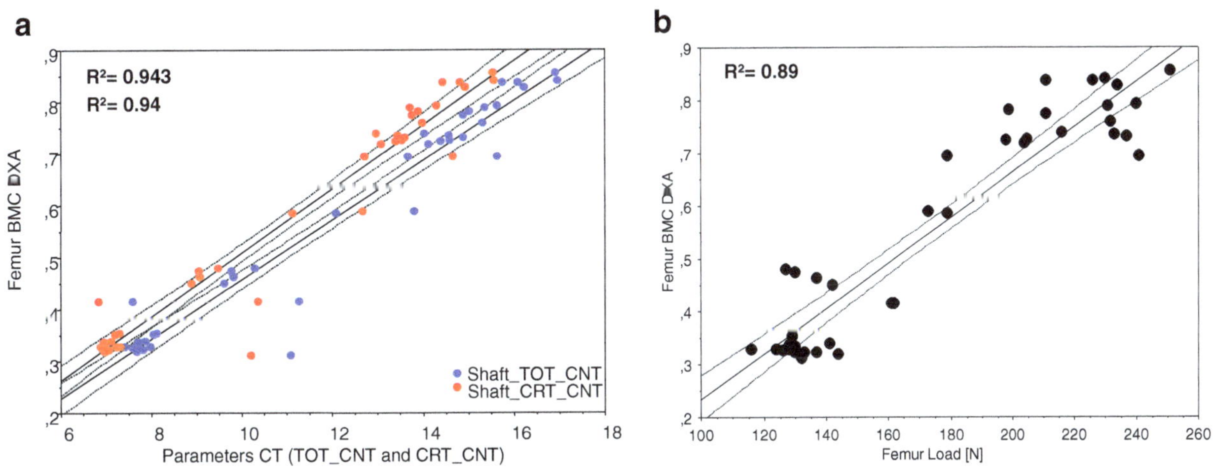

Fig. 3 Correlation graphs (Bivariate Scattergrams with regression lines and 95% confidence bands). **a** Femoral DXA BMC (bone mineral content in g) versus pQCT total content (TOT_CNT, blue dots) and cortical content (CRT_CNT, red dots) show a strong correlation of both techniques. **b** Femoral DXA BMC (bone minerall content in g) versus failure load $R^2 = 0.89$. The correlation between pQCT – values (TOT_CNT and CRT_CNT) is identical

Table 2 Summary, biomechanical data, comparison between fixed and individualized bending setup

	Fixed Span $N = 20$	Individualized $N = 18$	Fixed vs. Individualized
Weight (g)	634.5(±26.9)	641.9 (±55.5)	$p = 0.59$
Length (mm)	42.9(±1.1)	43.1(±1.6)	$p = 0.63$
Failure Load (N)	205.5 (±30.36)	221.0 (±18.95)	$p = 0.07$
Stiffness (N/mm)	498.5 (±104.8)	358.1 (±34.64)	$p < 0.0001$

Means and standard deviations of weight, length, failure load and stiffness. Subgroups of femurs tested with a fixed span and heavy animals tested by the individualized setting. Both groups are not statistically significant different concerning weight or length. Though the fixed-span subgroup seems more homogenous concerning weight and lengths of the femurs, failure loads (tendency) and stiffness values (stat. significant) are more homogenous in the individualized-setting group

loads. As approximations of the failure/braking load are displayed by $F = 48*E*I*d/L^3$ (F = breaking load, E = Young's modulus, I = second moment of area, L = length between the supporting bars, d = deformation), naturally, modifications of the distance between the supporting bars provides major impact on the actual failure load [9]. By comparing failure load and stiffness measured with a fix span with the results of the individualised setting we could clearly demonstrate, that not only the absolute values were altered, moreover and more important, the variance within the samples was reduced significantly.

To reach consistent and reliable results, the aspect ratio (span of the lower supports / diameter of the bone at midshaft) of the tested bone should be maximized [30]. By doing so, shear forces are reduced to a minimum and bending as main component of the deflection of bone pronounced. That brings the tested specimen close to fulfilling the ideal beam criteria, which means the least amount of measurement error and the optimal condition for biomechanical characterization of the whole bone. Thus, the span between the lower supports should be increased as much as the bone allows, which is another advantage of an individualised testing protocol and favours results that are more accurate and consistent.

Adapting the biomechanical setup to the bone has been proposed before [9, 31, 32]. By introducing relative sizing (percentage) with respect to the whole bone, another step towards comparability and standardisation was presented in this study. In all specimens the percentage values corresponded well to the natural supporting surfaces of each bone directly supracondylar and directly below the lesser trochanter, which facilitated positioning of the bones on the supporting bars. Precise definition of these sections facilitated radiographic analysis exactly at the given distances and thus favoured correlation with biomechanical data [19].

In general, we reached high and consistent correlations of the BMC assessed by DXA and the pQCT parameters total content and cortical content measured at the shaft with the actual failure load of the bone. In previous studies a strong and positive correlation between biomechanics of bone and microstructural parameters obtained by pQCT and DXA have been reported for femurs of inbred mice [33] and for the human radius [34], both emphasizing the predictive value of the radiologic analysis. The work of Bagi et al. [35] shows similar results to our study. They evaluated cortical microstructural parameters of the unfractured rat femur by μCT, pQCT and DXA and were able to predict cortical bone strength for some of them. Compared to our results, their coefficients of determination (R^2), regardless of the actual method or parameter, remained relatively low (e.g. correlation between bone strength of the femoral midshaft done by three-point bending and bone mineral density of the whole femur determined by DXA: $R^2 = 0.34$; in our study $R^2 = 0.89$) [35]). As their biomechanical bending setup implicated a fix span of 15 mm, this might be an argument indicating that better

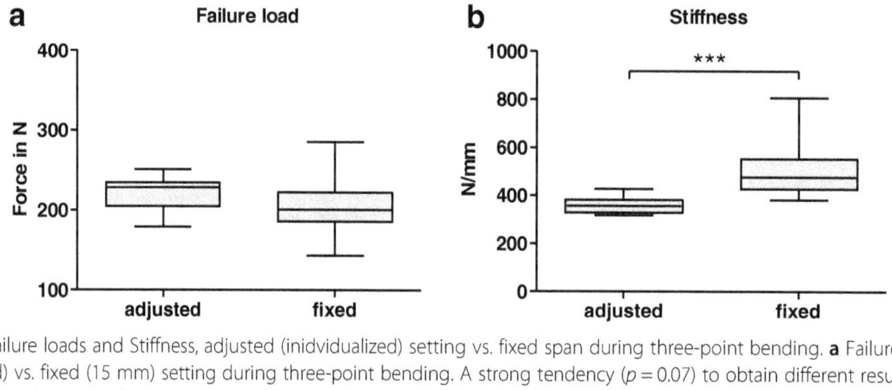

Fig. 4 Box Plots, Failure loads and Stiffness, adjusted (inidvidualized) setting vs. fixed span during three-point bending. **a** Failure loads of individual (adjusted) vs. fixed (15 mm) setting during three-point bending. A strong tendency ($p = 0.07$) to obtain different results by altering the setup was evident. Furthermore, the standard deviation within the sample was lowered by individual adjusted loading bars (18.95 N vs. 30.4 N, see Table 2). **b** Stiffness values of individual (adjusted) vs. fixed (15 mm) setting during three-point bending. Highly significant difference ($p <$ 0.0001), the standard deviation of the adjusted sample was only about one third compared to fixed bars (34.6 N/mm vs. 104.8 N/mm)

correlations between radiological parameters and biomechanics can be achieved in an individualized setting.

The weight of the testing animal seems to be another factor influencing consistency of results within the trait. In our study, we observed slightly more interindividual differences concerning the failure loads in young and light specimens. Interestingly, intraindividual variance of failure loads (left vs. right) was lowest in this group, whereas mature animals showed only a weak correlation between the left and the right side and relatively large differences in lengths and failure loads between the two bones of one animal. Though not reaching statistical significance in our data, one possible explanation could be that in rats something like handedness evolves during the lifespan, resulting in one favoured side (preferentially used for example as leading leg in climbing) and causing biomechanically relevant differences. In that context, Cunha et al. were recently able to prove paw-preferences and dexterity in behavioural tests of Sprague-Dawley male rats [36]. As previous, biomechanical studies in goats, sheep and dogs did not find relevant right/left differences [37–39], the concept of handedness in animals seems to be underestimated in the past. This might be an issue to investigate or rethink in the future. Concerning the stiffness, we observed the same behaviour but less clearly pronounced. With respect to our data, small rats should potentially be more suitable for normalized examinations (failure load of the experimental side as ratio to healthy side).

The fixation method we used potentially limits transferability of the data [40, 41]. Although Linde and Sorensen did not find relevant changes in the biomechanical behaviour of human trabecular bone specimens stored in 70% methanol for 100 days [42] and Mick et al. stated no differences for ultimate bending of human cortical specimens after rehydration due to formalin or ethanol-fixation (96%) compared to fresh frozen bones [43], we do not know the relevance of possible modifications caused by our treatment protocol. Anyway, as the comparison between the groups is more significant than the absolute values and all bones were treated equally, this systematic failure should not affect the main deductions drawn by our study.

Conclusions

Knowledge on natural fluctuation within a test population influences the sample size and limits the verifiability of any experimental result [4]. The given study focuses a systematic assessment of the biomechanical and morphological characteristics of femurs of the male Wistar-rat to improve accurate and unbiased sample size calculations in future experiments. Ruling out that functional relevance of morphological variations causes a methodological gap to obtain a level of significance, we furthermore aimed to close this gap with a methodological variation of biomechanical testing by respecting the individual length of every specimen. Furthermore, our results show that relevant, intraindividual side-differences potentially relate to dexterity in rat femurs of heavy (old) animals. Nevertheless, using paired specimens seems applicable, especially in small animals. By adapting the setting of the biomechanical testing to the individual length of the bone, interindividual variation could be reduced significantly. To achieve consistent results and to compare different studies, an individualized setting of biomechanical testing would be beneficial.

Abbreviations

AP: Anterioposterior; BMC: Bone mineral content; BMD: Bone mineral density; DXA: Dual energy X-ray absorptiometry; pQCT: Peripheral quantitative computed tomography

Acknowledgements

We would like to thank Dr.-Ing. Eduardo Grande Garcia (Biomechanics Laboratory, Department of Orthopaedics and Sportsorthopaedics at Klinikum rechts der Isar) for excellent support during biomechanical testing.

Authors' contributions

PMP and DB drafted the study. PMP, DB, PF, KK, RB and TT took part in the design and conception of the experiments. PMP, DB, PF, KK and HP conducted the biomechanical experiments. AS, RER, OB and TT conducted the radiological experiments. The manuscript was written by PMP, DB, PF, TT and RB. All authors read and approved the final version of the manuscript.

Consent for publication

Not applicable.

Competing interests

The authors declare that they have no competing interests.

Author details

[1]Klinik für Orthopädie und Sportorthopädie, Klinikum rechts der Isar der Technischen Universität München, Ismaninger Straße 22, 81675 Munich, Germany. [2]Abteilung für Fuß- und Sprunggelenkchirurgie, Klinik Volkach, Volkach, Germany. [3]Abteilung für Biomechanik, Klinik für Orthopädie und Sportorthopädie, Klinikum rechts der Isar der Technischen Universität München, Munich, Germany. [4]Klinik für Mund-, Kiefer- und Gesichtschirurgie, Universitätsklinikum Hamburg Eppendorf, Hamburg, Germany. [5]Orthopädische Klinik, Universitätsklinikum Düsseldorf, Heinrich-Heine-Universität, Düsseldorf, Germany. [6]Abteilung für Sportorthopädie, Klinik für Orthopädie und Sportorthopädie, Klinikum rechts der Isar der Technischen Universität München, Munich, Germany. [7]Klinik für Mund-, Kiefer- und Gesichtschirurgie, Klinikum rechts der Isar der Technischen Universität München, Munich, Germany. [8]Orthopädische Klinik und Poliklinik der Universität Rostock, Rostock, Germany.

References

1. Kaspar K, et al. An easily reproducible and biomechanically standardized model to investigate bone healing in rats, using external fixation. Biomed Tech (Berl). 2007;52(6):383–90.
2. Nunamaker DM. Experimental models of fracture repair. Clin Orthop Relat Res. 1998;(355 Suppl):S56–65.

3. Prodinger PM, et al. Does anticoagulant medication Alter fracture-healing? A morphological and biomechanical evaluation of the possible effects of rivaroxaban and enoxaparin using a rat closed fracture model. PLoS One. 2016;11(7):e0159669.
4. Leppanen OV, Sievanen H, Jarvinen TL. Biomechanical testing in experimental bone interventions–may the power be with you. J Biomech. 2008;41(8):1623–31.
5. O'Loughlin PF, et al. Selection and development of preclinical models in fracture-healing research. J Bone Joint Surg Am. 2008;90(Suppl 1):79–84.
6. Bissinger O, et al. A biomechanical, micro-computertomographic and histological analysis of the influence of diclofenac and prednisolone on fracture healing in vivo. BMC Musculoskelet Disord. 2016;17(1):383.
7. Kolk A, et al. A novel nonviral gene delivery tool of BMP-2 for the reconstitution of critical-size bone defects in rats. J Biomed Mater Res A. 2016;104(10):2441–55.
8. Jamsa T, et al. Comparison of three-point bending test and peripheral quantitative computed tomography analysis in the evaluation of the strength of mouse femur and tibia. Bone. 1998;23(2):155–61.
9. Jarvinen TL, et al. Dual-energy X-ray absorptiometry in predicting mechanical characteristics of rat femur. Bone. 1998;22(5):551–8.
10. Pautke C, et al. Characterization of eight different tetracyclines: advances in fluorescence bone labeling. J Anat. 2010;217(1):76–82.
11. Jarvinen TL, et al. Revival of bone strength: the bottom line. J Bone Miner Res. 2005;20(5):717–20.
12. Akman S, et al. Effect of diclofenac sodium on union of tibial fractures in rats. Adv Ther. 2002;19(3):119–25.
13. Bosemark P, Isaksson H, Tagil M. Influence of systemic bisphosphonate treatment on mechanical properties of BMP-induced calluses in a rat fracture model: comparison of three-point bending and twisting test. J Orthop Res. 2014;32(5):721–6.
14. Hak DJ, Stewart RL, Hazelwood SJ. Effect of low molecular weight heparin on fracture healing in a stabilized rat femur fracture model. J Orthop Res. 2006;24(4):645–52.
15. Krischak GD, et al. Effects of diclofenac on periosteal callus maturation in osteotomy healing in an animal model. Arch Orthop Trauma Surg. 2007; 127(1):3–9.
16. Sen C, et al. Effects of diclofenac and tenoxicam on distraction osteogenesis. Arch Orthop Trauma Surg. 2007;127(3):153–9.
17. Bigham-Sadegh A, Oryan A. Selection of animal models for pre-clinical strategies in evaluating the fracture healing, bone graft substitutes and bone tissue regeneration and engineering. Connect Tissue Res. 2015; 56(3):175–94.
18. Reifenrath J, et al. Replacement, refinement, and reduction: necessity of standardization and computational models for long bone fracture repair in animals. J Biomed Mater Res A. 2014;102(8):2884–900.
19. Prodinger PM, et al. Whole bone testing in small animals: systematic characterization of the mechanical properties of different rodent bones available for rat fracture models. Eur J Med Res. 2018;23(1):8.
20. Eckstein F, et al. Insulin-like growth factor-binding protein-2 (IGFBP-2) overexpression negatively regulates bone size and mass, but not density, in the absence and presence of growth hormone/IGF-I excess in transgenic mice. Anat Embryol (Berl). 2002;206(1–2):139–48.
21. Lochmuller EM, et al. In situ femoral dual-energy X-ray absorptiometry related to ash weight, bone size and density, and its relationship with mechanical failure loads of the proximal femur. Osteoporos Int. 2000; 11(4):361–7.
22. Schmidt C, et al. Precision and accuracy of peripheral quantitative computed tomography (pQCT) in the mouse skeleton compared with histology and microcomputed tomography (microCT). J Bone Miner Res. 2003;18(8):1486–96.
23. Jepsen KJ, et al. Establishing biomechanical mechanisms in mouse models: practical guidelines for systematically evaluating phenotypic changes in the diaphyses of long bones. J Bone Miner Res. 2015;30(6):951–66.
24. Turner CH, Burr DB. Basic biomechanical measurements of bone: a tutorial. Bone. 1993;14(4):595–608.
25. Pawlak D, et al. The association between elevated levels of peripheral serotonin and its metabolite - 5-Hydroxyindoleacetic acid and bone strength and metabolism in growing rats with mild experimental chronic kidney disease. PLoS One. 2016;11(10):e0163526.
26. Peric M, et al. The rational use of animal models in the evaluation of novel bone regenerative therapies. Bone. 2015;70:73–86.
27. Bonnarens F, Einhorn TA. Production of a standard closed fracture in laboratory animal bone. J Orthop Res. 1984;2(1):97–101.
28. Shefelbine SJ, et al. Intact fibula improves fracture healing in a rat tibia osteotomy model. J Orthop Res. 2005;23(2):489–93.
29. Histing T, et al. Small animal bone healing models: standards, tips, and pitfalls results of a consensus meeting. Bone. 2011;49(4):591–9.
30. Schriefer JL, et al. A comparison of mechanical properties derived from multiple skeletal sites in mice. J Biomech. 2005;38(3):467–75.
31. Creecy A, et al. Changes in the fracture resistance of bone with the progression of type 2 diabetes in the ZDSD rat. Calcif Tissue Int. 2016; 99(3):289–301.
32. Leppanen O, et al. Three-point bending of rat femur in the mediolateral direction: introduction and validation of a novel biomechanical testing protocol. J Bone Miner Res. 2006;21(8):1231–7.
33. Voide R, van Lenthe GH, Muller R. Bone morphometry strongly predicts cortical bone stiffness and strength, but not toughness, in inbred mouse models of high and low bone mass. J Bone Miner Res. 2008;23(8):1194–203.
34. Hudelmaier M, et al. Can geometry-based parameters from pQCT and material parameters from quantitative ultrasound (QUS) improve the prediction of radial bone strength over that by bone mass (DXA)? Osteoporos Int. 2004;15(5):375–81.
35. Bagi CM, et al. The use of micro-CT to evaluate cortical bone geometry and strength in nude rats: correlation with mechanical testing, pQCT and DXA. Bone. 2006;38(1):136–44.
36. Cunha AM, et al. Pawedness trait test (PaTRaT)-a new paradigm to evaluate paw preference and dexterity in rats. Front Behav Neurosci. 2017;11:192.
37. Bramer JA, et al. Representative assessment of long bone shaft biomechanical properties: an optimized testing method. J Biomech. 1998; 31(8):741–5.
38. Jonsson U, Stromberg L. Uniformity in mechanics of long bones at torque. A dog experiment. Acta Orthop Scand. 1984;55(3):347–8.
39. van Haaren EH, et al. Effect of long-term preservation on the mechanical properties of cortical bone in goats. Acta Orthop. 2008;79(5):708–16.
40. Unger S, Blauth M, Schmoelz W. Effects of three different preservation methods on the mechanical properties of human and bovine cortical bone. Bone. 2010;47(6):1048–53.
41. Vesper EO, et al. Even with rehydration, preservation in ethanol influences the mechanical properties of bone and how bone responds to experimental manipulation. Bone. 2017;97:49–53.
42. Linde F, Sorensen HC. The effect of different storage methods on the mechanical properties of trabecular bone. J Biomech. 1993;26(10):1249–52.
43. Mick E, et al. Influence of short-term fixation with mixed formalin or ethanol solution on the mechanical properties of human cortical bone. Curr Dir Biomed Eng. 2015;1:335–9.

10

Biologic plating of unstable distal radial fractures

Jae-Man Kwak[1] and Gu-Hee Jung[2*]

Abstract

Background: Volar locking plating through the flexor carpi radialis is a well-established technique for treating unstable distal radial fractures, with few reported complications. In certain circumstances, including metaphyseal comminuted fractures, bridge plating through a pronator quadratus (PQ)-sparing approach may be required to preserve the soft tissue envelope. This study describes our prospective experience with bridge plating through indirect reduction.

Methods: Thirty-three wrists (four 23A2, six 23A3, 15 23C1, and eight 23C2) underwent bridge plating through a PQ-sparing approach with indirect reduction from June 2006 to December 2010. Mean patient age was 56.8 years (range, 25–83 years), and the mean follow-up period was 47.5 months (range, 36–84 months). Changes in radiologic parameters (volar tilt, radial inclination, radial length, and ulnar variance) were analyzed, and functional results at final follow-up were evaluated by measuring the Modified Mayo Wrist Score (MMWS) and Modified Gartland-Werley Score (MGWS).

Results: All wrists achieved bone healing without significant complications after a single operation. At final follow-up, radial length was restored from an average of 3.7 mm to 11.0 mm, as were radial inclination, from 16.4° to 22.5°, and volar tilt, from – 9.1° to 5.5°. However, radial length was overcorrected in three wrists, and two experienced residual dorsal tilt. Excellent and good results on the MGWS were achieved in 30 wrists (90.9%). The average MMWS outcome was 92.6 (range, 75–100).

Conclusion: Our experience with bridge plating was similar to that previously reported in the earlier publications. Compared with the conventional technique, bridge plating through a PQ-sparing approach may help in managing metaphyseal comminuted fractures of both cortices with a reduced radio-ulnar index.

Keywords: Distal radial fracture, Bridging plate, PQ-sparing technique

Background

The increasing incidence of complex fracture patterns after high-energy trauma and the demand for early return to activities of daily living have increased the number of patients requiring operative intervention to treat distal radial fractures. Fractures may be reduced directly and fixed with volar locking plates [1–3]. This method has also yielded lower complication rates, ranging from 7% to 24%, than other treatment modalities [4]. The development of an internal fixator with locking plate technology has increased the rate of biologic fixation through minimally invasive plate osteosynthesis (MIPO, bridge plating). This method preserves soft tissue around the fracture site and prevents surgical morbidities of direct reduction in treating comminuted fractures of the lower limbs [5, 6]. Less is known, however, about the results of bridge plating for distal radial fractures [7–9].

Many factors influence the management of distal radial fractures, including the low complication rate of the open method, lesion size, and the easy manipulation and restoration of anatomic continuity using closed maneuvers. In addition, the postoperative radiologic and clinical outcomes of MIPO and conventional plating for distal radial fractures did not differ significantly [9]. The only advantages of MIPO were reported to be the preservation of the pronator quadratus (PQ) muscle and

* Correspondence: jyujin2001@hotmail.com
[2]Department of orthopaedic surgery, Gyeongsang national university, college of medicine and Gyeongsang national university Changwon hospital, 555 Samjungja-Dong, Changwon-si 642-160, Republic of Korea

cosmesis, suggesting that conventional plating should be preferred to MIPO, provided that adequate reduction and sufficient fixation could be addressed [7–9]. Therefore, the clinical relevance of MIPO for distal radial fracture remains unclear.

Because MIPO involves indirect reduction through separate incisions, there are technical issues involved, with optimal results depending on anatomic restoration of the articular surface and extra-articular realignment [6]. However, few reports have assessed the indirect reduction technique involving MIPO for distal radial fractures [10]. This retrospective analysis of prospectively enrolled patients describes our experiences with bridge plating of distal radial fractures using a PQ-sparing approach, including the reduction technique, focusing on the usefulness and suggested indications of this method.

Methods

The study protocol was approved by the ethics committee of our institution. Consecutive subjects with unstable distal radial fractures were enrolled prospectively from June 2006 to December 2010, and the results of bridge plating using a PQ-sparing approach were analyzed retrospectively. All patients with distal radial fracture were initially managed in the emergency room with closed reduction and splinting. This study excluded patients aged < 18 years, those with concomitant upper extremity injuries (e.g., carpal bone injury, forearm fracture, elbow, and humeral fractures), patients with pathologic fractures, patients who had previously undergone surgical treatment of the same wrist, and those whose fractures were fixed with a 3.5 mm T-plate. The 2.4 mm volar distal radius plating system (LDRS®; Synthes, Oberdorf, Switzerland) was used in all cases of volar plate fixation. Each patient was followed up for more than 36 months after surgery.

The plain radiographs and CT scans of all patients were reviewed by two investigators using the Picture Archiving and Communication System (PACS), with their classifications verified according to the AO comprehensive classification system (AO/OTA) [11]. All subjects provided uniform informed consent that the choice of direct fixation or bridge plating through a PQ-sparing approach for each distal radial fracture would be determined intraoperatively based on several factors, including the quality of intraoperative reduction, an unexpected fracture line, and unknown causes.

Intraoperative decision on bridge plating or direct fixation

Once surgery was indicated, all wrists underwent secondary evaluation by multidetector CT with multiplanar reformation, which has been used to determine the approach and implant for distal radial fractures [12, 13]. Radiologic parameters were measured by PACS, including changes in radial length and volar tilt, the site of joint involvement in the articular fractures, the length of the distal fragment, and the width of metaphyseal comminutions in both cortices. Once it was decided to use a single volar plate, manual traction was applied to the wrist, followed by manipulation under anesthesia with an image intensifier to restore radiologic parameters except for radial length. The fracture was provisionally fixed with K-wires from the radial styloid to maintain the reduction (Fig. 1). If reduction was acceptable, except in radial length, bridge plating through a PQ-sparing approach was chosen.

Bridge plating through the PQ-sparing approach with indirect reduction

Bridge plating through a PQ-sparing approach has been described in detail [10]. Once provisionally fixed, an image intensifier was used to archive the saved images of the contralateral wrist, which were used as reference guides to the restoration of radiologic parameters, including radial length and volar tilt, in the injured wrist. The tendon sheath was distally incised using a flexor carpi radialis (FCR) approach, allowing separate incisions for bridge plating, followed by exposure of the watershed line and distal margin of the PQ muscle and a proximal incision based on the length of the expected plate (Fig. 2). The plate was slid under the PQ muscle in a distal-to-proximal direction, and the optimal position of the plate on the distal radius was secured by inserting K-wires through the proximal and distal holes. After provisionally positioning the volar plate, radiologic parameters and conformity of the volar plate were thoroughly assessed. The plate was fixed with two or three screws in the distal hole and with a temporary K-wire in the proximal hole, thereby maintaining plate alignment. After securing the distal subchondral row with two or three screws, intraoperative fluoroscopy was performed to ensure that the distal locking screws were no more than 3–4 mm from the joint line and did not penetrate the joint surface. If the radial length was not restored, an additional screw was inserted proximally beyond the plate. Using a spreader, a distractive force was applied to restore radial length, comparing it with the saved image of the opposite wrist under the control of an image intensifier (Fig. 3, spreader). After verifying all the radiologic parameters, the empty holes on the plate were fixed and the wounds were closed.

Outcome evaluations and statistical analysis

Wrists were evaluated radiologically by measuring the volar tilt (dorsal tilt is expressed as a negative value), radial inclination, and radial length (the distance between the most proximal point of the articular surface of the radius and the ulnar head, with positive values when the

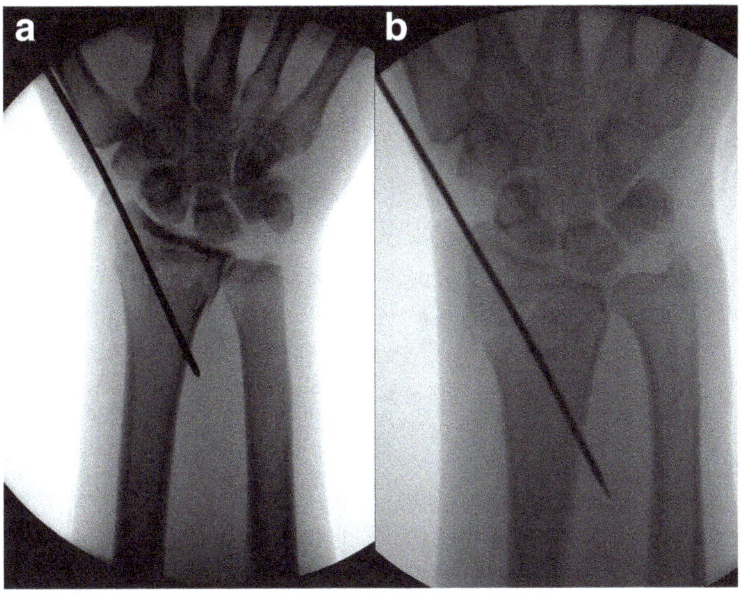

Fig. 1 **a** After manual traction and manipulation of the injured wrist, the distal radial fracture was reduced with the restoration of radial length, with the reduction maintained by provisionally fixed K-wires from the radial styloid. **b** Although radial length was not restored, a provisional K-wire could be applied because of the distractive technique

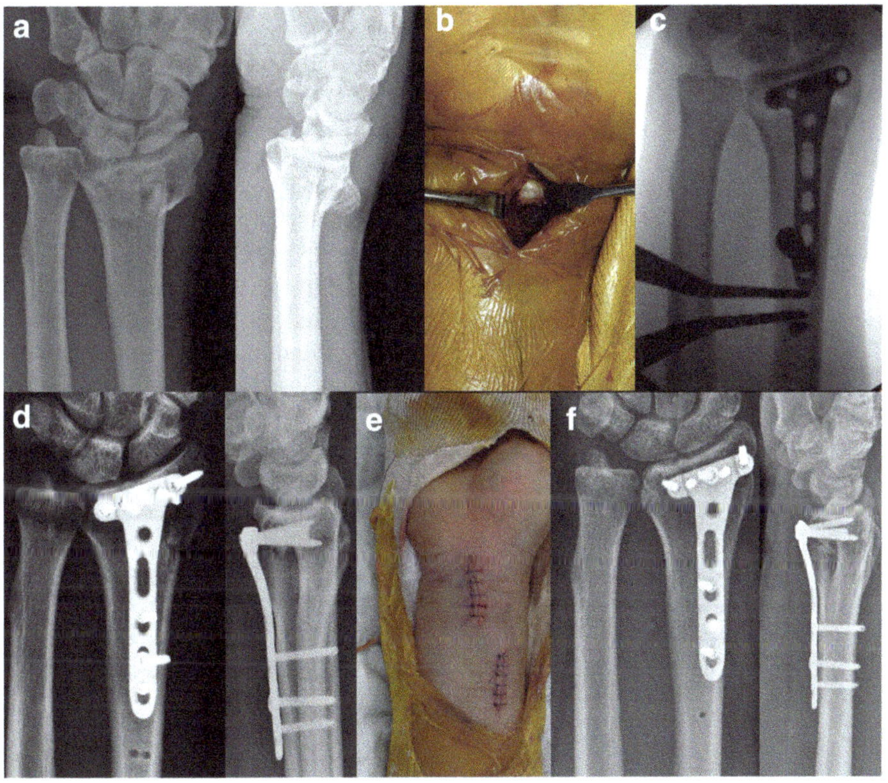

Fig. 2 **a** Simple radiographs, showing a distal radial fracture with metaphyseal comminution and radial shortening. **b** A distal incision around the flexor carpi radialis tendon, exposing the distal margin of the PQ muscle. **c** Sliding of the plate through a PQ-sparing approach and the distractive technique to restore radial length using the spreader. **d** Postoperative radiographs showing good realignment of the distal radial fracture. **e** Two separated incisions. **f** After 16 weeks, the distal radial fracture was well healed without radial length shortening

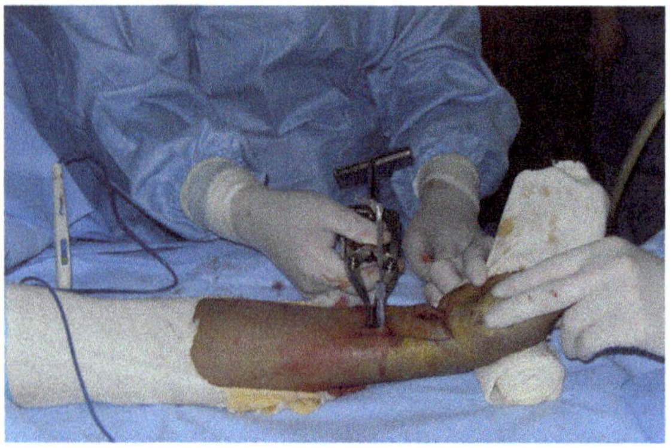

Fig. 3 Application of a spreader for distraction using a screw outside the plate

ulna is more distal than the radius and negative values when the ulna is more proximal than the radius) [14, 15]. Radiological parameters were measured preoperatively, immediately after surgery, and at the final follow-up visit using PACS, based on standard anteroposterior and lateral projection radiographs. These radiographs were compared with those of the non-injured wrist (Table 1). Activities of daily living at final follow-up were evaluated using the Modified Mayo Wrist Score (MMWS) and the Modified Gartland-Werley Score (MGWS) [16].

For statistical analysis, the radiologic results were expressed as mean and range, and their normal distribution was assessed using the Shapiro-Wilk test. Normally distributed parameters, including volar tilt and radial inclination, were compared using paired t-tests. Non-normally distributed parameters, including radial length and radio-ulnar index, were compared using Wilcoxon signed rank tests. A P-value < 0.05 was considered statistically significant. All statistical analyses were performed using SAS 9.2 software (SAS Institute, Cary, NC, USA).

Results

This study enrolled 33 wrists of 28 patients, 12 men, and 16 men. Their mean age at surgery was 56.8 years (range, 25–83 years) and their mean follow-up duration was 47.5 months (range, 36–67 months). Two patients were lost during follow-up because of death (one suicide and one car accident). One patient underwent emergency surgery on the day of injury, but most underwent surgery about 7 days after injury. The causes of injury to the 28 patients included falling ($n = 1$), traffic accident ($n = 12$), industrial trauma ($n = 2$), and falling while standing ($n = 13$).

Of the 33 fractures, ten were type 23A, including four 23A2 and six 23A3 fractures, and 23 were type 23C, including 15 23C1 and eight 23C2 fractures. There were two open fractures, one Gustilo-Anderson (GA) type I and one GA type IIIA. The GA type I fracture was treated as a closed fracture on the day of the injury, whereas the type IIIA fracture underwent emergency surgery and application of a spanning external fixator because the distal ulnar head was protruding through the open wound.

Of the 33 fractures enrolled, none required intraoperative conversion to direct open reduction. Twenty-six patients (31 fractures) were managed with a single-stage operation, which included a surgical delay for conditioning the soft tissue around the injured wrist. However, the remaining two patients (two fractures) underwent staged definitive fixation as soon as the status of the soft tissue permitted. The average time from injury to surgery was 5.8 days (range, 0–16 days). One patient with an open fracture was initially treated with emergency irrigation and debridement in the operating room, followed 16 days later by definitive fixation, after recovery of the soft tissue envelope. The other patient presented with a crush injury, which resulted in comminuted fractures of the distal radius and ulna with severe swelling. This patient was initially treated with plate fixation of the ulna and application of the spanning external fixator. The time interval from the first operation to definitive fixation was 7 days. The mean operative time for all bridge plating procedures was 61 min (range, 33–98 min), and all 33 fractures were united without secondary procedure to promote bone healing.

Despite closed maneuvers and a surgical delay of more than 2 weeks in four patients, extra-articular realignment was achieved using the above technique, with all articular fractures showing restoration of joint incongruity to < 2 mm and significant restoration of all radiologic parameters (Table 1) sufficient for statistical significance. The radio-ulnar index (RUI) [14] was changed to a negative

Table 1 Radiologic results after bridge plating of distal radius fracture

	Non-injured	Preop	Postop	Final FU
Volar tilt (°)	9.2 ± 4.3	− 9.1 ± 11.9	5.9 ± 11.0 ($p = 0.0004$)	5.5 ± 11.3 ($p = 0.0004$)
Radial inclination (°)	25.4 ± 3.9	16.4 ± 3.1	22.6 ± 8.1 ($p = < 0.0001$)	22.5 ± 9.1 ($p = < 0.0001$)
Radial length (mm)	9.8 ± 2.8	3.7 ± 4.9	11.2 ± 3.9 ($p = < 0.0001$)	11.0 ± 4.2 ($p = 0.0004$)
Radioulnar index (mm)		1.9 ± 2.1		−0.6 ± 2.6 ($p = < 0.0001$)

Data are mean ± standard deviation

Preop preoperative results, *Postop* postoperative results, *Final FU* final results at last follow-up value by distraction using a spreader. Radiographs taken at the final visit revealed that the radiologic parameters were well maintained, except for slight losses of radial length and radial inclination in some wrists. Of the 23 wrists with articular fractures, 15 23C1 and eight 23C2, all but one with a C2 fracture had articular gaps < 2 mm. The patient with significant articular incongruity did not wish to undergo a second operation because of associated injury to the head and abdomen.

At final evaluation, all patients had achieved nearly full finger range of motion; that is, they were able to touch their palms with the fingertips and to fully extend their fingers to a neutral position. In addition, all patients achieved wrist flexion, as assessed by a goniometer, having > 90% motion compared with the uninjured wrist [17]. The average MMWS score was 92.6 points (range, 75–100 points), and 30 wrists (90.9%) showed excellent and good MGWS results. Overall outcomes were excellent in 15 patients, good in 10, and fair in three. None of these patients had residual wrist pain or sleep disturbance due to pain, and all were able to perform daily activities without restriction. During follow-up, however, three patients with excessive radial length experienced mild pain in the distal radio-ulnar joint at the first outpatient follow-up visit. Compared with the average RUI, the RUIs differed after surgery in these patients by 4.0, 4.0 and 5.0 mm, differences that were significant. Pain in all three of these patients resolved within 6 months.

None of these patients experienced deep infections or wound complications that required additional surgery. No patient complained of plate-related symptoms or underwent plate removal [18]. Five patients developed postoperative complications related to indirect reduction (Table 2). Two had insufficient reduction of the distal articular angle that was not fully restored to volar tilt by indirect methods, whereas three experienced transient pain in the distal radio-ulnar joint due to radial length overcorrection. None of these patients, however, experienced other conventional complications of volar plating, such as extensor tendon rupture, injury of the median nerve, or loosening.

Table 2 Complications related with bridge plating through pronator-sparing approach in distal radius fractures

Details	Cases No.
Indirect reduction	
intraoperative conversion	–
symptomatic over-correction of radial length	3
insufficient correction of volar tilt	2
Volar plate fixation	
Intra-articular screw placement	–
loosening of screw	–
loss of reduction & fixation	–
deep infection	–
Tendon problems	
tendon irritation or rupture	–
FCR adhesion	–
Carpal tunnel syndrome	–
Reoperation	
bone graft	–
plate removal	–

complications from subsequent fracture collapse rather than from time of surgery

Discussion

Use of a volar locking plate has advantages in treating unstable fractures of the distal radius, as it is accompanied by osteosynthesis. The volar locking plate has expanded the indications for operative treatment of these fractures and greatly improved their clinical and radiologic outcomes [1, 3]. However, despite the popularity of bridge plating to treat complex fractures of the lower limbs, only a few reports have described the use of this technique to treat distal radius fractures [7–10, 19–21]. Although bridge plating using a PQ-sparing approach may have the advantage of PQ muscle preservation, the use of small incisions can prevent acceptable fracture reduction [7, 8]. Sen MK et al. indicated that this technique should not be used if it compromises the adequacy of reduction or fixation of the distal radius and that it be performed only in carefully selected patients [8].

Despite the proven benefits of direct reduction and anatomic fixation for distal radial fracture, the authors have adopted the concept of extra-articular realignment during prospective enrollment, especially for indirect reduction of metaphyseal fragments in accordance with MIPO technique. Compared with the concept of conventional anatomical reduction, extra-articular realignment is more focused on realignment of the injured limb by restoring the alignment index (length, rotation, and axis) rather than by anatomic reduction of the fracture fragments (Fig. 4). The reduction of distal radial fractures should focus on the restoration of radial length because most problems occurred in patients who achieved fair or poor restoration of radial length after conservative management [14]. Radial length was found to be automatically re-established upon restoration of anatomic continuity of the volar cortex through direct reduction [22]. Automatic restoration should not be expected, however, if a volar cortex is comminuted at the metadiaphyseal area or the fracture surfaces could not be opened, such as in the PQ-sparing approach, and an additional procedure might be needed to achieve the original length. A distractive technique using a spreader could be easily applied, similar to a femoral distractor

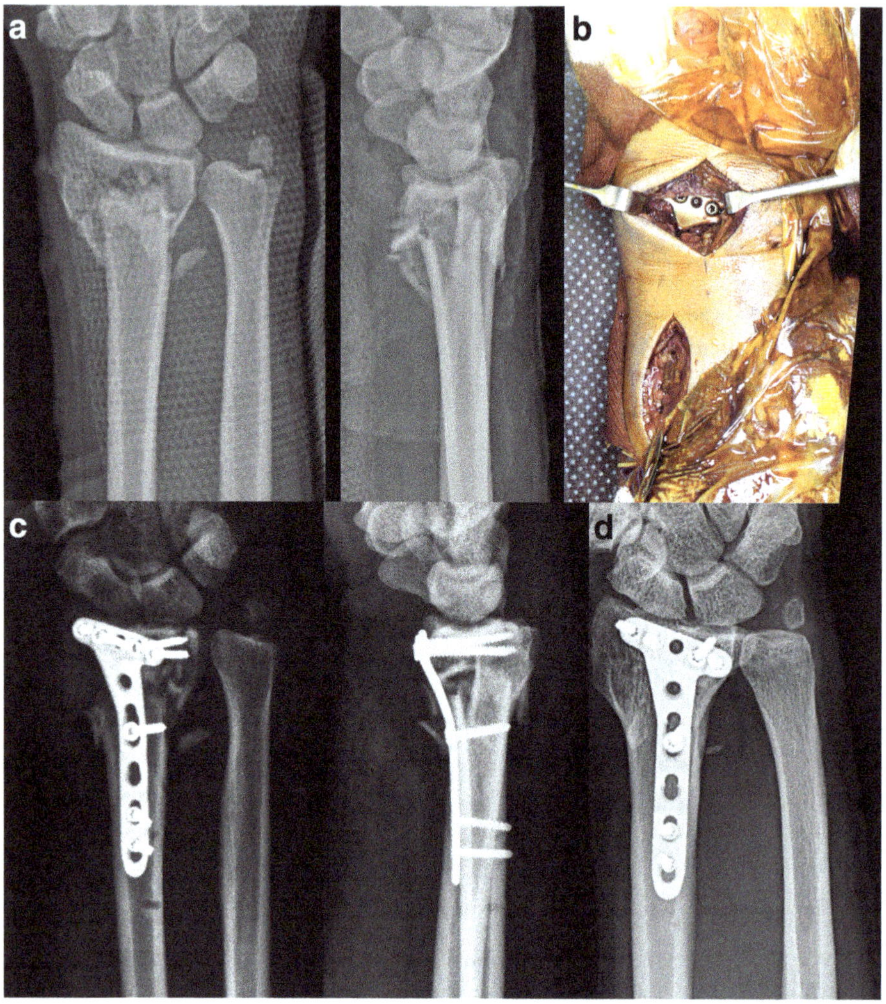

Fig. 4 a A 34-year-old man fell from a height of 5 m. Simple radiographs showed metaphyseal comminution in both cortices. **b** Bridge plating through a PQ-sparing approach was performed with a distractive technique to fix a single volar plate. **c** Postoperative radiographs showing the restoration of radiologic parameters, including radial length, volar tilt, and radial inclination. **d** Radiographs after 24 months showing sound union without complications

[10]. Compared with the use of a large distractor or provisional external fixator to restore limb length [23], bridge plating with distractive technique has several benefits. That is, the reduction force could be controlled gradually by the surgeon and verified in the coronal and sagittal planes using an image intensifier in real time. Five wrists, however, experienced complications related to reduction obstacles, including two with undercorrection of the volar/residual dorsal tilt and three with overcorrection of radial length. Compared with the uninjured wrist, the average radial length of the injured wrist, which is strongly associated with clinical outcomes [24], was restored from 3.7 mm preoperatively to 11.2 mm at last follow-up. Although the effects of shortened radial length are widely known, the effects of overlengthening have never, to our knowledge, been reported. Although the prognosis of wrists with overlengthening has not been determined, none of the patients in the present study experienced any complications related to the procedure until final follow-up.

Following the introduction of the 2.4 mm volar locking plate system, five locking screws could be inserted into the subchondral row of the distal fragment [1]. Thus, indications for this procedure may be expanded to include extra-articular fractures with metaphyseal comminutions in both cortices, regardless of the size of the distal fragment (Fig. 4). Single volar plating of an articular fracture requires the articular fragment to be of sufficient size, large enough for at least two screws of the 2.4 mm locking plate system [25]. We found that, following satisfactory reduction of the articular surface, the indications were similar for bridge plating and conventional options in the treatment of articular fractures. However, it is very important to verify the reduction status of the radial

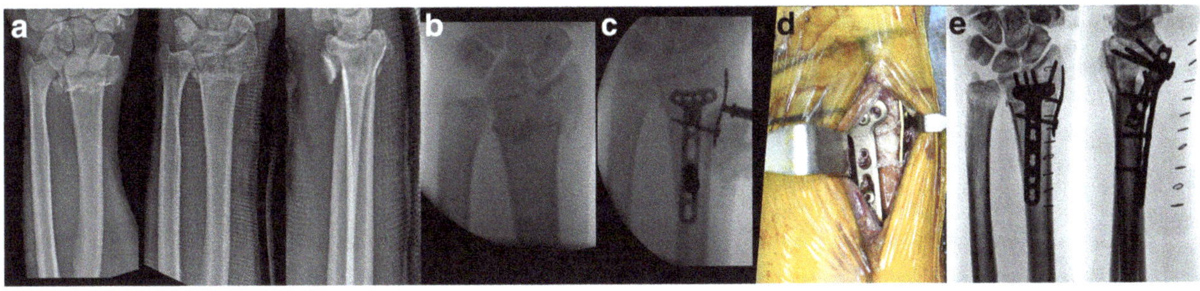

Fig. 5 a Plain radiographs showing a metaphyseal comminuted fracture of the distal radius with radial length shortening. **b** Despite manipulations of the injured wrist under anesthesia, articular congruity was not restored because the radial styloid fragment was not reduced. **c** Use of the conventional flexor carpi radialis approach by splitting the PQ muscle from its origin to buttress the radial styloid fragment with the plate. **d** Orthogonal plate fixation of the distal radius through the conventional approach. **e** Postoperative radiographs showed the restoration of articular congruity and radial length

styloid fragment, which is closely related to articular step-off and radial inclination. Thus, single volar plate fixation using the PQ-sparing approach could be performed if the radial styloid fragment of the articular fracture was sufficiently large for the fixation of two or three screws and if articular congruity was restored by indirect reduction and percutaneous maneuvers. However, if reduction cannot be obtained, it is better to switch to ORIF (Fig. 5).

Our experience clearly demonstrated that the term biologic fixation through bridge plating (BFBP) is more accurate than MIPO, since the two incisions might be larger in size than those of the conventional technique. In addition, this retrospective analysis indicates that BFBP has several potential limitations. First, the use of two incisions may lead to cosmetic problems, especially in younger patients. Second, the operation time was longer and radiation exposure was greater with BFBP than with the conventional technique. Third, the PQ-sparing technique was not compared directly with the conventional technique [20]. Nevertheless, our study, as well as others [19–21], reported satisfactory outcomes with the PQ-sparing technique, suggesting that the latter may reduce postoperative pain, enable motion exercises to be started sooner after surgery, and maintain the muscular envelope of the distal radius, thus potentially avoiding postoperative complications. As this study was not adequately powered due to the lack of a direct comparison group, further studies are required to optimize plate removal and the degree of radiation exposure, as well as to directly compare the PQ-sparing and conventional techniques.

Conclusions

A combination of bridge plating through a PQ-sparing approach and the distractive technique results in good reduction, with restoration of radial length and reasonable long-term functional outcomes. Compared with the conventional technique, the PQ-sparing technique, despite disadvantages such as technical difficulties, increased radiation exposure, and cosmetic problems, may be helpful in managing metaphyseal comminuted fractures of both cortices with reduced RUI.

Abbreviations

BFBP: Biologic fixation through bridge plating; FCR: Flexor carpi radialis; GA: Gustilo-Anderson; MGWS: Modified Gartland-Werley Score; MIPO: Minimally invasive plate osteosynthesis; MMWS: Modified Mayo Wrist Score; PACS: Picture archiving and communication system; PQ: Pronator quadratus; RUI: Radio-ulnar index

Funding

The authors, their immediate families, and any research foundation with which they are affiliated have not received any financial payments or other benefits from any commercial entity related to the subject of this article.

Authors' contributions

GHJ designed and analyzed data and serves as the corresponding author. JMK was a major contributor in writing the manuscript as the first author. All authors read and approved the final manuscript.

Competing interests

The authors declare that they have no competing interests.

Author details

[1]Department of Orthopaedic Surgery, Asan Medical Center, University of Ulsan, Seoul, Republic of Korea. [2]Department of orthopaedic surgery, Gyeongsang national university, college of medicine and Gyeongsang national university Changwon hospital, 555 Samjungja-Dong, Changwon-si 642-160, Republic of Korea.

References

1. Larson AN, Rizzo M. Locking plate technology and its applications in upper extremity fracture care. Hand Clin. 2007;23(2):269–78. vii
2. Ruch DS, Weiland AJ, Wolfe SW, Geissler WB, Cohen MS, Jupiter JB. Current concepts in the treatment of distal radial fractures. Instr Course Lect. 2004; 53:389–401.
3. Jupiter JB, Marent-Huber M, Group LCPS. Operative management of distal radial fractures with 2.4-millimeter locking plates. A multicenter prospective case series. J Bone Joint Surg Am. 2009;91(1):55–65.
4. McKay SD, MacDermid JC, Roth JH, Richards RS. Assessment of complications of distal radius fractures and development of a complication checklist. J Hand Surg Am. 2001;26(5):916–22.

5. Perren SM. Basic aspects of internal fixation. In: Müller ME, Allgöwer M, Schneider R, Willenegger H, editors. Manual of internal fixation. 3rd ed. New York: Springer-Verlag; 1991. p. 1–112.
6. Oh CW, Kyung HS, Park IH, Kim PT, Ihn JC. Distal tibia metaphyseal fractures treated by percutaneous plate osteosynthesis. Clin Orthop Relat Res. 2003; 408:286–91.
7. Imatani J, Noda T, Morito Y, Sato T, Hashizume H, Inoue H. Minimally invasive plate osteosynthesis for comminuted fractures of the metaphysis of the radius. J Hand Surg Br. 2005;30(2):220–5.
8. Sen MK, Strauss N, Harvey EJ. Minimally invasive plate osteosynthesis of distal radius fractures using a pronator sparing approach. TechHand Up ExtremSurg. 2008;12(1):2–6.
9. Zenke Y, Sakai A, Oshige T, Moritani S, Fuse Y, Maehara T, Nakamura T. Clinical results of volar locking plate for distal radius fractures: conventional versus minimally invasive plate osteosynthesis. J Orthop Trauma. 2011;25(7):425–31.
10. Jung GH, Cho CH, Kim JD. Distractive bridge plating in metaphyseal comminuted fractures of the distal radius through a pronator sparing approach. Eur J Orthop Surg Traumatol. 2012;22(7):613–9.
11. Marsh JL, Slongo TF, Agel J, Broderick JS, Creevey W, DeCoster TA, Prokuski L, Sirkin MS, Ziran B, Henley B, et al. Fracture and dislocation classification compendium - 2007: Orthopaedic trauma association classification, database and outcomes committee. J Orthop Trauma. 2007;21(10 Suppl):S1–133.
12. Martineau PA, Berry GK, Harvey EJ. Plating for distal radius fractures. Orthop Clin North Am. 2007;38(2):193–201. vi
13. Kim RY, Rosenwasser MP. Internal fixation of distal radius fractures. Am J Orthop (Belle Mead NJ). 2007;36(12 Suppl 2):2–7.
14. Altissimi M, Antenucci R, Fiacca C, Mancini GB. Long-term results of conservative treatment of fractures of the distal radius. Clin Orthop Relat Res. 1986;206:202-210.
15. Gartland JJ Jr, Werley CW. Evaluation of healed Colles' fractures. J Bone Joint Surg Am. 1951;33-A(4):895–907.
16. Souer JS, Lozano-Calderon SA, Ring D. Predictors of wrist function and health status after operative treatment of fractures of the distal radius. J Hand Surg Am. 2008;33(2):157–63.
17. Lattmann T, Meier C, Dietrich M, Forberger J, Platz A. Results of volar locking plate osteosynthesis for distal radial fractures. J Trauma. 2011;70(6):1510–8.
18. Turner RG, Faber KJ, Athwal GS. Complications of distal radius fractures. Orthop Clin North Am. 2007;38(2):217–28. vi
19. Itoh S, Yumoto M, Kanai M, Yoshida W, Yoshioka T. Significance of a pronator Quadratus-sparing approach for volar locking plate fixation of comminuted intra-articular fractures of the distal radius. Hand (NY). 2016;11(1):83–7.
20. Haberle S, Sandmann GH, Deiler S, Kraus TM, Fensky F, Torsiglieri T, Rondak IC, Biberthaler P, Stockle U, Siebenlist S. Pronator quadratus repair after volar plating of distal radius fractures or not? Results of a prospective randomized trial. Eur J Med Res. 2015;20:93.
21. Chen CY, Lin KC, Yang SW, Renn JH, Tarng YW. Clinical results of using minimally invasive long plate osteosynthesis versus conventional approach for extensive comminuted metadiaphyseal fractures of the radius. Arch Orthop Trauma Surg. 2015;135(3):361–7.
22. Orbay JL, Fernandez DL. Volar fixation for dorsally displaced fractures of the distal radius: a preliminary report. J Hand Surg Am. 2002;27(2):205–15.
23. Baumgaertel F, Dahlen C, Stiletto R, Gotzen L. Technique of using the AO-femoral distractor for femoral intramedullary nailing. J Orthop Trauma. 1994;8(4):315–21.
24. Trumble TE, Schmitt SR, Vedder NB. Factors affecting functional outcome of displaced intra-articular distal radius fractures. J Hand Surg Am. 1994;19(2):325–40.
25. Helmerhorst GT, Kloen P. Orthogonal plating of intra-articular distal radius fractures with an associated radial column fracture via a single volar approach. Injury. 2012;43(8):1307–12.

11

Association of wrist and forearm range of motion measures with self-reported functional scores amongst patients with distal radius fractures

Zixian Yang[1*], Peggy Poh Hoon Lim[1], Sing Hwee Teo[2], Huiwen Chen[3], Huaying Qiu[4] and Yong Hao Pua[5]

Abstract

Background: Patients with distal radius fractures (DRF) often have limited range-of-motion (ROM) in multiple planes of movement. No studies have comprehensively examined the impact of various ROM limitations on physical function.

Methods: We performed a multi-center, longitudinal study of 138 patients with conservatively managed DRF. ROM measures were taken at initial evaluation, and at 4 and 8 weeks later. Self-reported physical function was indexed by the Quick Disabilities of the Arm, Shoulder and Hand (QuickDASH).

Results: Wrist extension, active thumb opposition and a full composite grip were amongst the strongest ROM measures associated with functional scores over time. However, wrist radial deviation and forearm pronation were non-significantly associated with functional scores.

Conclusion: Given that ROM is potentially modifiable, the identification of important ROM measures associated with QuickDASH scores can potentially facilitate patient education and refine interventions to optimize functional recovery. Well-designed randomized intervention studies are however needed to confirm these association findings.

Keywords: Rehabilitation, Occupational therapy, Distal radius fractures, Range of motion, Function

Background

Distal radius fractures (DRFs) are a common occurrence in clinical practice and account for 20% of all fractures seen in emergency departments [1, 2]. Due to the involvement of the wrist joint, patients often have limited range of motion (ROM) in multiple planes of movement - namely, wrist flexion and extension, wrist radial and ulnar deviation, forearm supination and pronation. As the wrist joint is imperative for proper function of the hand, fundamental hand functions such as making a full composite grip and thumb opposition are also often affected [3] despite not being injured. These can adversely impact on one's ability to perform activities of daily living (ADLs), work or leisure, which causes loss of productive work hours, school in-attendance, loss of independence, and even lasting disability – extending beyond the direct healthcare costs [4–6]. Hence, occupational therapists and patients spend considerable amount of time addressing these multiple ROM impairments with the aim of functional restoration.

To our knowledge, the published literature on the relationship between the various ROM measures and physical function amongst patients with conservatively managed DRFs is limited to 2 small cross-sectional studies [7, 8]. Kilic et al. ($n = 29$) examined ROM measures as a total (combined) arc-of-motion in the planes of wrist flexion/extension and forearm supination/pronation and thus, could not tease apart the isolated associations of the specific ROM measures with physical function [7]. The other study by Tremayne et al. ($n = 20$) examined only one ROM measure (wrist extension) [8]. Although several

* Correspondence: yang.zixian@sgh.com.sg
[1]Department of Occupational Therapy, Singapore General Hospital, Singapore, Singapore
Full list of author information is available at the end of the article

longitudinal studies have described the ROM measures and functional scores over time [9–11], these studies were largely descriptive and did not formally examine the associations between the specific ROM measures and physical function using adequately controlled multivariable analyses. Thus, we believe that a consistent and comprehensive examination of the ROM-physical function association in patients with conservatively managed DRFs has not been previously presented.

As ROM is potentially modifiable, the identification of important ROM measures associated functional scores can facilitate patient education and help refine rehabilitation interventions to optimize functional outcomes. Thus, the aim of this study was to examine the longitudinal associations of 8 forearm, wrist and hand ROM measures with self-reported functional scores amongst patients with non-complicated, conservatively managed DRFs. Specifically, the ROM measures include wrist flexion and extension; wrist radial and ulnar deviation; forearm supination and pronation; active thumb opposition and the ability to make a full composite grip.

Methods

Design

This study was a retrospective, longitudinal, multi-center study involving four major outpatient occupational therapy hand clinics in Singapore. Patients were evaluated at three time points. Specifically, the baseline time point was taken to be at the commencement of active mobilization, and the subsequent two time points were set at the commencement of passive and strengthening exercises, respectively.

Participants and setting

All patients with conservatively managed, unilateral DRFs who were referred to four outpatient occupational therapy hand clinics during the period of April to June 2015 were included in the study. Patients were excluded if there were other upper limb fractures, bilateral injuries, or associated complicating injuries such as tendon, ligament or nerve injuries. Patients who had been treated by other institutions as well as those who developed complex regional pain syndrome (CRPS) subsequently were also excluded. The study received ethics approval from all participating institutions. Demographic and clinical information such as age, gender, injured side, handedness (the preferred hand for performing certain unimanual tasks [12]), edema, time from injury to first therapy session were collected from therapy records of the patients involved in the study. Of note, edema was measured with a soft measuring tape, using a figure-of-eight method [13].

Treatment providers

Patients included in this study were treated by 34 occupational therapists across four hand clinics. There was an equal distribution of therapists who had 5 or more years of clinical experience in hand therapy ($n = 17$), and those who had less than 5 years ($n = 17$). Across the four hand clinics, the average number of years of clinical experience was 6.78 years. 8 therapists were masters/postgraduate level occupational therapists.

Range of motion

Wrist goniometers (Smith & Nephew; Kinetec; North Coast Medical; Baseline) were used to measure active range of motion (ROM) of wrist flexion, extension, radial and ulnar deviation as well as forearm supination and pronation in the injured upper limb. Wrist flexion and extension were measured with the forearm in neutral on a stable surface, and the goniometer on the radial aspect of the wrist, aligned along the third metacarpal. Wrist radial and ulnar deviation were measured with the forearm in pronation on a flat surface and elbow slightly flexed. Goniometer measurements were taken along the line of the third metacarpal and the radius bone. Forearm supination and pronation measurements were performed with elbow flexed at 90 degrees, at the side of the body and goniometer readings aligned to the imaginary line between the radial and ulnar styloids. Active thumb opposition was recorded using the modified Kapandji score [14]. Measurements of distance from tip of finger to distal palmar crease (DPC) were performed using flat edge goniometers (Roylan; Jamar; Sammon Preston; North Coast Medical), where 0 cm indicates a full composite grip. All methods of measurement were standardized across all four hand clinics and were performed by occupational therapists at the commencement of active and passive mobilization as well as strengthening phases.

The QuickDASH outcome measure

The QuickDASH is a shortened version of the original 30-item Disabilities of the Arm, Shoulder and Hand (DASH) questionnaire [15]. Developed to measure physical function and symptoms in people with musculoskeletal disorders of the upper limb, the QuickDASH is an 11-item self-administered questionnaire scored on a 5-point scale. The QuickDASH score ranges between 0 and 100, where a lower score indicating lower disability levels. A QuickDASH score would not be generated if more than 10% of the items were left blank [16]. Noteworthy, the QuickDASH is a well-accepted patient-reported outcome [17] and we chose a self-report measure because it is easier for patient to express their perception of the impact of their injury on function as well as making it easier for the clinician to analyse [18].

Statistical analysis

Continuous variables were presented as means with standard deviations (SD) for normally distributed data, and medians with interquartile ranges (IQRs) for non-normally distributed data, whilst categorical variables were presented as frequencies with percentages. We modeled the time course of the QuickDASH scores using a generalized least-squares model that included all available observations from all time points, and we accounted for within-patient correlation over time using a first order autoregressive covariance structure [19, 20]. To avoid assuming linear time trends, actual assessment dates were used and time (weeks since baseline time point) was modeled flexibly as a restricted cubic spline [19, 21].

To assess the independent associations of QuickDASH with the various ROM measures, these measures were each used as a time-varying independent variable in separate models and the covariates included age, sex, edema, hand dominance, time since fracture, and treatment center. To evaluate whether the associations of the ROM measures with QuickDASH changed over time, we considered their first-order interactions with time. To facilitate interpretation and comparison of the results, we scaled the regression coefficients of the ROM measures by their IQRs such that the coefficients may be interpreted as comparing patients with relatively high (75th percentile) versus low (25th percentile) ROM on the QuickDASH scores [19]. Besides allowing valid comparisons, IQR regression coefficients represented a more clinically meaningful distinction than the conventional one-unit (1° or 1 cm) change in the ROM values.

We assessed the appropriateness of all models using residual plots and we used *R* software, version 3.2.3 (http://www.r-project.org), for all analyses.

Results

Sample characteristics and time course of physical measures

A total of 138 patients were included in the study. Table 1 shows the baseline characteristics of the total sample. Mean age was 59 years (SD 16) and women accounted for more than half (67%) of the sample. Nearly half of the sample injured their dominant hand and the median time since injury to the first occupational therapy session was slightly more than a month. Majority of the distal radius fractures were as a result of a low energy fall (88%).

Table 1 Baseline characteristics

Participants demographics (n = 138)	
Age in years, mean (SD)	59 (16)
Gender, male	45 (33%)
Injured dominant hand	68 (49%)
Injury due to low energy fall	121 (88%)
Weeks from injury to first occupational therapy session, median (IQR)	5.3 (4.4–7.0)
Weeks from baseline session to PROM phase, median (IQR)	4.1 (2.9–6.0)
Weeks from baseline session to strengthening phase, median (IQR)	8.0 (6.0–11.8)

Table 2 shows the mean values of all physical measures at all time points, except that of the QuickDASH scores which were expressed as medians with IQRs. Overall, there was improvement in all physical measures and QuickDASH scores from baseline to the commencement of strengthening phase.

Association of physical measures with QuickDASH scores over time

Table 3 shows results of the generalized least squares models of QuickDASH for the various ROM measures. None of the ROM-by time interactions were statistically significant, indicating that the associations between ROM and QuickDASH were consistent across time. Wrist extension ROM (8.95 [CI -4.94 to – 12.95] lower QuickDASH scores per IQR increase in wrist extension ROM), active thumb opposition (IQR-β, – 8.9 [– 2.73 to – 15.07]) and the ability to make a full composite grip (IQR-β, 7.64 [3.6 to 11.69]) were among the strongest ROM measures associated with QuickDASH scores. Other ROM measures that were statistically significantly associated with QuickDASH included wrist flexion (IQR-β, – 6.70 [– 11.50 to – 1.89]), forearm supination (IQR-β, – 6.57 [– 9.81 to – 3.33]) and wrist ulnar deviation (IQR-β, – 4.06 [– 7.21 to – 0.90]). In contrast, the associations of forearm pronation (IQR-β, – 0.63 [– 2.66 to – 3.93]) and wrist radial deviation (IQR-β, – 2.43 [1.28 to – 6.15]) were not statistically significantly associated with QuickDASH scores over time.

Discussion

In a sample of 138 patients with non-complicated, conservatively managed distal radius fracture, we examined the longitudinal associations of 8 forearm, wrist and hand ROM measures with QuickDASH scores. Adjusting for covariates, we found that wrist extension, active thumb opposition (using modified Kapandji scores) and the ability to make a full composite grip (measured by the distance of finger tips to distal palmar crease) were among the strongest ROM measures associated with QuickDASH scores. In contrast, forearm pronation and wrist radial deviation were weakly and non-significantly associated with QuickDASH scores. To our knowledge, this study is the first comprehensive evaluation of the ROM measures associated with changes in self-reported functional recovery in a relatively large cohort of patients with DRF.

Table 2 Physical measures at active, passive mobilization and strengthening phases

Physical measures	AROM[a] (1) mean (SD)	PROM[b] (2) mean (SD)	Strengthening (3) mean (SD)	1 vs 2	2 vs 3
Wrist flexion, degrees	28 (11)	39 (14)	44 (14)	< 0.001	< 0.001
Wrist extension, degrees	35 (15)	49 (12)	56 (11)	< 0.001	< 0.001
Wrist radial deviation, degrees	11.5 (7.5)	16.4 (7.9)	17.7 (6.6)	< 0.001	0.041
Wrist ulnar deviation, degrees	21 (8.5)	27 (10)	28.7 (9.4)	< 0.001	0.035
Forearm supination, degrees	62 (22)	78 (13)	81.5 (8.7)	< 0.001	0.039
Forearm pronation, degrees	65 (21)	75 (14)	78 (13)	< 0.001	0.041
Distance to distal palmar crease (DPC)[c], cm	1.9 (2.1)	1.0 (1.6)	0.52 (1.06)	< 0.001	< 0.01
Active thumb opposition[d]	5.3 (2.1)	6.4 (1.9)	7.0 (1.4)	< 0.001	< 0.001
Edema, cm	1.11 (1.46)	0.78 (1.10)	0.53 (0.86)	< 0.001	0.02
QuickDASH[e] Scores, median (IQR)	39 (24–64)	27 (16–41)	14 (5–25)	< 0.001	< 0.001

[a]Active mobilization phase
[b]Passive mobilization phase
[c]The lesser the distance, the tighter the composite grip
[d]Using the modified Kapandji score
[e]Quick Disability of the Arm, Shoulder & Hand Questionnaire

Ability to make a full composite grip and thumb opposition

Previous studies evaluating outcomes of distal radius fractures were often limited to the examination of wrist and forearm ROM measures, as well as functional outcomes such as DASH or the Patient-Rated Wrist Evaluation (PRWE) [7–9, 22–24]. Little is known about the impact of hand ROM measures following a distal radius fracture [25]. In a study that evaluated 260 patients following distal radius fractures, it was found that the development of hand stiffness was associated with poorer functional outcomes [25]. Stiffness was defined as fingertip to DPC distance greater than 1 cm for any one finger and functional outcome was indexed by the DASH questionnaire [25]. Similarly, our study found strong associations between hand-related ROM measures – such as the ability to make a full composite grip and thumb opposition – and physical function over time. It is possible that the amount of edema in the hand may have contributed to both limited hand mobility and poor physical function but our findings persisted after adjustment for edema and other potential confounders in the multivariable analyses (Table 3). As hand function is often altered due to the involvement of the wrist joint post DRF, it may be overlooked frequently in post DRF rehabilitation, where the focus is usually targeted specifically at wrist ROM. Our study highlights the imperative need to maintain finger and thumb ROM during immobilization due to the detrimental effects on function when ROM is lost. Hence, occupational therapists

Table 3 Association of physical measures with QuickDASH scores over time[a]

Physical measures	Percentile[b]		Difference (95% CI)	*P*-value
	25th	75th		
Wrist flexion, degrees	25	45	−6.70 (−11.50, −1.89)	< 0.01
Wrist extension, degrees	35	55	−8.95 (−12.95, −4.94)	<.0001
Wrist radial deviation, degrees	10	20	−2.43 (−6.15, 1.28)	0.20
Wrist ulnar deviation, degrees	20	30	−4.06 (−7.21, −0.90)	0.01
Forearm supination, degrees	65	85	−6.57 (−9.81, −3.33)	< 0.001
Forearm pronation, degrees	65	85	−0.63 (−3.93, −2.66)	0.71
Distance to distal palmar crease (DPC)[c], cm	0	2.5	7.64 (3.60, 11.69)	< 0.001
Active thumb opposition[d]	4	8	−8.90 (− 15.07, − 2.73)	< 0.01

[a]Results shown are from separate multivariable generalized least-squares models for QuickDASH scores during follow-up, adjusted for age, sex, edema, hand dominance, time since first therapy session, time since fracture, and treatment center. None of the interactions between the ROM measures and time (weeks since first therapy session) were statistically significant
[b]Adjusted differences in QuickDASH scores reflect a comparison between the 75th vs. the 25th percentile values of each physical measure. For example, with all covariates kept equal, patients with wrist extension at the 75th percentile (55 degrees) would have, on average, 9.0 points (95% confidence interval [95% CI] 4.9 to 13.0 points) lower QuickDASH scores than patients with wrist extension at the 25th percentile (35 degrees). This scaling is done to facilitate the interpretation and comparison of effect sizes of various ROM measures that are measured on different units
[c]The lesser the distance, the tighter the composite grip
[d]Using the modified Kapandji score

need to intervene and educate patients with DRF during the immobilization phases to optimize function post DRF.

Wrist and forearm ROM measures

In our study, we found that wrist flexion, wrist extension, ulnar deviation, and forearm supination were statistically significantly associated with QuickDASH scores over time. Specifically, on average, an IQR increase in these ROM measures was associated with 4.1 to 9.0 points lower QuickDASH scores (Table 3). Using a different outcome measure such as the QuickDASH, our results expand on previous findings [26] indicating that wrist extension and ulnar deviation ROM were correlates of functional activities. Our interpretation of these findings is that wrist extension and ulnar deviation form part of the dart thrower's motion, which describes a direction of oblique wrist motion from radial extension to ulnar flexion [27]. As the dart thrower's motion is highly functional and is required in a variety of occupational, household, and sporting activities [28–30], our results are not surprising.

On the other hand, our results appear to contrast with those reported by Karnezis & Fragkiadakis (2002), who found that neither the wrist flexion-extension arc nor the forearm supination-pronation arc movements were significantly associated with functional scores [31]. However, it may be difficult to compare our results with those of Karnezis & Fragkiadakis (2002) due to differences in study population (unstable versus stable distal radius fractures), study design (cross-sectional versus longitudinal), outcome measures (Patient-Rated Wrist Evaluation versus QuickDASH) and sample sizes (31 versus 138). More research is needed to elucidate the reasons for the discrepant findings.

Wrist radial deviation and forearm pronation

In our study, forearm pronation and wrist radial deviation were weakly associated with QuickDASH scores, and these findings were not reported in previous studies. Nevertheless, to explain this null finding, we reason that limited forearm pronation may be compensated by elbow and shoulder movements during daily activities. Supporting this, Sardelli and colleagues (2011) reported a maximal forearm pronation range of 65 degrees required for typing on a keyboard which was still lesser than the maximal amount of supination (77 degrees) required in opening a door [32].

Study limitations

Our study has limitations. First, the retrospective nature of our study implies that we were unable to standardize (i) the timing of referral from injury to the first occupational therapy session and (ii) the time intervals for the follow-up assessments (Table 1). Although we have adjusted our results for these time variables using continuous-time regression models, we acknowledge that the ideal study would have standardized these variables to optimize the internal validity of the results. Second, to facilitate data collection, we have chosen a self-report measure of physical function (QuickDASH). However, given the poor concordance between self-reported measures versus actual performance of functions [31, 33], we acknowledge that our findings could be strengthened and complemented by examining performance-based measures of ADL tasks such as the Jebsen Test of Hand Function.

Conclusion

To summarize, in 138 patients with conservatively managed DRFs, we found that the various ROM measures have differential influence on upper limb physical function, with wrist extension, active thumb opposition and ability to make a full composite grip amongst the strongest ROM measures associated with QuickDASH over time. The results of this study have potential implications on efforts in providing treatment and outcome assessments amongst people with DRFs. They also highlight the need for intervention and education of patients with DRFs to maintain hand-related ROM during the immobilization phase, to optimize function post DRF. That said, well-designed randomized intervention studies are needed to confirm these association findings, and future studies should explore how ROM measures interplay with muscle strength and pain levels to influence function post DRF.

Abbreviations

ADLs: Activities of daily living; CRPS: Complex regional pain syndrome; DASH: Disabilities of the Arm, Shoulder and Hand; DPC: Distal palmar crease; DRF: Distal radius fracture; IQR: Interquartile range; PRWE: Patient-Rated Wrist Evaluation; QuickDASH: Quick Disabilities of the Arm, Shoulder and Hand; ROM: Range of motion; SD: Standard deviation

Acknowledgements

We thank the occupational therapists of the upper limb rehabilitation services from the participating institutions for their assistance in retrieving data. We also acknowledge the support from the various Heads of Department of Occupational Therapy in the four institutions. This research did not receive any specific grant from funding agencies in the public, commercial, or not-for-profit sectors.

Funding

This research received no specific grant from any funding agency in the public, commercial, or not-for-profit sectors.

Authors' contributions

Study conception and design, as well as data acquisition were done by YZ, LPH, TSH, CH and QH. Statistical analysis and interpretation of data were done by PYH. YZ wrote the first draft of the manuscript. All authors reviewed and edited the manuscript, and approved the final version of the manuscript.

Competing interests

The authors declare that they have no competing interests.

Author details

[1]Department of Occupational Therapy, Singapore General Hospital, Singapore, Singapore. [2]Department of Occupational Therapy, Tan Tock Seng Hospital, Singapore, Singapore. [3]Department of Occupational Therapy, Changi General Hospital, Singapore, Singapore. [4]Department of Occupational Therapy, Ng Teng Fong General Hospital, Singapore, Singapore. [5]Department of Physiotherapy, Singapore General Hospital, Singapore, Singapore.

References

1. Chung KC, Spilson SV. The frequency and epidemiology of hand and forearm fractures in the United States. J Hand Surg. 2001;26(5):908–15.
2. Simic PM, Weiland AJ. Fractures of the distal aspect of the radius: changes in treatment over the past two decades. J Bone Joint Surg. 2003;85(3):552–64.
3. de Bruijn HP. Functional treatment of Colles fracture. Acta Orthop Scand. 1987;58(sup223):1–95.
4. Steffen T, Eugster T, Jakob RP. Twelve years follow-up of fractures of the distal radius treated with the AO external fixator. Injury. 1994;25:SD44–54.
5. Thompson PW, Taylor J, Dawson A. The annual incidence and seasonal variation of fractures of the distal radius in men and women over 25 years in Dorset, UK. Injury. 2004;35(5):462–6.
6. Krischak GD, Krasteva A, Schneider F, Gulkin D, Gebhard F, Kramer M. Physiotherapy after volar plating of wrist fractures is effective using a home exercise program. Arch Phys Med Rehabil. 2009;90(4):537–44.
7. Kilic A, Ozkaya U, Kabukcuoglu Y, Sokucu S, Basilgan S. The results of non-surgical treatment for unstable distal radius fractures in elderly patients. Acta Orthop Traumatol Turc. 2009;43(3):229–34.
8. Tremayne A, Taylor N, Mcburney H, Baskus K. Correlation of impairment and activity limitation after wrist fracture. Physiother Res Int. 2002;7(2):90–9.
9. Arora R, Gabl M, Gschwentner M, Deml C, Krappinger D, Lutz M. A comparative study of clinical and radiologic outcomes of unstable colles type distal radius fractures in patients older than 70 years: nonoperative treatment versus volar locking plating. J Orthop Trauma. 2009;23(4):237–42.
10. MacDermid JC, Richards RS, Roth JH. Distal radius fracture: a prospective outcome study of 275 patients. J Hand Ther. 2001;14(2):154–69.
11. Hurov JR. Fractures of the distal radius: what are the expectations of therapy?: a two-year retrospective study. J Hand Ther. 1997;10(4):269–76.
12. Clerke A, Clerke J. A literature review of the effect of handedness on isometric grip strength differences of the left and right hands. Am J Occup Ther. 2001;55(2):206–11.
13. Maihafer GC, Llewellyn MA, Pillar WJ, Scott KL, Marino DM, Bond RM. A comparison of the figure-of-eight method and water volumetry in measurement of hand and wrist size. J Hand Ther. 2003;16(4):305–10.
14. Kay S, Haensel N, Stiller K. The effect of passive mobilisation following fractures involving the distal radius: a randomised study. Aust J Physiother. 2000;46(2):93–101.
15. Kennedy CA, Beaton DE, Solway S, McConnell S, Bombardier C. Disabilities of the arm, shoulder and hand (DASH), The DASH and QuickDASH outcome measure User's manual. Third ed. Toronto: Institute for Work & Health; 2011.
16. The QuickDASH outcome measure [http://www.dash.iwh.on.ca/sites/dash/files/downloads/quickdash_info_2010.pdf]. Accessed 30 Apr 2015.
17. Ritting AW, Wolf JM. How to measure outcomes of distal radius fracture treatment. Hand Clin. 2012;28(2):165–75.
18. Skinner KM, Miller DR, Lincoln E, Lee A, Kazis LE. Concordance between respondent self-reports and medical records for chronic conditions: experience from the veterans health study. J Ambul Care Manag. 2005;28(2):102–10.
19. Harrell F: Regression modeling strategies: with applications to linear models, logistic and ordinal regression, and survival analysis: Springer International Publishing; 2015.
20. Pinheiro J, Bates D: Mixed-effects models in S and S-PLUS: Springer Verlag New York; 2006.
21. Durrleman S, Simon R. Flexible regression models with cubic splines. Stat Med. 1989;8(5):551–61.
22. Nielsen TL, Dekkers MK. Progress and prediction of occupational performance in women with distal radius fractures: a one-year follow-up. Scand J Occup Ther. 2013;20(2):143–51.
23. Young BT, Rayan GM. Outcome following nonoperative treatment of displaced distal radius fractures in low-demand patients older than 60 years. J Hand Surg. 2000;25(1):19–28.
24. Batra S, Gupta A. The effect of fracture-related factors on the functional outcome at 1 year in distal radius fractures. Injury. 2002;33(6):499–502.
25. Egol KA, Karia R, Zingman A, Lee S, Paksima N. Hand stiffness following distal radius fractures. Bull Hosp Joint Dis. 2014;72(4):288–93.
26. Wilcke MKT, Abbaszadegan H, Adolphson PY. Patient-perceived outcome after displaced distal radius fractures: a comparison between radiological parameters, objective physical variables, and the DASH score. J Hand Ther. 2007;20(4):290–9.
27. Moritomo H, Apergis EP, Herzberg G, Werner FW, Wolfe SW, Garcia-Elias M. 2007 IFSSH committee report of wrist biomechanics committee: biomechanics of the so-called dart-throwing motion of the wrist. J Hand Surg. 2007;32(9):1447–53.
28. Crisco JJ, Heard WM, Rich RR, Paller DJ, Wolfe SW. The mechanical axes of the wrist are oriented obliquely to the anatomical axes. J Bone Joint Surg. 2011;93(2):169–77.
29. Palmer AK, Werner FW, Murphy D, Glisson R. Functional wrist motion: a biomechanical study. J Hand Surg. 1985;10(1):39–46.
30. Ryu J, Cooney WP, Askew LJ, An K-N, Chao EYS. Functional ranges of motion of the wrist joint. J Hand Surg. 1991;16(3):409–19.
31. Karnezis IA, Fragkiadakis EG. Association between objective clinical variables and patient-rated disability of the wrist. J Bone Joint Surg Br. 2002;84(7):967–70.
32. Sardelli M, Tashjian RZ, MacWilliams BA. Functional elbow range of motion for contemporary tasks. J Bone Joint Surg Am. 2011;93(5):471–7.
33. Adams BD, Grosland NM, Murphy DM, McCullough M. Impact of impaired wrist motion on hand and upper-extremity performance. J Hand Surg. 2003; 28(6):898–903.

12

Is fast reversal and early surgery (within 24 h) in patients on warfarin medication with trochanteric hip fractures safe?

Leif Mattisson[1*], Lasse J. Lapidus[1] and Anders Enocson[1,2]

Abstract

Background: Hip fracture patients in general are elderly and they often have comorbidities that may necessitate anticoagulation treatment, such as warfarin. It has been emphasized that these patients benefit from surgery without delay to avoid complications and reduce mortality. This creates a challenge for patients on warfarin and especially for those with trochanteric or subtrochanteric hip fractures treated with intramedullary nailing, as this is associated with increased bleeding compared to other types of hip fractures and surgical methods.
The aim of the study was to evaluate if early surgery (within 24 h) of trochanteric or subtrochanteric hip fractures using intramedullary nailing is safe in patients on warfarin treatment after fast reversal of the warfarin effect.

Methods: A retrospective case-control study including 198 patients: 99 warfarin patients and 99 patients without anticoagulants as a 1:1 ratio control group matched for age, gender and surgical implant. All patients were operated within 24 h with a cephalomedullary nail due to a trochanteric or subtrochanteric hip fracture. All patients on warfarin were reversed if necessary to INR ≤ 1.5 before surgery using vitamin K and/or four-factor prothrombin complex concentrate (PCC). Per- and postoperative data, transfusion rates, adverse events and mortality was compared.

Results: There were no significant differences in the calculated blood-loss, in-house adverse events or mortality (in-house, 30-day or 1-year) between the groups. There were no significant differences in the pre- or peroperative transfusions rates, but there was an increased rate of postoperative transfusions in the control group ($p = 0.02$).

Conclusion: We found that surgical treatment with intramedullary nailing within 24 h of patients with trochanteric or subtrochanteric hip fractures on warfarin medication after reversing its effect to INR ≤ 1.5 using vitamin K and/or PCC is safe.

Keywords: Hip fracture, Surgical treatment, Warfarin, Anticoagulation treatment, Intramedullary nailing

Background

In Sweden about 1.8% of the population is on warfarin medication [1]. Despite a current trend in favour of using Novel Oral Anticoagulants (NOAKs), warfarin is still the most widely prescribed oral anticoagulant for indications such as mechanical heart valves, atrial fibrillation or high grade renal insufficiency and thromboembolic disorder [2, 3]. Hip fracture patients in general are elderly and often have comorbidities that may necessitate anticoagulation treatment, such as warfarin. Now days it is recommended that hip fracture patients should be operated without delay to reduce postoperative complications and mortality [4]. This creates a challenge when surgical treatment of the hip fracture is necessary and the patient is on warfarin medication. It is especially relevant for the management of patients with trochanteric or subtrochanteric hip fractures treated with intramedullary nailing, as these fractures are associated with increased bleeding compared to other types of hip fractures and surgical methods [5, 6].

* Correspondence: leif.mattisson@sll.se
[1]Department of Clinical Science and Education, Stockholm South General Hospital, Karolinska Institutet, Unit of Orthopaedics, S-118 83 Stockholm, Sweden

One of the strategies to reduce the bleeding in these patients is to temporary postpone the warfarin administration and then wait until the anticoagulation effect of the warfarin has subsided, measured as a normal (non-therapeutic) level of the International Normalized Ratio (INR) [7]. However, this may take up to 4 days [8] and according to previous literature this delay can explain up to 8% of all hip fracture surgical delays [9]. Another faster strategy is reversing the effect of the warfarin using vitamin K or four-factor prothrombin complex concentrate (PCC). This may allow surgery without major delay [10]. However, little is published in the literature on this topic and most of the authors who have studied the surgical management of patients on warfarin do not differentiate between different types of hip fractures or surgical methods [7, 11].

The aim of the study was to evaluate if early surgery (within 24 h) of trochanteric or subtrochanteric hip fractures treated with intramedullary nailing is safe in patients on warfarin treatment after fast reversal of the warfarin effect.

Methods

All patients on warfarin medication operated at our institution with an intramedullary nail due to a trochanteric or a subtrochanteric hip fracture from January 2011 to December 2014 were identified. To be included in the study patients should be: > 60 years of age, have sustained an acute non-pathological trochanteric or subtrochanteric femoral fracture due to a low-energy trauma without other injuries demanding acute surgery or causing major bleeding. Only patients operated within 24 h, calculated from the hospital admission to the start of the surgery were selected. Patients with late presentation to the hospital (> 24 h from injury) were excluded.

A 1:1 ratio control group matched for age, gender and surgical implant (long or short nail), operated within 24 h, was identified. These patients were operated at our institution during the same time period due to non-pathological trochanteric or subtrochanteric fractures after low-energy trauma and had no anticoagulation medication at all.

Patients' records were searched in order to find information including demographic data, medication, pre- and postoperative data and adverse events occurring during the hospital stay. Mortality data was obtained from the Swedish national Cause of Death Register. Follow-up time was 1 year. Calculation of blood-loss was based on the haemoglobin (Hb) level (g/dL) and the estimated blood volume (BV). The latter was calculated according to gender, weight and height using the formulae [12]: BV (l) = height (m)^3 × 0.356 + weight (kg) × 0.033 + 0.183 for women, and BV (l) = height (m)^3 × 0.367 + weight (kg) × 0.032 + 0.604 for men. In assumption that the BV on day 2–4 after surgery was the same as that before surgery and that all the red blood cell (RBC) transfusion units contained the same number of cells (a unit of RBC contains approximately 250 ml and 45 g Hb). The loss of Hb (in grams) was then estimated according to the formula: $Hb_{loss} = BV \times (Hb_{adm} - Hb_{fin}) + Hb_{trans}$. The Hb_{loss} is the calculated total Hb loss (g), Hb_{adm} is the haemoglobin value (g/dL) on admission, Hb_{fin} is the final recorded Hb value (g/dL) on day 2–4 after surgery, and Hb_{trans} is the total amount of haemoglobin (g) in the transfused RBC units before the measurement of Hb_{fin}. We finally estimated the Blood loss (BL) using the following formula: BL (mL) =1000 × (Hb_{loss} / Hb_{adm}).

Before the operation all patients on warfarin with an INR > 1.5 were reversed to ≤1.5 using vitamin K (Konakion®), four-factor prothrombin complex concentrate (PCC) (Ocplex®) or both. All operations were performed on a radiolucent traction table and spinal anaesthesia was the standard method for anaesthesia. Implants used were a short, or a long, Gamma3 cephalomedullary nail (Stryker Howmedica, Kalamazoo, MI, USA). Cloxacillin 2 g administered within 30 min before the operation was used as antibiotic prophylactics. Starting on the evening after the operation, a minimum of 2 h after wound closure, low molecular-weight heparin (5000 U dalteparin or 4500 U tinzaparin) was given subcutaneously once daily as thromboprophylactics. Thromboprophylactic therapy was continued until INR was on a therapeutic level for the warfarin patients and for 4 weeks for the control patients. No strict transfusion protocol was used, but the patients were given RBC transfusion based on their current Hb level and a cut off level of 10 g/dL was mostly used. However, the decision whether to transfuse or not was always made on an individual basis with consideration of several factors such as ongoing cardiac disease, blood pressure and other factors were taken into consideration in addition to the Hb value. Patients were mobilised the day after the surgery using necessary walking aids and usually allowed full weight-bearing.

Statistical methods

The Mann-Whitney U-test was used for comparisons of nonparametric variables in independent groups. The Student's t-test was used for comparisons of normally distributed variables in independent groups. Normality was tested with the Kolmogorov-Smirnov test. Nominal variables were tested by the Chi-square test or Fisher's exact test. All tests were two-sided. The results were considered significant at $p < 0.05$. The statistical software used was IBM SPSS Statistics, Version 23 for Windows (SPSS Inc., Chicago, Illinois).

Results

A total of 198 patients were included in the study: 99 patients on warfarin and 99 patients in the matched control group without anticoagulants. Age, gender and implant type were similar between the groups, as these were the matching variables. The warfarin patients in general had an impaired state of health compared with the control patients, displayed as a lower number of patients with ASA class 1–2 ($n = 5$ versus 18, $p = 0.007$) and a higher mean (±SD) Charlson comorbidity index (5.4 ± 1.3 versus 5.0 ± 1.2, $p = 0.1$). The warfarin patients also had a higher mean (±SD) weight (69 ± 14 versus 64 ± 12 kg, $p = 0.02$), but similar height. All patients were operated within 24 h after admission, but the mean (±SD) time to surgery was shorter for the control group (14 ± 5.6 h) compared to the warfarin patients (16 ± 4.8 h) ($p = 0.04$). All patients except one, (a warfarin patient), was operated under spinal anesthesia. There was no difference in the time of surgery between the groups. Details on patient demographics and surgical data are given in Table 1.

Warfarin patients

The most common indications for warfarin treatment were: atrial fibrillation ($n = 55/99$), atrial fibrillation with previous stroke ($n = 21/99$) or previous embolism ($n = 7/99$) (Table 2). One warfarin patient was treated with low-dose ASA (75 mg) and one patient with dipyridamol in addition. No other anticoagulants were used by the warfarin patients. The initial mean (±SD, range) INR of the warfarin patients was 2.5 (±0.6, 1.2–4.4). Before the surgery patients with INR > 1.5 were reversed to ≤1.5 using vitamin K ($n = 33/99$), PCC ($n = 14/99$) or both ($n = 45/99$). No plasma was used for reversing the warfarin effect (Table 2).

Adverse events and mortality

The total number of adverse events was 58: 27 in the warfarin group and 31 in the control group ($p = 0.6$). The most common adverse event was a urinary tract infection ($n = 28$), followed by a pressure ulcer ($n = 20$) or a pneumonia ($n = 16$), a myocardial infarction (n = 1) in warfarin group and a stroke (n = 1) in control group, no other thromboembolic disorders, such as pulmonary embolism or deep venous thrombosis, were reported in any group. There were no differences in the numbers of the different types of adverse events between the groups (Table 3). The total in-house mortality was 3.5% ($n = 7/198$), the total 30-day mortality 8.1% ($n = 16/198$) and the total 1-year mortality 26% ($n = 52/198$). There were no differences between the groups when comparing in-house, 30-day or 1-year mortality (Table 3). The mean (±SD, range) length of stay was 4.9 (±2.6, 1–15) days for the warfarin patients and 4.9 (±2.6, 1–16) days for the control group ($p = 0.9$). There was no difference in number of the re-admissions within 30 days between the warfarin patients (9.1%, $n = 9/99$) and the control group (16%, $n = 16/99$) ($p = 0.2$).

Table 1 Demographic and surgical data for all patients

	Warfarin patients (*n* = 99)	Control group (*n* = 99)	*P*-value
Age (years), mean (±SD)	86 (7.4)	86 (7.1)	0.8
Gender, female *n* (%)	69 (70)	69 (70)	1.0
Height (cm), mean (±SD)	167 (10)	166 (10)	0.3
Weight (kg), mean (±SD)	69 (14)	64 (12)	0.02
Charlson comorbidity index, mean (±SD)	5.4 (1.3)	5.0 (1.2)	0.1
ASA class 1 or 2, *n* (%)	5 (5.1)	18 (18)	0.007
Fracture type			
Trochanteric, *n* (%)	68 (69)	66 (67)	0.9
Subtrochanteric, *n* (%)	31 (31)	33 (33)	
Implant type			
Short nail, *n* (%)	66 (67)	66 (67)	1.0
Long nail, *n* (%)	33 (33)	33 (33)	
Time to surgery (hours), mean (±SD)	16 (4.8)	14 (5.6)	0.04
Anaesthesia type			
Spinal, *n* (%)	98 (99)	99 (100)	1.0
General, *n* (%)	1 (1.0)	0	
Time of surgery (min), mean (±SD)	65 (16)	64 (14)	0.8

ASA = American Society of Anesthesiologists

Table 2 Details on warfarin patients

Indication for warfarin	*n* (%)
Atrial fibrillation	55 (56)
Atrial fibrillation with previous stroke	21 (21)
Previous embolism	7 (7.1)
Mechanical valve replacement	6 (6.1)
Atrial fibrillation with biological valve replacement	4 (4.0)
Atrial fibrillation with ischemic heart disease	3 (3.0)
Previous stroke	3 (3.0)
Methods for reversing warfarin preoperative	*n* (%)
Vitamin K + PCC	45 (46)
Vitamin K	33 (3.0)
PCC	14 (14)
None	7 (7.1)

PCC = four-factor prothrombin complex concentrate

Transfusions and blood-loss

The mean (±SD) preoperative (on arrival) Hb was lower in the control group (12.3 ± 1.5 g/dL) compared to the warfarin group (12.8 ± 1.6 g/dL) ($p = 0.03$) as was the mean (±SD) postoperative Hb (9.9 ± 1.4 g/dL) compared to (10.4 ± 1.2 g/dL) ($p = 0.01$). There were no differences in the late (day 2–4) Hb or the calculated blood-loss between the groups (Table 4). The total rate of patients given any RBC transfusion was 65% ($n = 128/198$). There was a greater proportion of control group patients who received postoperative transfusions (71%, $n = 70/99$) compared to warfarin patients (54%, $n = 53/99$) ($p = 0.02$). There were no differences in the pre- or intraoperative transfusion rates, or the mean total number of units given between the groups (Table 4). Four patients, 3 in the warfarin and 1 in the control group, were given plasma postoperatively.

Discussion

The major finding of this study was that patients with trochanteric and subtrochanteric hip fractures on warfarin and operated within 24 h with an intramedullary nail after fast reversal of the warfarin effect displayed no increased risk for adverse events or increased mortality compared to a matched control group of patients without anticoagulant medication.

Now days most treatment guidelines, local or national, advocate early surgery for hip fracture patients [4, 13–17]. However, this endeavor for early surgery creates a challenge when the patient is on warfarin medication. Lawrence et al. in 2016 [18] showed an association between warfarin therapy with prolonged time to surgery (mean 46 h versus 24 h for the control group), and an increased 1-year mortality rate in hip fracture patients. In an observational study by Dettoni et al. in 2011 [19] including 875 consecutive hip fracture patients they reported that the presence of two critical factors: warfarin therapy and a delay in time to surgery, was associated with a significantly higher risk for complications and mortality compared to all other patients. They concluded that the "discontinue drug and delay surgery" strategy is not suitable for hip fracture patients on warfarin therapy. Obviously, the choice of the way to overcome the anticoagulation effect of the warfarin will influence and sometimes delay the time to surgery. Instead of passively wait until the warfarin effect has faded out, a more active approach can be used. Bhatia et al. in 2010 [20] described that using intravenous vitamin K is a safe and effective treatment to avoid delay in the treatment in this group of patients. Despite this statement they still reported at least 2 days (mean 38 h) delay to surgery in the warfarin group. Similarly, Moores et al. in 2015 [21] described that using

Table 3 Adverse events and mortality for all patients

	Warfarin patients (*n* = 99)	Control group (*n* = 99)	*P*-value
Myocardial infarction, *n* (%)	1 (1.0)	0	1.0
Stroke, *n* (%)	0	1 (1.0)	1.0
Pulmonary embolism, *n* (%)	0	0	
Deep venous thrombosis, *n* (%)	0	0	
Sepsis, *n* (%)	0	1 (1.0)	1.0
Pneumonia, *n* (%)	6 (6.1)	10 (10)	0.4
Urinary tract infection, *n* (%)	14 (14)	14 (14)	1.0
Pressure ulcer, *n* (%)	10 (10)	10 (10)	1.0
Any adverse event, *n* (%)	27 (27)	31 (31)	0.6
In-house mortality, *n* (%)	5 (5.1)	2 (2.0)	0.4
30-day mortality, *n* (%)	9 (9.1)	7 (7.1)	0.8
1-year mortality, *n* (%)	26 (26)	26 (26)	1.0

Table 4 Blood-loss and transfusions for all patients

	Warfarin patients ($n = 99$)	Control group ($n = 99$)	P-value
Preoperative Hb (g/dL), mean (±SD)	12.8 (1.6)	12.3 (1.5)	0.03
Postoperative Hb (g/dL), mean (±SD)	10.4 (1.2)	9.9 (1.4)	0.06
Day 2–4 Hb (g/dL), mean (±SD)	10.7 (1.1)	10.7 (1.0)	0.7
Calculated blood loss (ml), mean (±SD)	1306 (960)	1285 (588)	0.5
Patients given preoperative transfusion, n (%)	5 (5.1)	1 (1.0)	0.2
Patients given intraoperative transfusion, n (%)	8 (8.1)	12 (12)	0.5
Patients given postoperative transfusion, n (%)	53 (54)	70 (71)	0.02
Patients given any[a] transfusion, n (%)	56 (57)	72 (73)	0.03
Transfusions per transfused patient, mean (±SD, range)	2.8 (2.8, 1–19)	2.8 (1.4, 1–8)	0.2

[a]Patients given transfusion pre- and/or intra- and/or postoperative

vitamin K is a safe method but they still had a time to surgery of 36–48 h in their study. Another option is administration of PCC which shows an effect within 30 min that lasts for at least 6 h. The co-administration of vitamin K will give a stable and rapid reversal of anticoagulation and prevent rebound increases in INR [22, 23]. In our study, almost all the warfarin patients were actively reversed preoperatively and the combination of vitamin K and PCC was the most commonly used method. As we found no statistical difference in the calculated blood loss, no increase in transfusion rate and no decrease in Hb level in the warfarin group we conclude that using vitamin K and/or PCC as mentioned above minimize bleeding.

As known from other studies the extra-capsular (trochanteric and subtrochanteric) hip fractures, which are especially studied in this paper, are associated with increased bleeding tendency in comparison with the intra-capsular hip fractures [24, 25]. In addition, other studies found that intramedullary nailing compared with other surgical techniques was associated with an increased rate of RBC transfusions [6, 26, 27]. In 2006 Foss et al. [6] found that the median calculated total peri-operative blood loss in patients that had undergone intramedullary nailing was increased compared to patients that were operated with arthroplasty due to a hip fracture (1.86 L versus 1.30 L, respectively). Similarly, in a recent study by Cohn et al. in 2017 [28] they found significantly lower preoperative Hb in patients undergoing intra medullary nailing (extra-capsular fractures) and a greater blood loss in the warfarin group compared with a control group (1.22 L versus 1.19 L) but this was not statistically significant. In contrast we found no difference in the calculated blood-loss when comparing warfarin patients with the control patients. One reason could be that we used a more active approach when reversing the warfarin effect that resulted in a pronounced shorter time to surgery in comparison with Cohn et al. (mean 16 versus 47 h). Cohn et al. furthermore reported that their warfarin patients were delayed to surgery (mean 29 versus 47 h) and had a longer hospital stay (mean 5.6 versus 8.6 days) when comparing control patients with warfarin patients. This indicates the superiority of using vitamin K and/or PCC to reduce the INR level to ≤1.5 and operate these patients without delay within 24 h.

We found no difference in the frequency of adverse events or mortality up to 1 year between warfarin patients and the control group. This is in line with Cohn et al. but unfortunately, they do not report mortality beyond the discharge from the hospital.

Somewhat to our surprise we found a lower postoperative RBC transfusion rate in the warfarin group. We speculate that this is because a prolonged effect of the reversing agents administered preoperatively. We found a high transfusion rate in both the warfarin and control cohorts. However, this is in line with other published literature such as Desai et al. [5] who found that 52% of intertrochanteric fractures treated with an intramedullary nail were transfused. In addition Fazal et al. [29] recently reported a transfusion rate of 53% in 79 patients who underwent nailing surgery and among those the transfusion rate was 72% for the 32 patients that were treated with a long nail. Finally, Boone et al. [30] reported a transfusion rate of 57% and 40% for long and short nails respectively.

One obvious limitation of this study is its retrospective design. Ideally this topic should be investigated within the context of a randomized controlled trial. However, the current knowledge and opinion would hardly ethically allow a study that compared early and late surgery in these fragile patients. Another limitation is that we lack information on late complications (after hospital discharge). However, this is to some extent compensated for by that we do have accurate mortality data up to 1 year after surgery. Most of the patients in our cohort had relatively benign indications for warfarin, such as atrial fibrillation. Therefore, the safety of active warfarin reversal in patients on warfarin for reasons other than atrial fibrillation remain unaddressed in this study. The major strengths of the study are the large and homogenous groups, both the study group and the control group. This limits the influence of confounding factors on the results.

Conclusion

We found that the surgical treatment with intramedullary nail within 24 h for patients with trochanteric or subtrochanteric hip fractures on warfarin medication after fast reversing its effect to INR ≤ 1.5 using vitamin K and/or PCC is safe.

Abbreviations

ASA class: American Society of Anesthesiologists classification; BL: Blood loss; BV: Estimated blood volume; Hb_{adm}: The haemoglobin value on admission; Hb_{fin}: The final recorded Hb value; Hb_{loss}: The calculated total Hb loss; Hb_{trans}: The total amount of haemoglobin (g) in the transfused RBC units before the measurement of Hb_{fin}; Hb: Haemoglobin; INR: International normalized ratio; NOAKs: Novel oral anticoagulants; PCC: Prothrombin complex concentrate; RBC: Red blood cell

Acknowledgements

The authors wish to thank Evelina Wärle at the Department of Orthopaedics, Stockholm South General Hospital, Stockholm, Sweden for valuable contribution with data collection.

Authors' contributions

LM: study design and planning. Data collection and analysis. Writing of the manuscript. LJL: study design and planning. Writing of the manuscript. AE: study design and planning. Data collection and analysis. Writing of the manuscript. All authors have read and approved the final manuscript.

Consent to publication

Not applicable.

Competing interests

The authors declare that they have no competing interests.

Author details

[1]Department of Clinical Science and Education, Stockholm South General Hospital, Karolinska Institutet, Unit of Orthopaedics, S-118 83 Stockholm, Sweden. [2]Department of Molecular Medicine and Surgery, Karolinska University Hospital, Karolinska Institutet, Stockholm, Sweden.

References

1. Anticoagulation's therapy in atrial fibrillation – National Swedish guidelines.
2. The new guidelines from European Society of Cardiology (ESC) 2016. [Internet].
3. Anticoagulation's therapy in atrial fibrillation – treatment recommendation: Information from the Swedish Medical Products Agency, 2017;28(1):12–31. [Internet].
4. Simunovic N, Devereaux PJ, Sprague S, Guyatt GH, Schemitsch E, Debeer J, et al. Effect of early surgery after hip fracture on mortality and complications: systematic review and meta-analysis. CMAJ. 2010;182(15):1609–16.
5. Desai SJ, Wood KS, Marsh J, Bryant D, Abdo H, Lawendy A-R, et al. Factors affecting transfusion requirement after hip fracture: can we reduce the need for blood? Can J Surg. 2014;57(5):342–8.
6. Foss NB, Kehlet H. Hidden blood loss after surgery for hip fracture. Bone Joint Surg Br. 2006;88(8):1053–9.
7. Ashouri F, Al-Jundi W, Patel A, Mangwani J. Management of Warfarin Anticoagulation in patients with fractured neck of femur. ISRN Hematology. 2011;2011:294628.
8. White RH, McKittrick T, Hutchinson R, Twitchell J. Temporary discontinuation of warfarin therapy: changes in the international normalized ratio. Ann Intern Med. 1995;122(1):40–2.
9. Charalambous CP, Yarwood S, Paschalides C, Siddique I, Hirst P, Paul A. Factors delaying surgical treatment of hip fractures in elderly patients. Ann R Coll Surg Engl. 2003;85(2):117–9.
10. Tharmarajah P, Pusey J, Keeling D, Willett K. Efficacy of warfarin reversal in orthopedic trauma surgery patients. J Orthop Trauma. 2007;21(1):26–30.
11. Purmonen T, Törmälehto S, Säävuori N, Kokki H. Budget impact analysis of warfarin reversal therapies among hip fracture patients in Finland. Drugs in R&D. 2015;15(1):155–62.
12. Gao F-Q, Li Z-J, Zhang K, Sun W, Zhang H. Four methods for calculating blood-loss after Total knee arthroplasty. Chin Med J. 2015;128(21):2856–60.
13. Uzoigwe CE, Burnand HG, Cheesman CL, Aghedo DO, Faizi M, Middleton RG. Early and ultra-early surgery in hip fracture patients improves survival. Injury. 2013;44(6):726–9.
14. Moja L, Piatti A, Pecoraro V, Ricci C, Virgili G, Salanti G, et al. Timing matters in hip fracture surgery: patients operated within 48 hours have better outcomes. A meta-analysis and meta-regression of over 190,000 patients. PLoS One. 2012;7(10):e46175.
15. Aqil A, Hossain F, Sheikh H, Aderinto J, Whitwell G, Kapoor H. Achieving hip fracture surgery within 36 hours: an investigation of risk factors to surgical delay and recommendations for practice. J Orthop Traumatol. 2016;17(3):207–13.
16. Colais P, Di Martino M, Fusco D, Perucci CA, Davoli M. The effect of early surgery after hip fracture on 1-year mortality. BMC Geriatr. 2015;15:141.
17. Carretta E, Bochicchio V, Rucci P, Fabbri G, Laus M, Fantini MP. Hip fracture: effectiveness of early surgery to prevent 30-day mortality. Int Orthop. 2011;35(3):419–24.
18. Lawrence JE, Fountain DM, Cundall-Curry DJ, Carrothers AD. Do patients taking warfarin experience delays to theatre, longer hospital stay, and poorer survival after hip fracture? Clin Orthop Relat Res. 2017;475(1):273–9.
19. Dettoni F, Castoldi F, Giai Via A, Parisi S, Bonasia DE, Rossi R. Influence of timing and oral anticoagulant/antiplatelet therapy on outcomes of patients affected by hip fractures. European J Trauma and Emerg Surg : Official Publicof the European Trauma Soc. 2011;37(5):511–8.
20. Bhatia M, Talawadekar G, Parihar S, Smith A. An audit of the role of vitamin K in the reversal of international normalised ratio (INR) in patients undergoing surgery for hip fracture. Ann R Coll Surg Engl. 2010;92(6):473–6.
21. Moores TS, Beaven A, Cattell AE, Baker C, Roberts PJ. Preoperative warfarin reversal for early hip fracture surgery. J Orthop Surg (Hong Kong). 2015;23(1):33–6.
22. Asad EP, Nicole MA, Brian LE. Prothrombin complex concentrate for critical bleeding. Ann Pharmacother. 2011;45(7–8):990–9.
23. Palareti G. A guide to oral anticoagulant therapy. Italian Fed of Anticoagulation Clin Haemost. 1998;28(Suppl 1):1–46.
24. Kumar D, Mbako AN, Riddick A, Patil S, Williams P. On admission haemoglobin in patients with hip fracture. Injury. 2011;42(2):167–70.
25. Smith GH, Tsang J, Molyneux SG, White TO. The hidden blood loss after hip fracture. Injury. 2011;42(2):133–5.
26. Kadar A, Chechik O, Steinberg E, Reider E, Sternheim A. Predicting the need for blood transfusion in patients with hip fractures. Int Orthop. 2013;37(4):693–700.

13

Nordic Innovative Trial to Evaluate OsteoPorotic Fractures (NITEP-group): non-operative treatment versus surgery with volar locking plate in the treatment of distal radius fracture in patients aged 65 and over

Teemu P. Hevonkorpi[1*], Antti P. Launonen[2], Lauri Raittio[1], Toni Luokkala[3], Juha Kukkonen[4], Aleksi Reito[3], Bakir O. Sumrein[2], Minna K. Laitinen[2], Ville M. Mattila[1,2] and on behalf of the NITEP-group

Abstract

Background: In the literature, there are numerous studies that compare different surgical procedures in the treatment of distal radius fractures (DRF). It is, however, unknown whether operative treatment and better restoration of anatomy with volar locking plate yields a better functional outcome in the elderly population when compared with non-operative treatment.

Methods and design: This study is a prospective, randomized, controlled, multi-center trial. The purpose will be to compare the non-operative and operative treatment of initially or early malaligned distal radius fractures in patients aged 65 and older. The primary outcome in this study will be the patient rated wrist evaluation (PRWE) score measured after 1 and 2 years.

Discussion: We expect that initial operative treatment of a DRF with volar locking plate will not yield superior results when compared with non-operative treatment with cast immobilization in terms of functional outcome, pain, disability, quality of life, grip strength, and number of complications.

Trial registration: This trial is registered on clinicaltrials.gov, identifier NCT02879656, registration date 08/17/2016.

Keywords: Distal radius, Operative treatment, Non-operative treatment, Volar plating, Forearm fractures, Randomized controlled trial, RCT

* Correspondence: hevonkorpi.teemu.p@student.uta.fi
[1]School of Medicine, University of Tampere, 33014 Tampere, Finland
Full list of author information is available at the end of the article

Background

In the aging population, distal radius fracture (DRF) is one of the most common fractures and accounts for 4% of all fractures [1–4]. The age-adjusted overall incidence of DRF has varied between 100 to 300 per 100,000 person-years depending on sample, and it is more common (200 to 1200 per 100,000 person-years) in the elderly population [5, 6]. In Finland, the estimated annual number of DRFs among patients aged 60 and older is approximately 8000 to 9000.

In addition to the significant disability caused by DRFs among older individuals, these injuries are associated with a high economic impact. In general, the operative interventions, outpatient visits, and rehabilitation after a fracture put additional strains on scarce resources. The minimum direct cost of every operatively-treated fracture has been estimated to be approximately 1400 to 6800 € [7–9]. Considering the annual number of these fractures, it is essential that our limited resources are targeted at treatment methods with proven efficacy and cost-effectiveness.

Interestingly, some common orthopaedic operative interventions among older individuals, such as distal radius fracture surgery, are not based on well-established, high-quality scientific evidence [10]. In fact, there have been numerous studies that show the number of operative interventions for DRF is increasing, even though there is no high quality scientific evidence to support operative treatment [11, 12]. This is especially the case in patients aged over 60.

Treatment options for DRFs have varied between non-operative and operative, and numerous different surgical methods have been described over time. Operative treatment with a volar locking plate was introduced in the early 2000s, and since then the procedure has rapidly gained wide popularity. The aim of the procedure is to improve the repair of osteoporotic or comminuted fractures by providing a stable construction [12]. It has also been hypothesized that reducing the fracture to the normal anatomical position would produce a superior functional outcome [13]. Several other operative techniques, such as dorsal plates, fragment-specific plates, external fixators, metal wires and screws, have been proposed for treating DRFs. However, none of them have been shown to be superior to any other. According to several high-quality randomized controlled trials, percutaneous techniques, such as external fixator and metal wires, produced similar functional outcomes when compared with a volar locking plate [14, 15].

The most important question has, however, remained unanswered; whether operative treatment is superior to non-operative treatment in terms of functional outcome (based on Patient Rated Outcome Measures (PROMs)) and cost-efficiency in the older population. Undoubtedly, operative interventions result in fewer malunions compared with closed reduction and immobilization with a plaster cast [16]. However, non-operative treatment may be related to lower complication rates in terms of non-mechanical and mechanical problems, such as infection, wound breakage, and technical mistakes [17].

It has been shown that the functional outcome of a DRF correlates with the anatomical position of the articular surface in young, active patients. In the older population, however, the anatomic parameters correlate poorly with a positive long-term functional outcome [18, 19]. The challenge is to apply the results derived from the studies into clinical practice, especially with elderly patients. It is evident that not all people aged 65 and older are part of a homogeneous population of frail people with consistent low demands regarding physical activity. Indeed, contradicting reports have also been published regarding the correlation of anatomical parameters and functional outcome, and it has been suggested that there might be a subset of elderly patients who suffer from malunion. [20, 21] Setting a specific threshold on a continuum (i.e., age or a specific radiographic parameter) might therefore be arbitrary. The obvious challenge is to predict the subset of patients who are at risk from the majority of patients who do well.

Contrary to anatomic parameters, certain patient-related characteristics have been shown to correlate well with the outcome of the treatment [22]. These characteristics include variables, such as pain-related anxiety, catastrophic thinking related to pain, and the severity of acute pain, which can be measured by using the pain catastrophizing scale (PCS) [23]. The PCS has been used to measure trauma-related catastrophic thinking, and it has been found to associate with finger stiffness after the operative treatment of DRF, for instance [24].

Previous studies that have compared operative to non-operative treatment have had several study limitations that include small sample sizes, compromised outcome measures, and selection biases that have led to controversial conclusions about treatment [25]. Thus, the aim of this randomized prospective trial will be to compare the non-operative and operative treatment of initially or early malaligned distal radius fractures in patients aged 65 and older in terms of functional outcome.

Methods and design

Study design

The study will be a prospective, randomized, controlled, multi-center trial. The aim of the study will be to compare non-operative and operative treatment (open reduction and internal fixation with volar locking plate) of initially or early (5 to 10 days) malaligned distal radius fractures.

Aims of the study

The specific aims of this trial are as follows:

(i) to compare non-operative treatment to volar plating in the treatment of initially malaligned distal radius fractures in patients aged 65 and older in terms of functional outcome measured with PRWE
(ii) to compare non-operative treatment to volar plating in the treatment of distal radius fractures with early instability during follow-up, i.e., loss of reduction at 1 week (range 5 to 10 days) in patients aged 65 and older in terms of functional outcome measured with PRWE
(iii) to compare pain, disability, quality of life, grip strength, and the number of complications after non-operative treatment and the initial and delayed operative treatment of distal radius fracture
(iv) to assess the effect of pain catastrophizing score (PCS) on the functional outcome of non-operatively and operatively treated distal radius fracture
(v) to assess the association between physical activity and the number of wrist movements measured with Axivity accelerometer and functional outcome measured with PROMs of non-operatively and operatively treated distal radius fractures
(vi) to assess the effect of initial as well as the final radiological parameters on the functional outcome
(vii) to assess the correlation of probability of radiological malalignment estimated by clinical prediction rule (EWC) with functional outcome measured with PRWE and PASS

Primary outcome

The primary outcome will be the PRWE score measured after 1 and 2 years.

Secondary outcomes

The secondary outcomes measured will be disability [QuickDASH (disabilities of the arm, shoulder, and hand)], pain in the visual analogue scale (VAS), PCS, physical activity and the number of wrist movements measured with Axivity accelerometer, quality of life (15-D), complications, and the number of surgical interventions in the non-operatively treated group. Subgroup analysis will be performed to find out patient specific features indicating good or poor outcome. PCS will be used to assess whether mental susceptibility has an influence on the functional outcome. The Axivity accelerometer will be used for the objective evaluation of the patient's physical activity and movements of the fractured wrist in a subsample of patients. It will be used for 4 days at the 3-month and 1-year follow-up time points. EWC will be used to assess the probability of radiological malalignment from initial radiographs after injury, and its correlation with functional outcome and patient self-assessed state of symptom will be defined.

Hypotheses

Our primary hypotheses are as follows:

(i) Initial operative treatment of distal radius fracture with volar locking plates does not yield superior results compared with non-operative treatment.
(ii) Late operative treatment of distal radius fracture with volar locking plates does not yield superior results compared with continued non-operative treatment.
(iii) Initial or delayed operative treatment of malaligned distal radius fracture does not result in superior results compared with non-operative treatment with regard to pain, disability, quality of life, grip strength, and number of complications.
(iv) A high pain catastrophizing score predicts a poor functional outcome on the PRWE scale.
(v) A high level of physical activity and a high number of wrist movements predict good functional outcome on the PRWE scale and correlate negatively with the PCS.
(vi) Significant initial dislocation in radiographs (and high probability of malunion in EWC results) predicts a subset of poor functional outcomes on the PRWE scale and on PASS in patients between 65 to 74 years of age but not in patients aged 75 and older.

Study population

The eligible study population will comprise all consecutive patients aged over 64 treated for a DRF, either identified in the public or referred by the emergency rooms (ERs) of the participating hospitals (Tampere University Hospital, Finland; Central Finland Central Hospital, Finland; Satakunta Central Hospital, Finland; Viborg Regional Hospital, Denmark).

The following patient selection criteria will be used throughout the study:

Inclusion criteria:

- a low-energy, intra- or extra-articular, dorsally displaced DRF within 3 cm of the radiocarpal joint, diagnosed with lateral and posterior-anterior radiographs in ER
- > 10° dorsal tilt and/or over 2 mm step-off and/or over 3 mm ulnar variance before the closed reduction of the fracture

Exclusion criteria:

- Refusal to participate in the study

- Open fracture with a severity greater than Gustilo grade 1
- Patient aged under 65
- Chauffeur's or Barton's fracture
- Smith's fracture (volar angulation of the fracture)
- Patient does not understand written or spoken guidance in local languages
- Pathological fracture or a previous fracture in the same wrist or forearm

To improve patient involvement in this trial, we will interview patients with DRF before the onset of the trial. The aim of the interviews will be to move towards patient-centered medicine by taking into account the patients' preferences and beliefs for a good outcome. To identify the questions to ask and the outcomes to measure, we will involve patients by asking questions at the beginning of the treatment. The questionnaires that will be used for patient self-assessment are attached as additional files (consult Additional files 1 and 2). The questionnaires will be repeated after 1 year, and the difference or indifference between the primary and follow-up responses will be reported.

Randomization

Patients will be randomized with a random number matrix in block allocation fashion. The blocks will be age, site, and intra- vs. extra-articular dependent because, according to the literature, age, the presence of an intra-articular fracture, and functional outcome are associated [26, 27]. The treatment allocations derived from the matrix will be sealed in an envelope. After patient enrolment has been confirmed and informed consent has been obtained, randomization will be performed by a Tampere University Hospital research coordinator who will not otherwise attend the study. The physician responsible for the intervention or treatment will not participate in measurements or in obtaining the questionnaires. The research coordinator will monitor the study flow. An independent monitoring committee has been established.

Intervention

Phase 1

All patients visiting the ER with DRF will undergo a closed reduction under local anesthesia by means of a local infiltration of Lidocaine 1%. The technique of closed reduction will not be limited to some specific method. After reduction, radiographs will be taken to verify the position of the fracture.

Patients will be asked to visit the study doctor at the outpatient clinic 1 to 3 days after the reduction. During the visit, patients will be asked to participate in the study. Thereafter, enrollment will be confirmed and informed consent obtained. The post-reduction radiograph will be analyzed during the visit, and patient allocation will be as follows; If satisfactory position (< 10° dorsal tilt, less than 2 mm step-off and less than 3 mm ulnar variance) after closed reduction is achieved, the patient will be allocated to Cohort 2 and non-operative treatment will be performed as usual (study flow from Fig. 1). If satisfactory reduction is not achieved (> 10° dorsal tilt and/or > 2 mm step-off and/or > 3 mm ulnar variance), the patient will be allocated to Cohort 1. After allocation, the patient will be asked to fill in the PCS, 15-D, patient history, and self-assessment questionnaires. EWC will be used to assess the probability of radiological malalignment.

In Cohort 1, the patients will be randomized to either non-operative (=Arm 1) or operative treatment (=Arm 2). Patients allocated to non-operative treatment will undergo a standard treatment protocol with a dorsal cast for 5 weeks. Patients allocated to operative treatment will undergo surgery with a volar locking plate by modified Henry's volar approach. A dorsal cast will be used for 2 weeks. After cast removal, a physiotherapist will guide the patients in carrying out non-weight bearing, full range of motion exercises that will be continued until the 5-week follow-up appointment. After this, progressive weight bearing active and passive exercises will be conducted. From week 5 in the non-operative arm, the exercises will follow a similar exercise protocol as in the operative group.

Phase 2

After 1 week, the patients allocated to Cohort 2 will visit the orthopaedic outpatient clinic at the hospital where the treatment was initially started. This visit is part of the study protocol. If reduction is maintained, the patients will undergo standard follow-up visits (=Arm 4). If reduction is lost to fulfill the inclusion criteria for surgery (> 10° dorsal tilt and/or > 2 mm step-off and/ or > 3 mm ulnar variance) the patient will be asked to participate to phase 2 of the study. After enrollment of the patients has been confirmed and informed consent signed, the patients will be randomized to either non-operative (=Arm 3 N) or operative treatment (=Arm 3O). If allocated to non-operative treatment, patients will undergo the same protocol as those in Arm 1. Patients allocated to operative treatment will undergo surgery with a volar locking plate by modified Henry's volar approach as described above. In addition, physiotherapy and exercises will be conducted as described above.

Patients who decline to attend the intervention trial will be asked to join the external follow-up group. This group will be used as external validation; the group content and outcomes will be compared with the allocated intervention and control groups. The treatment of this

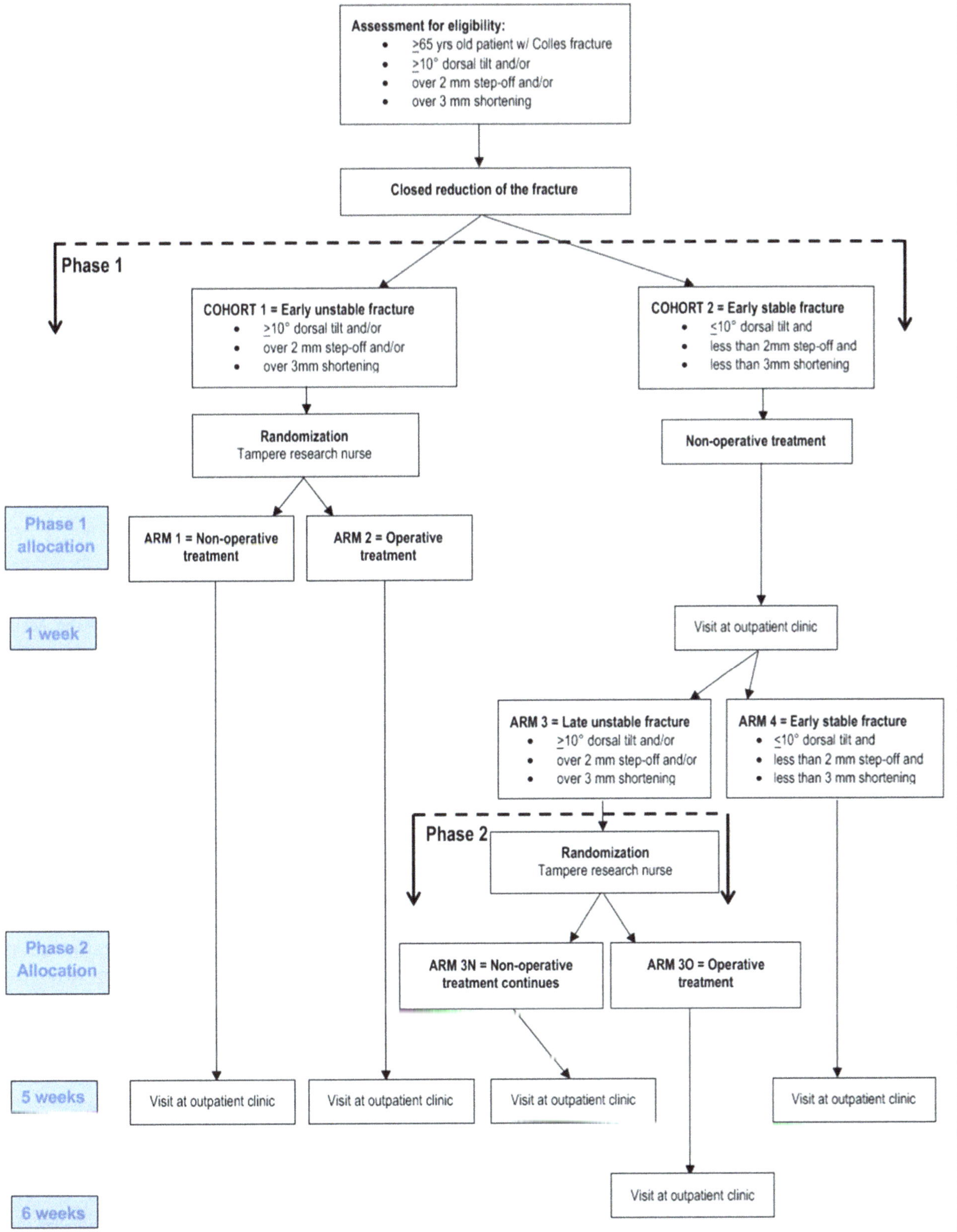

Fig. 1 Patient flow chart of the trial

group will be carried out in line with normal clinical practice, but the patients will have the same follow-up and asked to fill in the same questionnaires as the allocated patients.

Follow-up

Non-operatively treated patients in Arm 1 will be treated with cast immobilization. After 5 weeks, the cast will be removed and the patients will visit the orthopaedic outpatient clinic at the hospital for follow-up visits. During the visit, direct lateral and anteroposterior radiographs will be taken. Patients will visit the outpatient clinic again after 3 months and follow-up assessment will be performed by completing the PRWE, QuickDASH, VAS, PCS, and 15-D questionnaires. Radiographs will also be taken. Physical activity and the number of movements of the injured wrist will be evaluated with Axivity accelerometer in a subsample of patients. Operatively treated patients in Arm 2 will visit the clinic at 5 weeks and at 3 months, and the same follow-up protocol will be performed.

After the first week's visit to the clinic for phase 2 patients, the same follow-up protocol as in the Cohort 1 will be used.

For all patients, PRWE will be the primary outcome and will be measured at the 1 and 2-year follow-up time points by the Internet, post, or telephone query. PRWE, PCS, pain, QuickDASH, 15-D, and self-assessment will be measured (Table 1). At the 1-year follow-up, physical activity and the number of wrist movements will be measured with Axivity accelerometer in a subgroup of patients. Grip strength will also be measured. At the 1- and 2-year follow-up, patient files will be reviewed to detect complications.

Radiological analysis

Standard radiological parameters will be defined from initial as well as final (3 months) radiographs. These parameters will be as follows: 1) volar-dorsal angulation angle, 2) the presence of dorsal and volar comminution, 3) radioulnar inclination angle, 4) ulnar variance 5) intra-articular step-off, 6) intra-articular diastasis. Two musculoskeletal radiologists will separately evaluate the radiographs. The radiologists will be blinded to the final treatment method and outcome while performing their assessment of the initial radiographs. From the initial radiographs, the probability given by EWC will be defined. To be pragmatic, we will not measure ulnar variance from the radiographs of the uninjured side as in the original article [28]. Instead, we suppose neutral variance.

Power analysis

In this trial, a validated wrist specific PRWE-score will be used as the main outcome measure. In 2015, Wallenkamp and coworkers reported that the minimal clinically important difference in PRWE is 11 points and that SD is 14 [29]. Based on power calculations (Cl 95%, power 0.95, SD 14), the required sample size per group is 40 patients. Assuming a 30% drop-out rate based on possible surgical intervention during cast treatment, group size would be 57 per group (total 114). When two cohorts are taken into account, this would mean that a total of 228 patients is needed. Regardless of whether patients change to a different treatment group (cross-overs), the patients will be analyzed according to the intention-to-treat principle.

Statistical analysis

The differences between groups in continuous skewed main outcome variables will be analyzed by the Mann-Whitney U-test, and analyzed by the t-test when variables are unskewed. The results will be presented with 95% confidence intervals. Two-way tables with the chi-square test will be used for dichotomous variables. In subgroup analysis, the effect of age, sex, fracture group, and smoking will be evaluated against the scores and overall quality of life after fracture.

Analysis of covariance will be used to assess the effect of pain catastrophizing score on the outcome of cast treatment. PRWE will be used as the dependent variable, cast as independent variable, and pain catastrophizing score as covariate.

The effect of cast immobilization treatment on the PRWE will also be investigated in the multivariate manner. Multivariable analysis will be performed with linear regression analysis since the outcome variable PRWE is normally distributed. The main variables of interest included will be cast immobilization and age, sex, fracture

Table 1 Assessments and procedures

	Medical history	Radiograph	PRWE	EWC	PCS	Pain	Grip	Axivity	Quick-DASH	15-D	Self-assessment
Baseline	x	x		x	x					x	x
1 week (Cohort 2)	x	x									
5–6 weeks	(x)	x									
3 months	x	x	x		x	x	x	x	x	x	
1 year			x		x	x	x	x	x	x	x
2 years			x		x	x			x	x	x

group, and smoking, and other diseases will be used as confounding variables. Self-assessment questionnaires (Additional files 1 and 2) will be analyzed and compared to find out which parameters are of the most importance for patients at the beginning of the treatment, and if the same parameters are equally important after the 1 and 2-year follow-up periods.

Setting and recruitment

We need to recruit a total of 228 patients. Recruitment in Arm 3 will be challenging. As a single center, there is a risk that the required number of patients will not be achievable. This risk will be alleviated through Nordic collaboration by means of a multicenter study. When conducting a randomized controlled multicenter trial, the critical points are patient recruitment rate and key personnel stability. The collaboration between the different centers of the NITEP group has been found to be effective and reliable, and it has played crucial roles in the previous proximal humerus trial. This study will be carried out at Tampere University Hospital, Central Finland Central Hospital, Satakunta Central Hospital in Finland and Viborg regional Hospital in Denmark. We aim to maintain homogeneity between centers with solid trial designs, data, and project management including monitoring. Site personnel training has already started. We have been assisted by local research centers. The stability of the trial will be maintained with regular communications and bi-annual meetings.

Data management

Each patient will be assigned a unique trial identification number (TIN) that will be matched with the patient's identification number (ID). The matching key will be stored in a locked office at Tampere University Hospital, Finland, and the identification of each patient will only be possible after retrieving the matching key. Throughout the trial, the research data will be handled only with a TIN. The research data will be saved to a database with an online patient management program (PMP) located on a secure research server. The research data saved to the server will contain only anonymous TINs with a set of numbers acquired from the questionnaires, i.e., each question will be answered with a number. This will ensure the anonymity of each individual patient and that the identity of the patient will remain secret should the server data be revealed to third-parties.

All primary and secondary data will be acquired and stored on the study trial server. Data will be entered either by the patient during the control visits (via tablets) or by a researcher or study nurse when the questionnaires are mailed. The researchers from each hospital will have access to the secure study server where the trial research data is stored. The server has been approved by an information security committee at Tampere University Hospital. At the end of the trial, each researcher will have access to the data for further analyses. The questionnaires will be pre-programmed according to the PMP, and the individual patient data acquired at different time-points will be saved in Comma Separated Values (CSV) format, which is transferrable to, e.g., Microsoft Excel. All variables in the dataset will be described and suitable metadata standards will be used when available.

The copyright of the trial research data will be owned and created by the collaboration parties. The data will be shared freely among the collaboration parties. All participating researchers will receive access to the data after the trial is completed. Due to confidentiality and legal agreements, public data sharing will be restricted, (we have permission to store the data in the specific research server, but not to transfer the data). Under certain circumstances, e.g., when a new member joins the collaboration, we will grant access to the data. All data will be saved for 15 years after the end of the trial.

Schedule

The patient recruitment will start in February 2018. The recruiting time will be 2 years and the results will be analyzed after a 1-year and a 2-year follow-up period.

Discussion

Traditionally, the treatment decision (operative or non-operative) in fragility fractures has been based on the orthopaedic surgeon's experience and beliefs. A few decades ago, this view was challenged by evidence-based medicine. As previously stated, a significant proportion of common orthopaedic interventions are not based on high-quality scientific evidence [10, 30]. Since the 2000s, randomized controlled trials (RCT) have become the gold standard in medical research.

We expect that an initial operative treatment of a DRF with volar locking plate will not yield superior results compared with a non-operative treatment with cast immobilization in terms of functional outcome, quality of life, disability, pain, grip strength, and number of complications among patients aged 65 and older. Moreover, we expect that functional outcome after treatment of distal radius fracture is related more to physical activity and catastrophic thinking than treatment modality. We assume that the late operative treatment of displaced distal radius fractures observed during short-term follow up will offer no additional benefit to continued non-operative treatment.

After our results are published, our aim will be to support the creation and dissemination of trustworthy guidelines by health authorities and professional organizations. We expect that after demonstrating the clinical results of our trial and supporting the creation and dissemination of trustworthy guidelines for the treatment policies of this common orthopaedic complaint, Nordic countries will be substantially changed and will reflect the best current evidence.

Abbreviations

15-D: 15-dimensional; CI: Confidence interval; CSV: Comma separated values; DRF: Distal radius fracture; ER: Emergency room; EWC: Edinburgh wrist calculator; ID: Identification; NITEP: Nordic innovative trial to evaluate osteoporotic fractures; PASS: Patient self-assessed state of symptom; PCS: Pain catastrophizing score; PMP: Patient management program; PROM: Patient rated outcome measure; PRWE: Patient rated wrist evaluation; Quick-DASH: Quick- disabilities of arm, shoulder and hand; SD: Standard deviation; TIN: Trial identification number; VAS: Visual analogue scale

Acknowledgements

Not applicable.

Funding

This trial has received a research grant from the Academy of Finland. Other Nordic collaborators are responsible for their own costs.

Authors' contributions

TH, AL, AR, ML, TL, BS, LR, JK and VM have been involved in designing this RCT study. VM has calculated the power analysis of the study population. AL has designed the allocation blocks. AL will monitor and advise the methodological aspects of the trial. TH, AL, AR, ML, BS, LR, TL, JK and VM have written the manuscript. All authors have critically read and approved the final manuscript.

Consent for publication

Not applicable.

Competing interests

No competing interests declared.

Author details

[1]School of Medicine, University of Tampere, 33014 Tampere, Finland. [2]Department of Orthopaedics, Unit of Musculoskeletal Surgery, Tampere University Hospital, Teiskontie 35, PL2000, 33521 Tampere, Finland. [3]Central Finland Central Hospital, Keskussairaalantie 19, 40620 Jyväskylä, Finland. [4]Satakunta Central Hospital, Sairaalantie 3, 28500 Pori, Finland.

References

1. Lauritzen JB, Schwarz P, Lund B, McNair P, Transbol I. Changing incidence and residual lifetime risk of common osteoporosis-related fractures. Osteoporos Int. 1993;3(3):127–32.
2. Seeley DG, Browner WS, Nevitt MC, Genant HK, Scott JC, Cummings SR. Which fractures are associated with low appendicular bone mass in elderly women? The study of osteoporotic fractures research group. Ann Intern Med. 1991;115(11):837–42.
3. Court-Brown CM, Caesar B. Epidemiology of adult fractures: a review. Injury. 2006;37(8):691–7.
4. Larsen CF, Lauritsen J. Epidemiology of acute wrist trauma. Int J Epidemiol. 1993;22(5):911–6.
5. Flinkkila T, Sirnio K, Hippi M, Hartonen S, Ruuhela R, Ohtonen P, Hyvonen P, Leppilahti J. Epidemiology and seasonal variation of distal radius fractures in Oulu, Finland. Osteoporos Int. 2011; https://doi.org/10.1007/s00198-010-1463-3.
6. Brogren E, Petranek M, Atroshi I. Incidence and characteristics of distal radius fractures in a southern Swedish region. BMC Musculoskelet Disord. 2007;8:48.
7. Shauver MJ, Clapham PJ, Chung KC. An economic analysis of outcomes and complications of treating distal radius fractures in the elderly. J Hand Surg Am. 2011; https://doi.org/10.1016/j.jhsa.2011.09.039.
8. Pirkanmaan sairaanhoitopiiri. Tuotehinnasto. 2017. http://www.pshp.fi/download/noname/%7B2F6BDDB9-65DF-4F6A-81D0-F957E1D2737A%7D/51137.
9. Helsingin ja Uudenmaan sairaanhoitopiiri. Palveluhinnasto. 2018. http://www.hus.fi/hus-tietoa/talous/Hinnoittelu/Documents/HUS%20Palveluhinnasto%202018.pdf.
10. Lohmander LS, Roos EM. The evidence base for orthopaedics and sports medicine. BMJ. 2015; https://doi.org/10.1136/bmj.g7835.
11. Mattila VM, Huttunen TT, Sillanpaa P, Niemi S, Pihlajamaki H, Kannus P. Significant change in the surgical treatment of distal radius fractures: a nationwide study between 1998 and 2008 in Finland. J Trauma. 2011; https://doi.org/10.1097/TA.0b013e3182231af9.
12. Wilcke MKT, Hammarberg H, Adolphson PY. Epidemiology and changed surgical treatment methods for fractures of the distal radius: a registry analysis of 42,583 patients in Stockholm County, Sweden, 2004-2010. Acta Orthop. 2013; https://doi.org/10.3109/17453674.2013.792035.
13. Tarallo L, Mugnai R, Adani R, Catani F. Malunited extra-articular distal radius fractures: corrective osteotomies using volar locking plate. J Orthop Traumatol. 2014;15(4):285–90.
14. Esposito J, Schemitsch EH, Saccone M, Sternheim A, Kuzyk PRT. External fixation versus open reduction with plate fixation for distal radius fractures: a meta-analysis of randomised controlled trials. Injury. 2013; https://doi.org/10.1016/j.injury.2012.12.003.
15. Costa ML, Achten J, Parsons NR, Rangan A, Griffin D, Tubeuf S, Lamb SE, DRAFFT Study Group. Percutaneous fixation with Kirschner wires versus volar locking plate fixation in adults with dorsally displaced fracture of distal radius: randomised controlled trial. BMJ. 2014; https://doi.org/10.1136/bmj.g4807.
16. Grewal R, MacDermid JC. The risk of adverse outcomes in extra-articular distal radius fractures is increased with malalignment in patients of all ages but mitigated in older patients. J Hand Surg [Am]. 2007;32(7):962–70.
17. Wei J, Yang T, Luo W, Qin J, Kong F. Complications following dorsal versus volar plate fixation of distal radius fracture: a meta-analysis. J Int Med Res. 2013; https://doi.org/10.1177/0300060513476438.
18. Leung F, Ozkan M, Chow SP. Conservative treatment of intra-articular fractures of the distal radius–factors affecting functional outcome. Hand Surg. 2000;5(2):145–53.
19. Plant CE, Parsons NR, Costa ML. Do radiological and functional outcomes correlate for fractures of the distal radius? Bone Joint J. 2017; https://doi.org/10.1302/0301-620X.99B3.35819.
20. Kodama N, Takemura Y, Ueba H, Imai S, Matsusue Y. Acceptable parameters for alignment of distal radius fracture with conservative treatment in elderly patients. J Orthop Sci. 2014; https://doi.org/10.1007/s00776-013-0514-y.
21. Martinez-Mendez D, Lizaur-Utrilla A, de-Juan-Herrero J. Intra-articular distal radius fractures in elderly: a randomized prospective study of casting versus volar plating. J Hand Surg Eur Vol. 2017; https://doi.org/10.1177/1753193417727139.
22. Jiang Y, Sanchez-Santos MT, Judge AD, Murray DW, Arden NK. Predictors of patient-reported pain and functional outcomes over 10 years after primary Total knee arthroplasty: a prospective cohort study. J Arthroplast. 2017;32(1):92–100. e2; doi:https://doi.org/10.1016/j.arth.2016.06.009
23. Sullivan MJL, Bishop SR, Pivik J. The pain catastrophizing scale: development and validation. Psychol Assess. 1995;7(4):524–32.
24. Teunis T, Bot AGJ, Thornton ER, Ring D. Catastrophic thinking is associated with finger stiffness after distal radius fracture surgery. J Orthop Trauma. 2015; https://doi.org/10.1097/BOT.0000000000000342

25. Arora R, Lutz M, Deml C, Krappinger D, Haug L, Gabl M. A prospective randomized trial comparing nonoperative treatment with volar locking plate fixation for displaced and unstable distal radial fractures in patients sixty-five years of age and older. J Bone Joint Surg Am. 2011; https://doi.org/10.2106/JBJS.J.01597.
26. Anzarut A, Johnson JA, Rowe BH, Lambert RGW, Blitz S, Majumdar SR. Radiologic and patient-reported functional outcomes in an elderly cohort with conservatively treated distal radius fractures. J Hand Surg [Am]. 2004; 29(6):1121–7.
27. Batra S, Gupta A. The effect of fracture-related factors on the functional outcome at 1 year in distal radius fractures. Injury. 2002;33(6):499–502.
28. Mackenney PJ, McQueen MM, Elton R. Prediction of instability in distal radial fractures. J Bone Joint Surg Am. 2006;88(9):1944–51.
29. Walenkamp MMJ, de Muinck KR, Goslings JC, Vos LM, Rosenwasser MP, Schep NWL. The minimum clinically important difference of the patient-rated wrist evaluation score for patients with distal radius fractures. Clin Orthop. 2015; https://doi.org/10.1007/s11999-015-4376-9.
30. Lim HC, Adie S, Naylor JM, Harris IA. Randomised trial support for orthopaedic surgical procedures. PLoS One. 2014; https://doi.org/10.1371/journal.pone.0096745.

14

Open reduction and internal fixation with bone grafts for comminuted mason type II radial head fractures

Guanyi Liu[1,2†], Erman Chen[2†], Dingli Xu[1], Weihu Ma[1], Leijie Zhou[1], Jianming Chen[1] and Zhijun Pan[2*]

Abstract

Background: The use of bone graft for the radial head fractures has been previously described and occasionally used by other authors.This is the first paper, to my knowledge, dealing with the relevant issue about the importance that the use of an autologous bone graft can have on the radial head fractures.

Methods: From July 2010 to July 2014, 20 consecutive patients who underwent open reduction and internal fixation for a closed Mason type II radial head fracture were retrospectively reviewed. Patients with Mason type I, III, simple type II, and comminuted type II fractures treated without bone grafting were excluded. A clinical examination and radiographic evaluation were performed. The overall functional result was evaluated using the Mayo Elbow Performance Score (MEPS). The Broberg and Morrey classification was used to evaluate traumatic arthritis.

Results: The average follow-up duration was 31 months (range, 24–50 months). Bone union of the radial head fracture was achieved in all patients at an average of 13.5 weeks (range, 12–17 weeks). Postoperative radiographs showed no cases of postsurgical ligamentous instability, necrosis of the radial head, or internal fixation failure. The mean range of motion of the affected elbow was 128° ± 8.4° in flexion, 14.5° ± 11.1° in extension, 68.7° ± 14.1° in pronation, and 65.2° ± 18.2° in supination. The mean MEPS was 92 ± 7.9 points (range, 80–100); the outcome was excellent (90–100 points) in 13 patients and good (75–89 points) in 7 patients. The MEPS tended to be higher in patients with an isolated fracture ($p = 0.016$). Based on the Broberg and Morrey classification for radiographic assessment of post-traumatic arthritis, 15 elbows had no evidence of degenerative changes (grade 0), and 5 elbows had grade 1 changes.

Conclusion: Although radial head fractures may not be amenable to internal fixation, our findings suggest that open reduction and internal fixation with an autogenous bone graft from the lateral epicondyle of the humerus provides satisfactory elbow function in patients with comminuted Mason type II radial head fractures.

Keywords: Elbow, Radial head fracture, Internal fixation

Background

Radial head fractures are common injuries and usually classified according to the original Mason classification: type I, fissure fractures or marginal sector fractures without displacement; type II, partial articular fractures with displacement; and type III, comminuted fractures involving the whole head of the radius [1]. Type II actually includes simple and comminuted partial articular fractures (Fig. 1). The operative treatment of comminuted type II radial head fractures has been controversial because of conflicting evidence supporting resection, prosthetic replacement, and open reduction and internal fixation (ORIF) [1–8]. Improvements in operation techniques and implants such as low-profile mini-plates have increased the appeal of internal fixation treatment, especially for comminuted type II fractures of the radial head [5–7]. To our knowledge, ORIF with an autogenous bone graft from the lateral epicondyle of the humerus for comminuted Mason type II radial head fractures has rarely been

* Correspondence: zrpzj@zju.edu.cn
†Guanyi Liu and Erman Chen contributed equally to this work.
[2]Department of Orthopedics, the Second Affiliated Hospital, School of Medicine, Zhejiang University 88 Jiefang RoadHangzhou, Zhejiang 310009, People's Republic of China

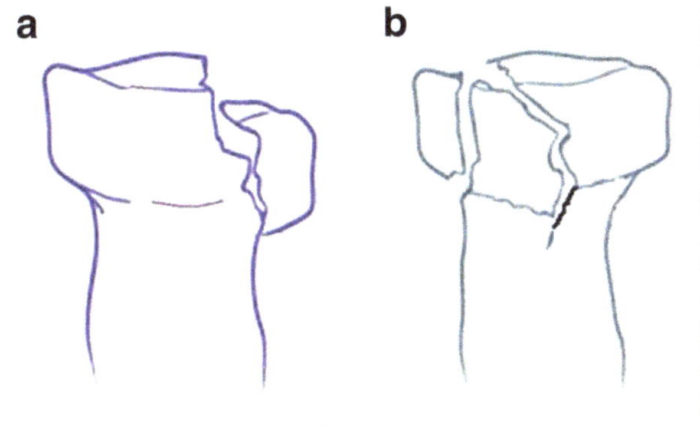

Fig. 1 Mason type II fractures of radial head include simple (**a**) and comminuted (**b**) partial articular fractures with displacement

reported. This technique was used to treat 20 patients in our study and produced desirable outcomes.

Methods

From July 2010 to July 2014, 40 consecutive patients who underwent ORIF of a closed Mason type II radial head fracture (simple fractures, $n = 11$; comminuted fractures, $n = 28$) performed by the senior author (G.Y.L.) at our institution were identified and retrospectively case studied. Of the 28 patients with comminuted fractures, 22 were treated by ORIF with an autogenous bone graft and 6 without. Patients with Mason type I, III, simple type II, and comminuted type II fractures treated without bone grafting were excluded.

The study protocol was approved by our institution's research ethics board. After reviewing the patients' medical records and radiographs in our electronic medical record and image databases, we invited the patients to our hospital for clinical and radiographic evaluations. Written informed consent was required for participation in this study. Two patients were lost to follow-up. Thus, the final study population comprised 20 patients.The patients comprised 12 men and 8 women with a mean age of 47 years (range, 20–65 years). They had 14 dominant injuries and 6 nondominant injuries. The mechanism of injury was a fall from a standing height in three patients, a fall from a greater height (> 3 m) in six patients, a traffic accident in eight patients, and a sports injury in three patients.

All patients had a comminuted Mason type II radial head fracture (a fracture involving the partial articular surface, splitting it into two or more fragments). According to the comprehensive classification of fractures, the patients had 3 type B fractures (all were B2.3) and 17 type C fractures (10 were C2.3 and 7 were C3.2). Three radial head fractures were isolated injuries; 17 were associated with a fracture-dislocation of the elbow joint (Mason–Johnston type IV) [1, 2]. Twelve patients had elbow terrible triad injuries, two had transolecranon fracture-dislocation of the elbow, two had Bado type II Monteggia fractures, and one had a radial head fracture combined with dislocation of the elbow [9]. The Bado type II fractures were subclassified based on the location of the ulnar fracture according to the Jupiter classification [10]. Both fractures were at the level of the coronoid process (type A). The coronoid fractures in patients with elbow terrible triad injuries were classified according to Regan-Morrey [11]. Three fractures were associated with minor coronoid avulsion fractures (Morrey type I), eight were associated with a Morrey type II fracture, and one was associated with a Morrey type III fracture.

Operative technique

The operative details varied depending on the indication for surgery and the numbers of fractures and injured ligaments. A brachial plexus block was used in all patients. Patients with an elbow terrible triad injury were placed in the supine position with the involved arm draped on the hand table. Patients with Monteggia fractures and transolecranon fracture-dislocation of the elbow were positioned in the lateral decubitus position with the limb supported over a bolster. Under pneumatic tourniquet control, the fracture was approached through an extended lateral approach for patients with an elbow terrible triad injury and through a midline longitudinal dorsal incision for those with Monteggia fractures and transolecranon fracture-dislocation of the elbow.

The radial head and lateral collateral ligament complex were exposed and checked. A longitudinal incision was made through the annular ligament and capsule, along the lateral collateral ligament. The radial head fracture was identified, and all pieces of the radial head were found following irrigation of the intra-articular hematoma. Care was taken to protect the synovium and periosteum overlying the fragments to preserve the vascular supply and facilitate reduction [12]. Once reduced, the fracture fragments were temporarily fixed with 1-mm Kirschner wires.

In this series, autogenous bone grafts from the lateral epicondyle were implanted in the bone defect of the radial head fractures. The donor site was located in the lateral metaphysis of the humerus and far away from the origins of the lateral collateral ligamentous complex and common extensor tendon. The size of the bone graft was commensurate with the injury. Both cancellous and corticocancellous bone were taken. Bone chips were implanted in the bone defect to maintain the reduction of fractures and/or buttress fragments of the articular surface.

Definitive fixation was then secured using countersunk head screws, Kirschner wires, mini locking plates, or combinations of these methods. The radial head fracture was fixed with Kirschner wires alone in one patient, with a low-profile mini-plate alone in six, with countersunk head screws alone in four, and with a combination of a plate and countersunk head screws in nine.

We used a low-profile T- or Y-shaped mini locking plate with a 0.55-mm profile height (F3 fragment plating system; Johnson & Johnson Co., New Brunswick, NJ, USA). The screws were 2.0 mm in diameter and could be countersunk into the plate. The plates were placed on the nonarticulating portion ("safe zone") of the radial head [13, 14]. The nonarticulating portion of the radial head exhibited a thinner band of yellowish cartilage relative to the wider, white, glistening cartilage of the articular portion of the radial head [15]. However, placement of mini-plates was not limited to the nonarticular portion of the radial head because they could be applied as a buttress from the radial shaft to the head or to the lower corner of the radial head [5]. Sometimes a fragment was too small to be fixed with a plate or screw and could only be fixed with 1-mm Kirschner wires (two patients).

Associated fractures of the coronoid process and olecranon were fixed concomitantly. After fixation, the stability of the fixation and the range of movement of forearm rotation were checked. The radial head and proximal radioulnar joint were examined by fluoroscopy to ensure extra-articular screw placement. The capsule and annular ligament were closed with absorbable sutures. Avulsion of the lateral collateral ligament occurred in 13 patients; reattachment to the lateral condyle was performed with a transosseous suture in 4 patients and with bone anchors (Johnson & Johnson Co., America) in 9 patients [16, 17]. Finally, stability of the elbow was tested by the hanging arm test in patients with terrible triad injuries [18]. If unacceptable instability persisted, then the medial collateral ligament was exposed and repaired (in two patients).

Postoperative management

Functional aftercare without immobilization was carried out in patients with isolated radial head fractures; otherwise, postoperative immobilization in a splint or cast was performed for an average of 2 weeks (range, 3 days to 3 weeks) followed by active exercises as tolerated by the patients. Partial weight bearing began at the sixth postoperative week. Full weight bearing was delayed until the fracture was healed and a callus appeared on radiographs.

Evaluation

The clinical examination and radiographic evaluation were performed by an independent observer. Flexion and extension of the elbow and wrist (forearm in neutral rotation) and the range of pronation and supination were measured. The overall functional result was evaluated using the Mayo Elbow Performance Score (MEPS) [19]. Follow-up radiographs, including anteroposterior and lateral projections of the elbow, were used to assess fracture union, congruity, post-traumatic osteoarthritis, and hardware-related problems. In patients with equivocal X-rays, reconstructed computed tomography scans were obtained for further assessment. The Broberg and Morrey classification was used to evaluate traumatic arthritis [19].

Statistical analysis

Data analyses were performed with SPSS 18.0 (SPSS Inc., Chicago, IL). Continuous variables are presented as mean ± standard deviation. A two-sample t test was performed to compare the ROM and MEPS between patients with an isolated fracture of the radial head and those with a more complex injury pattern. All p values were two-sided, and values < 0.05 were considered statistically significant.

Results

Result of the entire elbow injury

The clinical results are summarized in Table 1. All patients underwent operative treatment without neurovascular complications. The average follow-up duration was 31 months (range, 24–50 months). Postoperative radiographs showed no cases of postsurgical ligamentous instability and internal fixation failure. We found no serious persistent pain of the elbow, nerve impairment, complex regional pain syndrome, or infection.

The mean ROM of the affected elbow was 128° ± 8.4° in flexion, 14.5° ± 11.1° in extension, 68.7° ± 14.1° in pronation, and 65.2° ± 18.2° in supination with a flexion–extension arc of 113° ± 16.5° and pronosupination arc of 134° ± 28°. The mean MEPS was 92 ± 7.9 points (range, 80–100 points); the outcome was excellent (90–100 points) in 13 patients and good (75–89 points) in 7 patients. The MEPS tended to be higher in patients with an isolated fracture ($t = 3.155$, $p = 0.016$). Based on the Broberg and Morrey classification for the radiographic assessment of post-traumatic arthritis, 15 elbows had no evidence of degenerative changes (grade 0), and 5 elbows had grade 1 changes. There was no incidence of grade 2 or 3 changes at the final follow-up. Three of the 20 patients (15%) had evidence of periarticular ossification. In all three patients, the periarticular ossification was minimal.

Result of fractures of the radial head

Bone union of the radial head fractures was achieved in all patients at an average of 13.5 weeks (range, 12–17 weeks) (Fig. 2). No complications occurred in the donor site area. Postoperative radiographs showed no cases of necrosis of the radial head, reduction loss, or internal fixation failure.

Table 1 Characteristics of patients in the present series

Case	Age	Gender	Diagnosis	Follow-up(months)	Extension(°)	Flexion(°)	Pronation(°)	Supination(°)	MEPS
1	40	Male	radial head fracture	28	0	140	70	75	95
2	47	Male	radial head fracture	50	5	130	80	85	100
3	63	Male	radial head fracture	40	10	125	80	75	100
4	29	Female	radial head fracture and dislocation	35	10	120	80	65	95
5	62	Female	terrible triad injury	25	25	110	35	60	80
6	59	Male	terrible triad injury	29	35	125	60	40	85
7	49	Male	Monteggia fracture	30	25	125	75	55	95
8	51	Female	Monteggia fracture	26	15	135	75	70	95
9	65	Male	terrible triad injury	27	25	130	75	85	100
10	58	Male	terrible triad injury	24	25	120	60	30	80
11	43	Female	terrible triad injury	40	15	130	85	80	100
12	41	Female	terrible triad injury	39	5	135	55	45	85
13	46	Male	terrible triad injury	32	0	120	70	70	85
14	47	Female	terrible triad injury	27	5	125	65	50	85
15	29	Female	terrible triad injury	26	20	130	65	60	95
16	55	Male	transolecranon fracture-dislocation	24	15	135	70	75	100
17	65	Male	terrible triad injury	26	10	125	70	70	90
18	20	Male	terrible triad injury	40	25	135	60	55	95
19	28	Male	transolecranon fracture-dislocation	30	15	135	75	85	95
20	43	Female	terrible triad injury	28	5	130	70	75	85

No serious persistent pain and degenerative change of the lateral side of the elbow was found. None of these patients had a severe restriction of pronosupination or flexion–extension. Implant removal was performed in one patient.

Discussion

To our knowledge, this is the largest series of radial head fractures treated by ORIF with autogenous bone grafts. The main findings of the present study are as follows. (1) ORIF with an autogenous bone graft from the lateral epicondyle is an effective treatment for comminuted Mason type II radial head fractures. (2) Patients with an isolated fracture of the radial head tended to have better elbow function results. (3) Comminuted partial articular fractures of the radial head were more likely to be part of a serious complex injury pattern than to be isolated fractures.

The aim of the treatment of radial head fractures is to restore good elbow function. Radial head excision has been advised for comminuted fractures [3, 6]. However, excision of the radial head may be associated with proximal radial shaft migration and consequent disorders in the wrist [3, 6]. Radial head fractures combined with injury of the medial ligament of the elbow should not be treated by radial head excision [20–22]. Prosthetic replacement of the radial head is another alternative and is commonly performed when the head is fractured into more than three displaced fragments. However, complications associated with prosthetic replacement have been reported [25]. Flinkkilä et al. [23] reported that loosening of press-fit radial head prostheses was found in 12 of 37 patients (32.4%). van Riet et al. [24] reported that 47 elbows underwent removal of a failed metallic radial head replacement.

ORIF is the preferred treatment method for radial head fractures, particularly in young and active patients. Both biomechanical and clinical studies have proven that preservation of the radial head has a positive impact on elbow stability [25–27].

ORIF is good choice for treating type II fractures with a single fragment. However, Mason [1] recommended resection for type II partial articular fractures with more than one fragment because the risk of radial head necrosis and secondary loss of reduction seems high in comminuted radial head fractures. Heim et al. [28] encountered problems with healing or avascular necrosis in 5 of 11 comminuted fractures. Autogenous bone grafts are beneficial for both maintenance of reduction and healing of fractures. In the present series, no nonunion or avascular necrosis occurred after ORIF with a bone graft from the lateral epicondyle.

However, bone grafting has not been widely used in combination with ORIF for treatment of radial head fractures, and different donor sites have been reported

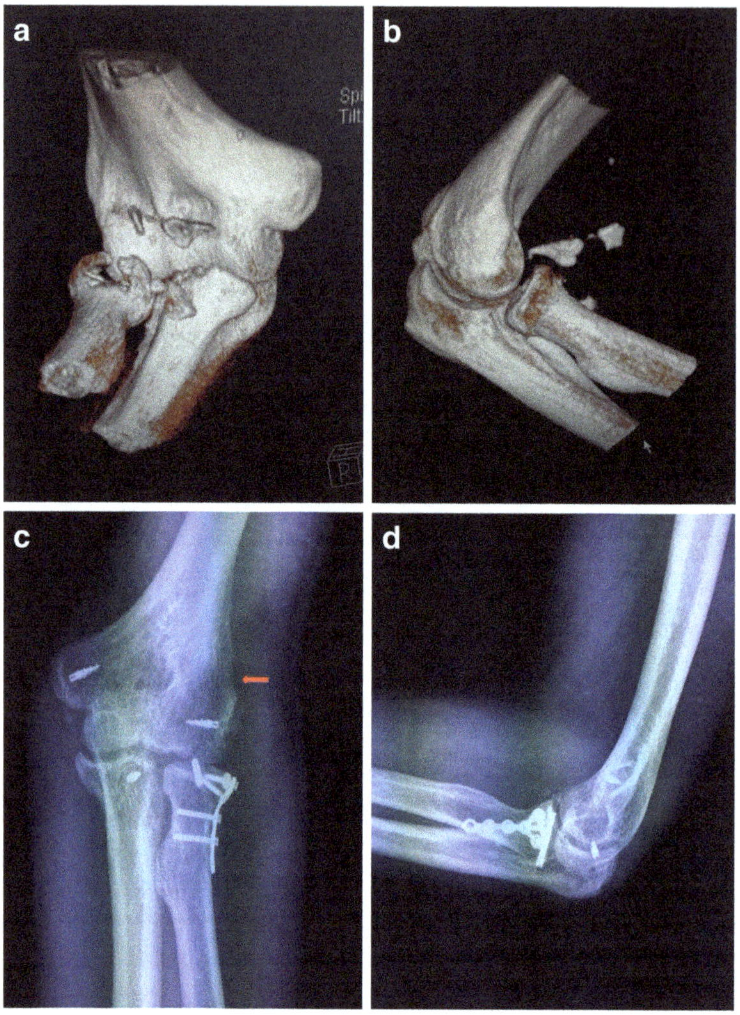

Fig. 2 A typical case. A 59-year-old man sustained a terrible triad elbow injury and was treated though a lateral approach combined with a medial approach (Case 9). Open reduction and internal fixation with a bone graft for the radial head fracture and repair of the lateral collateral ligament as well as fixation of the coronoid fracture and repair of the medial collateral ligament were performed. **a**, **b** Preoperative CT scans showed a comminuted Mason type II radial head fracture and a coronoid fracture. **c**, **d** Postoperative radiographs at the last follow-up demonstrated good bone union. The donor site could be seen on the anteroposterior radiograph of the elbow (red arrow)

in the literature [7, 29–31]. Ring et al. [7] applied ORIF with an autogenous bone graft to 1 of 30 patients with Mason type II fractures. Oztürk et al. [29] reported that 15 patients with radial head fractures underwent ORIF, and bone grafts from the distal part of the radius were used in 5 patients. Patel et al. [30] treated a severe comminuted fracture of the radial neck by ORIF with a tricortical iliac crest bone graft. Luenam et al. [30] reported that union was achieved in 9 of 10 patients who underwent an operation using an iliac crest bone graft for partial radial head reconstruction in the treatment of complex dislocation of the elbow. We prefer autografting from the lateral epicondyle of the humerus. The reasons for this choice are as follows: (1) taking bone chips from the same incision is convenient and induces less iatrogenic damage; (2) preparation of another sterile area for donation is not needed; and (3) the procedure is safe and has no adverse effects on elbow function.

Union of radial head fractures and good or excellent elbow function were achieved in all patients. The mean MEPS in this series was 92 points with a flexion–extension arc of 113° and pronosupination arc of 134°. The outcomes in our cohort were comparable with or better than other results reported in previous studies with similar patient populations. Ring et al. [7] reported a mean functional index of 92 points in 30 patients with Mason type II fractures using ORIF and a mean range of movement of 11° to 130° at the elbow (mean of 72° of pronation and 72° of supination). They found a trend toward unsatisfactory results with severe restriction of forearm rotation in patients with comminuted Mason type II fractures and unsatisfactory results in four patients. In our series, however, only two patients had forearm rotation of < 100° and none had fair or poor functional results. Both patients with restricted forearm rotation had a terrible triad injury of the elbow. Ring et al. [7] also found that patients with radial head fractures exhibiting a complex elbow dislocation pattern were more likely to have an unsatisfactory treatment result. We obtained the same finding in our series; patients with an isolated radial head fracture had a much higher MEPS than patients with a fracture and dislocation of the elbow.

Comminuted partial articular fractures of the radial head were more likely to be part of a complex elbow dislocation pattern. We noted that most such fractures (17 of 20 patients) were associated with fracture and dislocation of the elbow in this series. Pugh et al. [17] recommended prosthetic replacement for a radial head fracture with comminution or impaction in terrible triad injuries. Ring et al. [32] resected the radial head in 4 of 11 patients with terrible triad injuries, and 7 patients reported unsatisfactory results. All four patients with a satisfactory result were treated by ORIF for the radial head fracture. Ring et al. [7] suggested that when ORIF is impossible, resection of the radial head and prosthetic replacement should be considered for complex injury patterns. However, we consider that even when two or more fracture fragments are present, the primary goal is to fix the type II partial articular fracture. The radial head is important to elbow stability in this situation and therefore should not be resected. Prosthetic replacement should be performed when a radial head fracture is irreparable in complex injury patterns [17].

There are some limitations of this study. This is a retrospective study and has the biases of this study design with a small sample size. Future research with a randomized controlled trial may help to draw a conclusion of how much the bone graft can attribute to the obtained results. The accurate indications for ORIF with bone grafts for these fractures also need to be explored.

Conclusion

Although radial head fractures may not be amenable to internal fixation, our findings suggest that ORIF with an autogenous bone graft provides satisfactory elbow function in patients with comminuted Mason type II radial head fractures.

Abbreviations

MEPS: Mayo Elbow Performance Score; ORIF: open reduction and internal fixation; ROM: range of motion

Acknowledgements

We thank Angela Morben, DVM, ELS, from Liwen Bianji, Edanz Editing China (www.liwenbianji.cn/ac), for editing the English text of a draft of this manuscript.

Authors' contributions

GYL: Drafting the manuscript and surgical treatment. EMC: Data analysis and drafting the manuscript. DLX: Acquisition of the data. WHM: Analysis and interpretation of the data. LJZ: Patient review. JMC: Interpretation of the data. ZJP: Conception, design and manuscript revision. All authors read and approved the final manuscript.

Consent for publication

Not applicable.

Competing interests

The authors declare that they have no competing interests.

Author details

[1]Department of Orthopedics, Ningbo NO.6 Hospital, 1059 Zhongsandong Road, Ningbo, Zhejiang 315040, People's Republic of China. [2]Department of Orthopedics, the Second Affiliated Hospital, School of Medicine, Zhejiang University 88 Jiefang RoadHangzhou, Zhejiang 310009, People's Republic of China.

References

1. Mason ML. Some observations on fractures of the head of the radius with a review of one hundred cases. Br J Surg. 1954;42:123–32.
2. Johnston GW. A follow-up of one hundred cases of fracture of the head of the radius with a review of the literature. Ulster Med J. 1962;31:51–6.
3. Herbertsson P, Josefsson PO, Hasserius R, Besjakov J, Nyqvist F, Karlsson MK. Fractures of the radial head and neck treated with radial head excision. J Bone Joint Surg Am. 2004;86:1925–30.
4. Ikeda M, Oka Y. Function after early radial head resection for fracture: a retrospective evaluation of 15 patients followed for 3–18 years. Acta Orthop Scand. 2000;71:191–4.
5. Ikeda M, Yamashina Y, Kamimoto M, Oka Y. Open reduction and internal fixation of comminuted fractures of the radial head using low-profile mini-plates. J Bone Joint Surg Br. 2003;85:1040–4.
6. Ikeda M, Sugiyama K, Kang C, Takagaki T, Oka Y. Comminuted fractures of the radial head. Comparison of resection and internal fixation. J Bone Joint Surg Am. 2005;87:76–84.
7. Ring D, Quintero J, Jupiter JB. Open reduction and internal fixation of fractures of the radial head. J Bone Joint Surg Am. 2002;84:1811–5.
8. Lott A, Broder K, Goch A, Konda SR, Egol KA. Results after radial head arthroplasty in unstable fractures. J Shoulder Elb Surg. 2018;27:270–5.
9. Ring D. Monteggia fractures. Orthop Clin North Am. 2013;44:59–66.
10. Jupiter JB, Leibovic SJ, Ribbans W, Wilk RM. The posterior Monteggia lesion. J Orthop Trauma. 1991;5:395–402.
11. Regan W, Morrey B. Fractures of the coronoid process of the ulna. J Bone Joint Surg Am. 1989;71:1348–54.
12. Businger A, Ruedi TP, Sommer C. On-table reconstruction of comminuted fractures of the radial head. Injury. 2010;41:583–8.
13. Smith GR, Hotchkiss RN. Radial head and neck fractures: anatomic guidelines for proper placement of internal fixation. J Shoulder Elb Surg. 1996;5:113–7.
14. Soyer AD, Nowotarski PJ, Kelso TB, Mighell MA. Optimal position for plate fixation of complex fractures of the proximal radius: a cadaver study. J Orthop Trauma. 1998;12:291–3.
15. Caputo AE, Mazzocca AD, Santoro VM. The nonarticulating portion of the radial head: anatomic and clinical correlations for internal fixation. J Hand Surg Am. 1998;23:1082–90.
16. McKee MD, Pugh DM, Wild LM, Schemitsch EH, King GJ. Standard surgical protocol to treat elbow dislocations with radial head and coronoid fractures. Surgical technique. J Bone Joint Surg Am. 2005;87 Suppl 1(Pt 1):22–32.
17. Pugh DM, Wild LM, Schemitsch EH, King GJ, McKee MD. Standard surgical protocol to treat elbow dislocations with radial head and coronoid fractures. J Bone Joint Surg Am. 2004;86-A:1122–30.
18. Garrigues GE, Wray WH 3rd, Lindenhovius AL, Ring DC, Ruch DS. Fixation of the coronoid process in elbow fracture-dislocations. J Bone Joint Surg Am. 2011;93:1873–81.

19. Broberg MA, Morrey BF. Results of delayed excision of the radial head after fracture. J Bone Joint Surg. 1986;68A:669–74.
20. Charalambous CP, Stanley JK, Siddique I, Powell E, Ramamurthy C, Gagey O. Radial head fracture in the medial collateral ligament deficient elbow; biomechanical comparison of fixation, replacement and excision in human cadavers. Injury. 2006;37:849–53.
21. Hall JA, MD MK. Posterolateral rotatory instability of the elbow following radial head resection. J Bone Joint Surg Am. 2005;87:1571–9.
22. Jensen SL, Olsen BS, Sojbjerg JO. Elbow joint kinematics after excision of the radial head. J Shoulder Elbow Surg. 1999;8:238–41.
23. Flinkkilä T, Kaisto T, Sirniö K, Hyvönen P, Leppilahti J. Short- to mid-term results of metallic press-fit radial head arthroplasty in unstable injuries of the elbow. J Bone Joint Surg Br. 2012;94(6):805–10.
24. van Riet RP, Sanchez-Sotelo J, Morrey BF. Failure of metal radial head replacement. J Bone Joint Surg Br. 2010;92:661–7.
25. Morrey BF, Chao EY, Hui FC. Biomechanical study of the elbow following excision of the radial head. J Bone Joint Surg Am. 1979;61:63–8.
26. Epner RA, Bowers WH, Guilford WB. Ulnar variance. The effect of wrist positioning and roentgen filming technique. J Hand Surg Am. 1982;7:298–305.
27. Geel CW, Palmer AK. Radial head fractures and their effect on the distal radio-ulnar joint. A rationale for treatment. Clin Orthop Relat Res. 1992;275:79–84.
28. Heim U. Kombinierte Verletzungen von Radius und Ulna im proximalen Unterarmsegment. Hefte Unfallchir. 1994;241:61–79.
29. Oztürk K, Esenyel CZ, Orhun E, Ortak O, Durmaz H. The results of open reduction and internal fixation of radial head fractures. Acta Orthop Traumatol Turc. 2004;38:42–9.
30. Patel VR, Elliott DS. Salvage of the head of the radius after fracture-dislocation of the elbow. A case report. J Bone Joint Surg Br. 1999;81:306–8.
31. Luenam S, Kosiyatrakul A, Jangsombatsiri W, Pimpabootr N, Vathana T. Midterm outcome of partial radial head replacement with a contoured iliac crest bone graft in complex elbow dislocation. J Orthop Surg (Hong Kong). 2018;26 https://doi.org/10.1177/2309499017754105.
32. Ring D, Jupiter JB, Zilberfarb J. Posterior dislocation of the elbow with fractures of the radial head and coronoid. J Bone Joint Surg Am. 2002;84-A:547–51.

15

Efficacy of internal fixation with mini plate and internal fixation with hollow screw for Regan-Morrey type II and III ulna coronoid fractures

Hong-Wei Chen[1†], Hong-Hui He[2†] and Bin-Li Gao[3*]

Abstract

Background: Ulna coronoid fracture is a complicated injury and occurred in the coronal plane. Undeniably, there is no universally accepted approach for treating ulna coronoid fractures. Therefore, this study aimed at exploring the efficacy of different surgical treatments for Regan-Morrey type II and III ulna coronoid fractures.

Methods: A total of 164 patients with ulna coronoid fractures were admitted and treated in department of orthopedics at Yiwu Central Hospital, the Affiliated Yiwu Hospital of Wenzhou Medical University for retrospective analysis. The baseline features (age, gender, time from injury to surgery and so on) before the surgery and different conditions during the surgery were compared. Following that, the Visual Analogue Scale (VAS) pain score was employed to evaluate the severity of preoperative and postoperative pain experienced by the patients in each group. Afterwards, Broberg and Morrey elbow score was used to evaluate elbow joint function and surgical effect of the patients. Lastly, the postoperative recovery and complications were compared.

Results: It was firstly observed that internal fixation with mini plate and hollow screw compelled to lower average operation time and blood loss than Kirschner wire and steel wire suture. Next, the severity of postoperative pain was lessened in comparison with preoperative pain. Afterwards, mini plate and hollow screw improved elbow joint function more notable than Kirschner wire and steel wire suture, and Kirschner wire and steel wire suture resulted in higher incidence of complications and worse postoperative recovery.

Conclusion: Collectively, this study clarified that for the treatment of Regan-Morrey type II and III ulna coronoid fractures, internal fixation with mini plate and hollow screw has an overall superior surgical effect than internal fixation with Kirschner wire and steel wire suture.

Keywords: Ulna coronoid fracture, Regan-Morrey type II and III, Mini plate; hollow screw, Kirschner wire, Steel wire suture, Elbow joint function, VAS pain score

Background

Coronoid fractures are seldom isolated injuries and usually associated with other elbow injuries, which serve as three major instability patterns, including type I fractures (related to terrible triad injuries), type II fractures (related to varus posteromedial rotatory instability) and type III fractures (related to transolecranon fracture-dislocations) [1]. Ulna coronoid fractures play pivotal roles in providing ulnohumeral joint stability and are regarded as stabilizers against axial, varus, posteromedial, and posterolateral forces (articular laxity was noticed in the coronal or sagittal planes) [2]. The ulna coronoid fractures are important for maintaining the stability of elbows after dislocation and can be fractured, consequently leading to a coronoid fracture, an infrequent injury occurring in about 2–15% of patients with dislocated elbows [3]. A relation between coronoid fractures with specific patterns of traumatic

* Correspondence: Drgao_binli@163.com
[†]Hong-Wei Chen and Hong-Hui He contributed equally to this work.
[3]Department of Orthopedics, the Affiliated Hospital of Inner Mongolia Medical University, No. 1, Tongdao North Road, Hohhot 010050, The Inner Mongolia Autonomous Region, People's Republic of China

elbow instability has been reported [4]. Recent evidence has shown that coronoid fractures result from avulsing force of the brachialis muscle with a hyperextended position of the elbow joint, as well as shearing force acting upon the surface of the trochlear with posterior dislocation of the elbow joint [5]. At present, coronoid fractures are usually caused by traffic accidents, with some incidence from falls, explosions, and local trauma [6, 7]. Although ulna coronoid fractures are rare, they still negatively influence and impact the functional outcome if proper treatment is not administered [8]. Therefore, it is of great clinical significance to find an effective treatment option for ulna coronoid fractures.

Surgical treatment with open reduction and internal fixation has gained popularity recently [9]. A previous study supports surgical treatment of patients with elbow dislocations related to Regan-Morrey type II and III coronoid fractures for improved elbow reduction, stability, and early motion [10]. Another study suggested that rigid internal fixation could aid in treating significant displacement of coronoid process [11]. Besides, a recent study indicates that ulna coronoid fractures can be treated by internal fixation with frame shape plate and open reduction through anterior approach of the elbow, as it is an effective treatment option with minimal damage and strong fixation [12]. It has been previously reported that ulna coronoid fractures treated with internal fixation had better mechanical resistance than suture anchors for fixing small fragments and internal fixation with tension band wiring with steel wire is an excellent approach to treat coronoid fractures [13–15]. Internal fixation with mini plate is effective for early functional exercise as it provides sufficient stability and improves functional outcome [16]. Iannuzzi NP with 10 pairs of fresh frozen Regan-Morrey type II coronoid fractures cadaveric elbow found that screw fixation provided greater overall foundation with superior strength (405 N VS 207 N) and stiffness (284 thousand PA/mm VS 119 thousand PA/mm) compared to suture lasso fixation, and for the treatment of Regan-Morrey type II coronoid fractures, biomechanical property of screw fixation was superior than the property of suture lasso fixation [17]. Therefore, this study aims to compare the efficacy of internal fixation with mini plate, hollow screw, Kirschner wire and steel wire suture for the treatment of Regan-Morrey type II and III ulna coronoid fractures.

Methods

Ethics statement

The study was conducted with approval and under supervision of the Ethics Committee of Yiwu Central Hospital, the Affiliated Yiwu Hospital of Wenzhou Medical University. All subjects in this study were informed and all participants and their families signed informed consent in accordance with *Helsinki Declaration*. This experiment has been registered in the Chinese Clinical Laboratory Center.

Study subjects

With the aim of retrospective analysis, a total of 164 patients (male = 90; female = 74; average age = 36.2 ± 6.7) with ulna coronoid fractures were admitted and treated in department of orthopedics at Yiwu Central Hospital, the Affiliated Yiwu Hospital of Wenzhou Medical University from September 2012 to September 2016. Among these patients, there were 102 cases of falls and 62 cases of traffic injuries; 83 cases were of left side injuries while the remaining 81 cases were of right side injuries. The reported average time from injury to operation was 4.6 ± 1.2 days. According to the different internal fixation methods, the patients were grouped into four groups for retrospective analysis: mini plate group (31 cases), hollow screw group (44 cases), Kirschner wire group (62 cases), and steel wire suture group (27 cases). Inclusion criteria was as follows: (1) all patients were diagnosed with ulnar coronoid fractures by X-ray or CT examination and according to Regan-Morrey classification and there were 101 cases of type II coronoid fractures and 63 cases of type III coronoid fractures [18]; (2) all patients had closed fractures, and the operation was performed within 1 week after injury; (3) patients with in good physical condition for surgery; (4) patients can be trained and re-examined regularly after surgery. Exclusion criteria was as follows: (1) the injured elbow had been surgically operated upon once; (2) patients with old fracture, open fracture, comminuted fractures and their free articular fragments cannot be reset with a minimally invasive method; (3) patients with elbow joint dysfunction; (4) patients with significant nerve and vascular injury interfering with postoperative rehabilitation.

Surgical treatment

All patients were treated with routine auxiliary examination before surgery. The patients in supine position were administered a combination of intravenous inhaled anesthesia or brachial plexus anesthesia. After administering anesthesia, the C-arm X-ray machine was directed at the injured elbow and the injured elbow was adjusted to the right angle for traction reduction under observation of the C-arm X-ray machine. An anterior approach (repair of the distal biceps tendon) to the elbow joint was made. During the surgery, a longitudinal incision was made along the outside of the pronator circular muscle and a blunt tool was used to incise the subcutaneous tissue to protect the medial forearm dermatome and lateral forearm dermatome. Alongside, the circular muscles were pulled to the inside to protect the median nerve, as it was of great importance to avoid contact with the median nerve during the surgery. With the elbow joint flexed at 45°, the humeral muscle stop point and anterior elbow joint capsule as well as the ulna coronoid fractures were exposed. After operating upon the fracture, the coronoid was fixed with a mini plate, hollow screw, Kirschner wire and steel wire suture, respectively. Vital signs of the patients were monitored routinely after surgery and the patients were administered pain relief, detumescence and anti-infection treatments. After 3 days, the patients performed passive elbow flexion and elbow movement as well as active movement of wrists and fingers under the guidance of doctors.

Outcome evaluation

The patients' operation time and intraoperative blood loss were recorded (both the operator and the anesthetist measured intraoperative blood loss via visual method and estimated the amount of blood in the negative pressure bottle by weighing the amount of blood loss in the gauze.). The patients were followed up on 3 d, 1 month, 3 months, 6 months and 12 months after surgery (follow-up period from September 2016 to September 2017 for 1 year). Follow-up examination included X-ray (the fracture healing was evaluated by X-ray CT and the criterion for inclusion was the presence of the blurring fracture line with continuous osteophytes passing through the fracture line), fractures healing time, elbow joint activity, elbow joint stability, pain and complications. Broberg and Morrey elbow score was used to evaluate the function of elbow joint 1 year after surgery. This score is out of 100 points, with 40 points for elbow joint activity, 20 points for elbow joint strength, 5 points for elbow joint stability, and 35 points for pain; 95 ~ 100 points were regarded as excellent; 80 ~ 94 points were regarded as good; 60 ~ 79 points were regarded as medium; 0 ~ 59 points were regarded as poor [19]. Visual Analogue Scale (VAS) was used to evaluate the pain of patients 1 year after surgery (out of a score of 10 points): 0 point was no pain; 1–3 points signified mild and bearable pain; 4–6 points signified bearable pain which could affect sleep; 7–10 points signified gradually increasing and unbearable pain affecting appetite and sleep [20].

Statistical analysis

Statistical analysis was performed using the SPSS 21.0 statistical software (IBM Corp., Armonk, NY, USA). Measurement data were presented as mean ± standard deviation. Through homogeneity of variance test, *t*-test was employed for comparing between the two groups with homogeneity of variance, and Wilcoxon rank sum test was employed for comparing among multiple groups without homogeneity of variance and normal distribution. Enumeration data were expressed by constituent ratio or rate and examined by the chi square test. A one-way analysis of variance (ANOVA) with replicate measurement was used to compare data at a specific time points within a group, while multi-group data was compared using single factor ANOVA or multi-group chi-square test. A two-sided test was performed and a value of $p < 0.05$ was considered to be statistically significant.

Table 1 Comparison of clinical characteristics of patients with ulna coronoid fractures among the four groups

	Mini plate group ($n = 31$)	Hollow screw group ($n = 44$)	Kirschner wire group ($n = 62$)	Steel wire suture group ($n = 27$)	p
Gender (male/female)	19/12	23/21	36/26	12/15	0.557
Average age (year)	38.8 ± 6.1	35.0 ± 6.9	35.5 ± 6.6	36.1 ± 6.4	0.076
Time between injury and surgery (d)	4.5 ± 1.1	4.8 ± 1.3	4.3 ± 1.3	4.4 ± 1.0	0.217
Regan-Morrey type					
II	21	29	34	17	0.56
III	10	15	28	10	
Cause of injury					
Fall	17	23	44	18	0.186
Traffic injury	14	21	18	9	
Laterality of injury					
Left side	12	19	38	14	0.134
Right side	19	25	24	13	
Combined injury					
Dislocation of elbow joint	21	27	44	23	0.200
Simple ulna coronoid fractures	10	17	18	4	

Notes: Measurement data or counting data were presented as mean ± standard deviation or number of cases; one-way analysis of variance (ANOVA) with replicate measurement or chi square test were used to compare multi-group data; a value of $p < 0.05$ was considered to be statistically significant

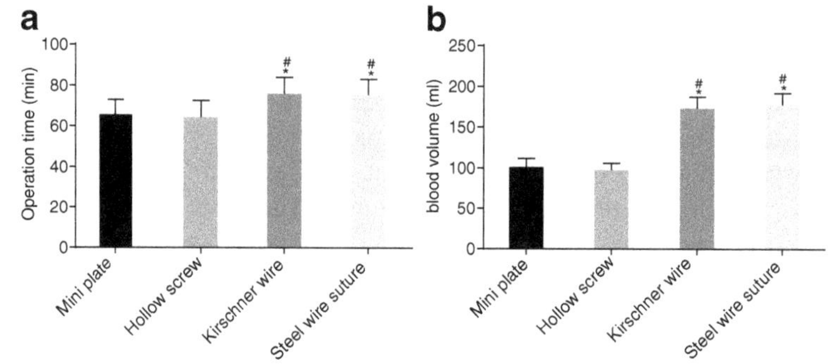

Fig. 1 Internal fixation with mini plate and hollow screw decreases average operation time and blood loss in comparison to Kirschner wire and steel wire suture. **a** comparison of operative time of patients between four groups; **b** comparison of intraoperative blood loss of patients between four groups. $n = 31$ in the mini plate group; $n = 44$ in the hollow screw group; $n = 62$ in the Kirschnner wire group; $n = 27$ in the steel wire suture group; measurement data was presented as mean ± standard deviation; multi-group data was compared using single factor ANOVA; *, vs. the mini plate group, $p < 0.05$; #, vs. the hollow screw group, $p < 0.05$

Results

Baseline characteristics of patients with ulna coronoid fractures in the four groups

Initially, the baseline characteristics of patients in each group were compared. The mini plate group (31 cases) included 9 males and 12 females with an average age of 38.8 ± 6.1 years. The hollow screw group (44 cases) included 23 males and 21 females with an average age of 35.0 ± 6.9 years. The Kirschner wire group (62 cases) included 36 males and 26 females with an average age of 35.5 ± 6.6 years. The steel wire suture group (27 cases) included 12 males and 15 females with an average age of 36.1 ± 6.4 years. No significant differences were observed in parameters of gender, average age, time from injury to surgery, Regan-Morrey type, cause of injury, laterality of injury and combined injury among the four groups ($p > 0.05$) (Table 1).

Internal fixation with mini plate and hollow screw caused lower average operation time and blood loss than Kirschner wire and steel wire suture

Following that, the different surgical conditions in four groups were compared. On comparing the operation time and intraoperative blood loss in the four groups, it was found that the mini plate group and the hollow screw group had significantly lower average operation time and average blood loss than the Kirschner wire group and the steel wire suture group (all $p < 0.05$). No significant differences were observed in the average operation time and average blood loss between the mini plate group and the hollow screw group (both $p > 0.05$). Similarly, no significant differences in average operation time and average blood loss were observed between the Kirschner wire group and the steel wire suture group, either (both $p > 0.05$) (Fig. 1). Altogether, patients undergoing internal fixation with mini plate and hollow screw had a shorter average operation time and lower blood loss than the patients with Kirschner wire and steel wire suture.

The postoperative VAS pain scores are lower than the preoperative VAS pain scores

Next, preoperative pain and postoperative pain of patients in four groups were compared. VAS pain score was used to evaluate the preoperative and postoperative pain of patients in the four groups. It was found that the VAS pain scores 3 days after surgery and 1 month after surgery were significantly lower than the score prior to surgery in the four groups (all $p < 0.05$). On the 3rd day after surgery, the Kirschner wire group and the steel wire suture group had an obviously higher VAS pain scores compared to the mini plate group and the hollow screw group (all $p < 0.05$). However, no significant differences were observed in

Table 2 Comparisons of preoperative and postoperative pain in the four groups

	Mini plate group ($n = 31$)	Hollow screw group ($n = 44$)	Kirschner wire group ($n = 62$)	Steel wire suture group ($n = 27$)
Before surgery	6.74 ± 0.77	6.41 ± 0.66	6.42 ± 0.62	6.63 ± 0.74
At 3 days after surgery	3.90 ± 0.75*	3.86 ± 0.46*	4.58 ± 0.67*#&	4.89 ± 0.51*#&
At 1 month after surgery	0.65 ± 0.49*	0.43 ± 0.50*	0.55 ± 0.50*	0.41 ± 0.50*

Notes: Measurement data were presented as mean ± standard deviation; one-way analysis of variance (ANOVA) with replicate measurement was used to compare data at different time points within-group, while multi-group data was compared using single factor ANOVA; n, number
*vs. the preoperative scores, $p < 0.05$; #vs. the mini plate group, $p < 0.05$; &vs. the hollow screw group, $p < 0.05$

Table 3 The function of elbow joint of patients with ulna coronoid fractures in the four groups

	Mini plate group ($n = 31$)	Hollow screw group ($n = 44$)	Kirschner wire group ($n = 62$)	Steel wire suture group ($n = 27$)
At 1 month after surgery	73.26 ± 10.49	78.45 ± 6.51	60.13 ± 12.42*#	60.59 ± 12.39*#
At 3 months after surgery	75.48 ± 10.62	85.84 ± 5.09*	63.94 ± 12.45*#	65.70 ± 10.81*#
At 6 months after surgery	80.48 ± 10.41	90.36 ± 5.16*	68.58 ± 12.54*#	70.41 ± 11.39*#
At 1 year after surgery	84.90 ± 11.23	94.39 ± 5.68*	73.48 ± 14.05*#	72.96 ± 13.74*#

Notes: Measurement data were presented as mean ± standard deviation; one-way analysis of variance (ANOVA) with replicate measurement was used to compare data at different time points within-group, while multi-group data was compared using single factor ANOVA
* vs. the mini plate group at the same time point, $p < 0.05$; #vs. the hollow screw group at the same time point, $p < 0.05$

the intensity of pain of patients among the four groups 1 month after surgery (all $p > 0.05$) (Table 2). In summary, the postoperative pain was alleviated compared to the preoperative pain.

Mini plate and hollow screw show better elbow joint function than Kirschner wire and steel wire suture

Following that, the elbow joint function of patients in the four groups was compared. Broberg and Morrey elbow score was used to evaluate the postoperative function of elbow joint in the four groups. The results showed that at each given time point after surgery, the Kirschner wire group and the steel wire suture group had notably lower Broberg and Morrey elbow scores than the mini plate group and hollow screw group (all $p < 0.05$). However, the hollow screw group presented significantly higher Broberg and Morrey elbow scores than the mini plate group at 3 months, 6 months and 1 year after surgery time points (all $p < 0.05$) (Table 3).

One year after surgery, the excellent and good functional outcomes of the mini plate group (54.8%) and the hollow screw group (90.9%) were significantly higher than those of the Kirschner wire group (29.0%) and the steel wire suture group (42.2%) (all $p < 0.05$), and the excellent and good functional outcomes of the hollow screw group was considerably higher compared to the outcomes of the mini plate group ($p < 0.05$). No significant difference was observed in the excellent and good functional outcomes between the Kirschner wire group and steel wire suture group ($p > 0.05$) (Table 4, Fig. 2).

Table 4 The surgical effect of patients with ulna coronoid fractures in the four groups

	Mini plate group ($n = 31$)	Hollow screw group ($n = 44$)	Kirschner wire group ($n = 62$)	Steel wire suture ($n = 27$)
Excellent	9	32	14	6
Good	8	8	4	0
Medium	12	4	36	17
Poor	2	0	8	4

Note: Counting data were presented as number of cases; chi square test was used to compare data at different time points within-group; a value of $p < 0.05$ was considered to be statistically significant

In conclusion, the elbow joint function was better in patients with Mini plate and hollow screw than the patients with Kirschner wire and steel wire suture.

Kirschner wire and steel wire suture cause higher incidence of complications and worse postoperative recovery

Finally, the postoperative recovery and complications were evaluated in the four groups. The findings indicated that the hollow screw group and the mini plate group had a significantly shorter fracture healing time and notably higher elbow flexion with better extension degree and forearm rotation degree than the Kirschner wire group and the steel wire suture group (all $p < 0.05$). No nonunion of fracture or delayed union was observed in the hollow screw group and the mini plate group. The hollow screw group had 2 cases of joint instability with 4.55% incidence of complications. The Kirschner wire group had 7 cases of delayed union, 5 cases of nonunion, 7 cases of failure of internal fixation, with 32.26% incidence of complications. The steel wire suture group had 2 cases of delayed union, 5 cases of heterotopic ossification, 4 cases of joint stiffness, with 37.04% incidence of complications. The patients in the Kirschner group and the steel wire suture group were at a higher risk for incidence of complications than the patients of the hollow screw group and mini plate group (Table 5). Therefore, higher incidence of complications and worse postoperative recovery were observable in patients with Kirschner wire and steel wire suture.

Discussion

Coronoid fractures have a low incidence and often occur in combination with other elbow joint injuries [6]. It is reported that the incidence of elbow dislocations is 5.21 per 100,000 people every year in America [21]. Previous evidence has shown that patients with proximal ulna fractures can restore a stable and functional elbow by means of open reduction and internal fixation [22]. Open reduction and internal fixation have been proven to be effective in treating anteromedial facet fracture of ulna coronoid by anatomical reduction and strong fixation [23]. In this study, it was found that internal fixation with mini plate and hollow screw had better efficacy than internal fixation

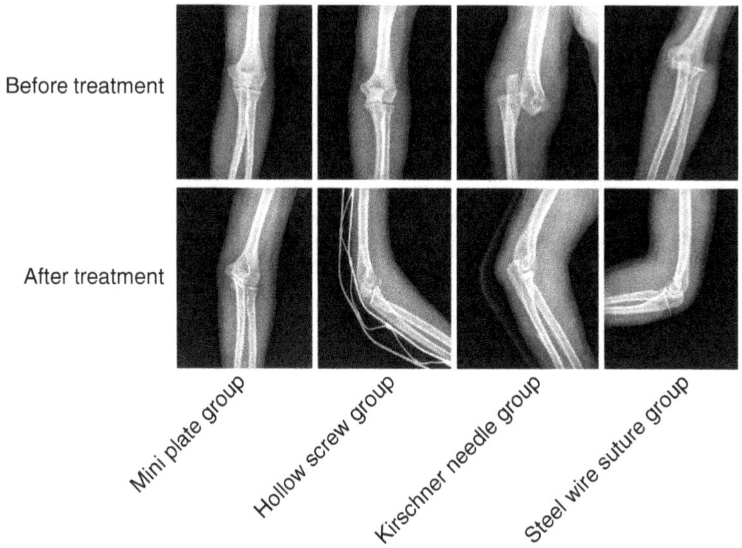

Fig. 2 Mini plate and hollow screw displays better elbow joint function than Kirschner wire and steel wire suture

with Kirschner wire and steel wire suture in treating Regan-Morrey type II and III ulna coronoid fractures.

The present study showed that internal fixation with mini plate and hollow screw had shorter average operation time, lower average blood loss, and less postoperative pain than internal fixation with Kirschner wire and steel wire suture while treating Regan-Morrey type II and III ulna coronoid fractures. A recent study showed that mini-locking plate fixation could be employed to treat Regan-Morrey type III coronoid fractures through elbow anterior approach, for satisfactory outcomes [24]. Another study also demonstrated that an anterior approach is effective for internal fixation of ulnar coronoid fractures because of minimal surgical dissection damage and clear visualization of ulnar coronoid fractures for reduction and internal fixation [25]. Moreover, among numerous surgical treatment techniques, mini plate and screw are superior options as they can stipulate rigid fixation important for progressive bone healing and early active finger motion [26]. In line with our study, Hanks et al. also confirmed that internal fixation of fracture of the coronoid process of the ulna is capable of restoring elbow stability [27]. Furthermore, a previous study has proven that mini-plate fixation as an effective treatment option for ulnar coronoid process fractures [28].

Additionally, our study also demonstrated that compared with internal fixation with Kirschner wire and steel wire suture, internal fixation with mini plate and hollow screw was more effective at restoring elbow joint function and lower incidence of complications after surgery. Another study also indicates that central tension plate internal fixation with sharp hook achieves excellent functional outcome in the treatment of intra-articular olecranon fracture as plate internal fixation is advantageous due to high union rate and low incidence of complications [29].

Conclusion

To conclude, this study found that internal fixation with mini plate and hollow screw was more effective

Table 5 Postoperative recovery and complications in the four groups

	Mini plate group ($n = 31$)	Hollow screw group ($n = 44$)	Kirschner wire group ($n = 62$)	Steel wire suture group ($n = 27$)
Fracture healing time (week)	10.1 ± 1.3	10.8 ± 1.0	13.4 ± 1.3*#	13.0 ± 1.6*#
elbow flexion and extension (°)	114.6 ± 6.5	115.4 ± 8.1	95.7 ± 8.1*#	94.4 ± 7.7*#
forearm rotation (°)	126.0 ± 7.3	127.7 ± 6.0	103.9 ± 4.2*#	102.5 ± 3.8*#
Incidence of complications	0 (0%)	2 (4.55%)	20 (32.26%)*#	10 (37.04%)*#

Notes: measurement data or counting data were presented as mean ± standard deviation or number of cases; one-way analysis of variance (ANOVA) with replicate measurement or chi square test were used to compare multi-group data

* vs. the mini plate group, $p < 0.05$; # vs. the hollow screw group, $p < 0.05$

than internal fixation with Kirschner wire and steel wire suture for treating Regan-Morrey type II and III ulna coronoid fractures. Thus, this study supports some superior treatments for Regan-Morrey type II and III ulna coronoid fractures. However, some other internal fixation methods such as internal fixation of tension band wiring with steel wire should be considered and studied in the future.

Abbreviations

ANOVA: Analysis of variance; VAS: Visual Analogue Scale

Acknowledgments

We would like show sincere appreciation to the reviewers for critical comments on this article.

Funding

This study was supported by Science Technology Department of Zhejiang Province (Grant No. 2013C33216), Health Bureau of Zhejiang Province (Grant No. 2014KYB296), Yiwu Science and Technology Project (Grant No. 2013-G3-02) and Yiwu High-Level Talents Research Project (Grant No. 201603).

Authors' contributions

HWC, HHH and BLG wrote the paper and conceived and designed the experiments; HHH and BLG analyzed the data; HWC and BLG collected and provided the sample for this study. All authors have read and approved the final submitted manuscript.

Competing interests

The authors declare that they have no competing interests.

Author details

[1]Department of Orthopedic Surgery, Yiwu Central Hospital, the Affiliated Yiwu Hospital of Wenzhou Medical University, Yiwu 322000, People's Republic of China. [2]Department of Joint Surgery and Sports Medicine, the Affiliated Nanhua Hospital, University of South China, Hengyang 421002, People's Republic of China. [3]Department of Orthopedics, the Affiliated Hospital of Inner Mongolia Medical University, No. 1, Tongdao North Road, Hohhot 010050, The Inner Mongolia Autonomous Region, People's Republic of China.

References

1. Budoff JE. Coronoid fractures. J Hand Surg Am. 2012;37:2418–23.
2. Shukla DR, Koehler SM, Guerra SM, Hausman MR. A novel approach for coronoid fractures. Tech Hand Up Extrem Surg. 2014;18:189–93.
3. Wells J, Ablove RH. Coronoid fractures of the elbow. Clin Med Res. 2008;6:40–4
4. Ring D, Horst TA. Coronoid Fractures. J Orthop Trauma. 2015;29:437–40.
5. Lee JM, Yi Y, Kim JW. Arthroscopically assisted surgery for coronoid fractures. Orthopedics. 2015;38:742–6.
6. Kiene J, Waldchen J, Paech A, Jurgens C, Schulz AP. Midterm results of 58 fractures of the coronoid process of the ulna and their concomitant injuries. Open Orthop J. 2013;7:86–93.
7. Samman M, Ahmed SW, Beshir H, Almohammadi T, Patil SR. Incidence and pattern of mandible fractures in the Madinah region: a retrospective study. J Nat Sci Biol Med. 2018;9:59–64.
8. Manidakis N, Sperelakis I, Hackney R, Kontakis G. Fractures of the ulnar coronoid process. Injury. 2012;43:989–98.
9. Steinmann SP. Coronoid process fracture. J Am Acad Orthop Surg. 2008;16:519–29.
10. Aksu N, Korkmaz MF, Gogus A, Kara AN, Isiklar ZU. Surgical treatment of elbow dislocations accompanied by coronoid fractures. Acta Orthop Traumatol Turc. 2008;42:258–64.
11. Kale TP, Aggarwal V, Kotrashetti SM, Lingaraj JB, Singh A. Mandibular coronoid fractures, how rare? J Contemp Dent Pract. 2015;16:222–6.
12. Yao S, Zhao C, Wu H, Cao Y. To cure coronoid process fractures of ulna through anterior approach of the elbow and frame shape plate internal fixation. Zhonghua Yi Xue Za Zhi. 2015;95:3678–80.
13. Garrigues GE, Wray WH 3rd, Lindenhovius AL, Ring DC, Ruch DS. Fixation of the coronoid process in elbow fracture-dislocations. J Bone Joint Surg Am. 2011;93:1873–81.
14. Clarke SE, Lee SY, Raphael JR. Coronoid fixation using suture anchors. Hand (N Y). 2009;4:156–60.
15. Mallard F, Hubert L, Steiger V, Cronier P. An original internal fixation technique by tension band wiring with steel wire in fractures of the coronoid process. Orthop Traumatol Surg Res. 2015;101:S211–5.
16. Kuang X, Cai H, Bao F, Huang H, Gong L, Lou Y, Chen X. Treatment of ulnar coronoid process fracture with mini-plate. Zhongguo Xiu Fu Chong Jian Wai Ke Za Zhi. 2010;24:1097–9.
17. Iannuzzi NP, Paez AG, Parks BG, Murphy MS. Fixation of Regan-Morrey type II coronoid fractures: a comparison of screws and suture lasso technique for resistance to displacement. J Hand Surg Am. 2017;42:e11-e4.
18. Regan W, Morrey B. Fractures of the coronoid process of the ulna. J Bone Joint Surg Am. 1989;71:1348–54.
19. Broberg MA, Morrey BF. Results of delayed excision of the radial head after fracture. J Bone Joint Surg Am. 1986;68:669–74.
20. Aitken RC. Measurement of feelings using visual analogue scales. Proc R Soc Med. 1969;62:989–93.
21. Stoneback JW, Owens BD, Sykes J, Athwal GS, Pointer L, Wolf JM. Incidence of elbow dislocations in the United States population. J Bone Joint Surg Am. 2012;94:240–5.
22. Melamed E, Danna N, Debkowska M, Karia R, Liporace F, Capo JT. Complex proximal ulna fractures: outcomes of surgical treatment. Eur J Orthop Surg Traumatol. 2015;25:851–8.
23. Huang HB, Ji XR, Fan SW, Bao F. Internal fixation for the treatment of anteromedial facet fracture of the coronoid process of ulna. Zhongguo Gu Shang. 2013;26:158–61.
24. Lian X, Zeng YJ. Mini-locking plates for the treatment of Regan-Morrey type III fracture of ulnar coronoid process through anterior approach of elbow joint. Zhongguo Gu Shang. 2017;30:9–13.
25. Yang X, Chang W, Chen W, Liu S, Zhu Y, Zhang Y. A novel anterior approach for the fixation of ulnar coronoid process fractures. Orthop Traumatol Surg Res. 2017;103:899–904.
26. Basar H, Basar B, Basci O, Topkar OM, Erol B, Tetik C. Comparison of treatment of oblique and spiral metacarpal and phalangeal fractures with mini plate plus screw or screw only. Arch Orthop Trauma Surg. 2015;135:499–504.
27. Hanks GA, Kottmeier SA. Isolated fracture of the coronoid process of the ulna: a case report and review of the literature. J Orthop Trauma. 1990;4:193–6.
28. Chen H, Pan J. Efficacy and outcome of open reduction and internal fixation with mini-plate in ulnar coronoid process fractures. Int J Clin Exp Med. 2016;9:8858–64.
29. Chen W, Zhang Q, Hou Z, Zhang Y. The application of central tension plate with sharp hook in the treatment of intra-articular olecranon fracture. BMC Musculoskelet Disord. 2013;14:308.

16

Epidemiology of Adult Ankle Fractures: 1756 cases identified in Norrbotten County during 2009–2013 and classified according to AO/OTA

Hans Juto*, Helena Nilsson and Per Morberg

Abstract

Background: The ankle fracture is one of the most common fractures, increasing in an ageing population, but not generally seen as an osteoporotic fracture. The aim of this study was to examine the relationship between different AO/OTA classes of ankle fractures, age, sex and type of trauma.

Methods: Ankle fractures, treated at any of the hospitals in Norrbotten County in Sweden between 2009 and 2013, were retrospectively identified and classified according to the AO/OTA-classification system. Information about the trauma mechanism was also obtained.

Results: In Norrbotten County, 1756 ankle fractures in 1735 patients aged 20 years or older were identified. This gave an incidence in the county of 179 per 100,000 person-years. Of these patients, 34.6% were 65 years or older, 58.4% were women and 68.2% of the trauma leading to a fracture was defined as low-energy. In 1.5% of the cases the fractures were open. Incidences of type B fractures increased substantially with age, from 62 (95% CI 50–77) at 30–39 years of age to 158 (95% CI 131–190) in patients older than 80 years of age per 100,000 person-years. Type B fractures showed a slightly higher proportion of low-energy trauma while type C showed a lower mean age and proportion of women.

Conclusions: This study shows an incidence of 179 adult ankle fractures annually per 100,000 persons. More than two thirds of the fractures were caused by a low-energy trauma and ankle fractures are more frequent among females. Females generally have an increased incidence during their life, mainly between the ages of 30 and 60. This is in contrast to men who have more of an even distribution throughout their life. Classification according to AO/OTA reveals some heterogeneity among the classes of ankle fractures in age and gender as well as the energy involved in the trauma.

Keywords: Ankle fracture, AO/OTA-classification, Epidemiology, Incidence, Osteoporosis

Background

Ankle fractures are one of the most common fractures among the adult population. It is the fourth most frequent fracture type after hip, wrist and hand fractures registered in the Swedish Fracture Register and it constitutes approximately every tenth fracture [1]. Similar numbers were found by Court-Brown et al. in the UK [2]. Ankle fractures are also the second most common fracture requiring hospitalization. However, the length of hospitalization decreases year-by-year [3, 4]. The incidence in different studies varies from 71 to 187 per 100,000 person-years [4–9]. It is generally accepted that the incidence of ankle fractures is rising, particularly among the elderly and female population [4–6, 8, 10].

Ankle fractures are commonly classified by the Danis-Weber, the Lauge-Hansen or the AO/OTA classification system [11]. The AO/OTA classification system of ankle fractures can be seen as a development of the Danis-Weber classification with both the height of the

* Correspondence: hans.juto@norrbotten.se
Sunderby Research Unit, Department of Surgical and Perioperative Sciences (orthopaedics), Umeå University, Umeå, Sweden

fibula fracture taken into account as well as the number of fractured malleoli and comminution of the fibula. The groups of the AO/OTA classification system can also be translated to the Lauge-Hansen system [12].

Ankle fractures are not regarded as the typical fracture associated with osteoporosis. While earlier studies on osteoporosis conclude that fractures of the wrist, humerus, vertebra and hip, for example have a significant relationship with low bone mass, ankle fractures do not [13, 14]. It is also stated that a general increase in age-related incidences is not found among ankle fractures [14, 15]. The majority of ankle fractures are found among patients under the age of 60. [2–4, 7]. In contrast to this, ankle fractures have been shown to increase the risk of a new fracture among postmenopausal women [16]. The epidemiology of ankle fractures is changing and while some earlier studies have reported a male predominance [6, 7] more recent studies now show a significantly higher incidence among females [4, 8, 17]. The age-adjusted incidence of ankle fractures in Finland amongst women over the age of 65 more than doubled between 1970 and 2000. [10]. The majority of studies show that there is a rise in incidence among women to the age of about 60 to 70 and thereafter it levels out or even declines. [3–7, 17–20]. Multimalleolar ankle fractures though, appear to increase with age amongst female patients [4, 5].

While ankle fractures are common, there are reasons to continue studying its epidemiology to better understand the fracture. The aim of this study is to examine the incidence of ankle fractures in Norrbotten County as well as the relationship between AO/OTA-classes of ankle fractures with age, gender and low-energy trauma.

Methods

Identification of fractures

Norrbotten County is the most northerly and sparsely-populated county in Sweden. Ankle fractures are treated at five emergency departments and six rural health care centres. The operative treatment of fractures is conducted at one main trauma hospital (Level II Trauma Centre) and another smaller hospital (Level III Trauma Centre). All hospitals and departments share the same computerized medical record system (VAS), where documentation and X-rays can be obtained. When a patient is treated in a hospital in Sweden there is a mandatory registration of the ICD-10 diagnosis linked to the appointment. Therefore, coverage of ankle fractures through VAS should be close to 100%.

Ankle fractures were identified in patients, 20 years of age or older, through a search in VAS using ICD-10 codes for open- and closed-ankle fractures (S82.50-S82.81). The ankle sprain injury has its individual ICD-10 code (S93.4) and was not included in the search.

To obtain information about the trauma mechanism, information in the referral text was mainly used, complemented in some cases with information from medical records. Low-energy trauma was defined in this study as a fall from a standing height or less, with an eventual physical activity not more than walking. The remaining fractures, including sports injuries and falls down stairs, were defined as non-low-energy trauma. All X-rays of the ankle fractures were extracted from the system, anonymized and numbered. The side (right or left) and date of X-ray was indicated. Patients who fractured their ankles more than once during the period of the study, or patients with a bilateral ankle fracture were identified similarly. Patients who had an ankle fracture diagnosis recorded in different years were checked in the medical record, to lower the risk of not detecting multiple injuries.

Due to the relatively high degree of injury misclassification, the search in VAS was extended by using ICD-10 codes for distal tibia fractures and isolated fibula shaft fractures. (S82.30–82.41). Before obtaining X-rays of these cases, an assessment was first conducted from the referral and medical records, as well as the X-rays, in order to detect if there were cases of ankle fractures misclassified as distal tibia or fibula shaft fractures.

Information about the patients' place of residence is continuously updated in VAS from the governmental residential information database (SPAR), and patients not residing in the county were identified by information in this database and in the medical records. Patients residing in the county, but injured and treated elsewhere, but followed up at home could also be identified.

Classification

The AO/OTA classification system for ankle fractures consists of three classes, nine groups and 27 subgroups. The A11 subgroup is defined as only a sprain and was therefore omitted. In addition to the subgroups, the cases could be defined as "no fracture", "other fracture than ankle" or "ankle fracture but not possible to classify".

Three different observers (HJ, HN and PM) classified the fractures into four levels according to the AO/OTA--system. The instructions at the AO foundation online surgery reference were used as guidelines for the classification [12]. The assessments were made by each observer independently, at their own pace and without access to each other's results. If there was agreement in at least two out of three assessments, the classification was considered final. In cases where there was total disagreement, the fracture was discussed at a final meeting and a majority decision finalized the classification.

Population

The mean adult population in the county during the study period was 196,351 people. The mean age of the total population in the county during the study was 43.3 years. Of the adult population, 49.5% were female [21].

Statistics

Descriptive Statistics in SPSS Statistics version 24 was used to calculate the number in each group, e.g. the number of females over 65 with a B2 fracture. The confidence interval of 95% was calculated in Openepi.com, using the Wilson method for binomial proportion and Mid-P exact test for incidence.

Results

Identified fractures

Between 2009 and 2013, 1851 unique patients aged 20 or older with ICD-10 S82.50-S82.81 (open or closed ankle fracture) were identified. Out of this group of patients, 145 resided outside of the county and were therefore excluded. Another 125 cases were classified from the X-rays, as non-ankle fractures and were also excluded. Thirty-eight of them were patients with diverse types of tibia fractures that had been incorrectly diagnosed as ankle fractures. Fifty were classified as either an avulsion fracture or as a sprain and accordingly excluded. Within the five-year time period of the study, seven patients had fractured both ankles in the same injury. In eleven cases the patients had sustained another (in one case two more) ankle fractures, leading to an additional 19 fractures.

An additional 154 unique patients with 156 ankle fractures within the study period were identified as incorrectly diagnosed with the ICD-10 code S82.30–82.41 (distal tibia or fibula shaft). This resulted in 1756 validated ankle fractures in 1735 patients, 20 years of age or older and resident in the county (Fig 1).

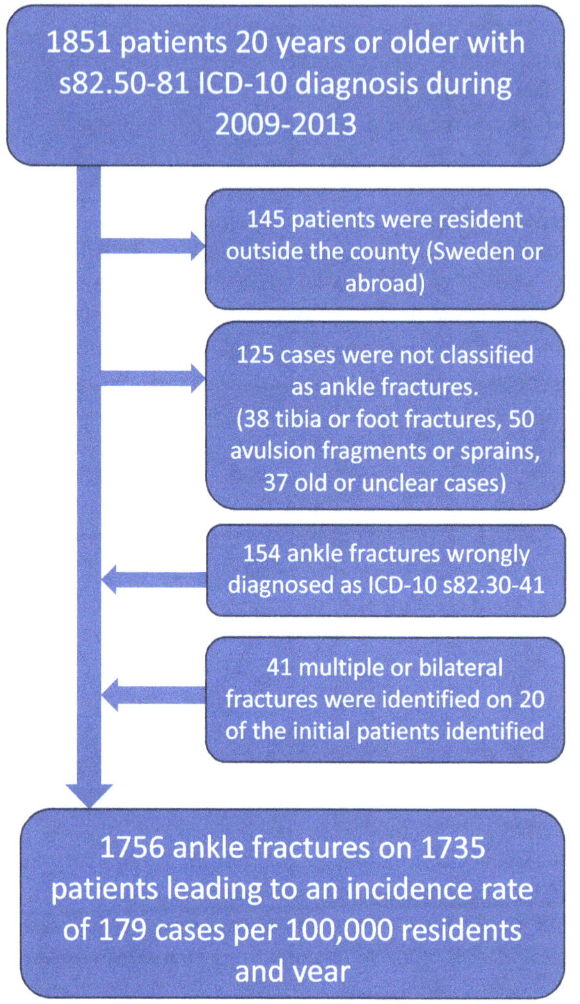

Fig. 1 Flow-chart identification of ankle fracture in computerized medical documentation system

Classification

All the ankle fractures were classified according to the AO/OTA-system by type, group and subgroup. Out of the initial cases (including other fractures and ankle fractures of non-residents, for example) there was complete agreement in the classification of the AO/OTA subgroup level between the three observers in 56% of the cases. In another 36% there were two observers against one and in 9% of the case there was total disagreement and those cases needed to be discussed at a meeting. The interobserver agreement amongst the raters was between 90 and 91% for AO/OTA type level, 75–81% for AO/OTA group and 65–75% for AO/OTA subgroup level.

Regarding ankle fractures, 19.8% were classified as a type A fracture, 66.2% as a type B and 10.6% as a type C fracture. The distribution between the subgroups was uneven and the five largest subgroups constituted 58.8% of all fractures. B11 was by far the largest subgroup with 484 (27.6%) cases while some subgroups like A31-A33, C12 and C32 included only very few cases (Table 1).

Incidence

The incidence of adult ankle fractures in Norrbotten County was 179 cases per 100,000 person-years during the study period. The lowest incidence was seen between 30 and 39 years of age. There was a rise in the incidence peaking at 60–69 years. A plateau with a small but non-significant decrease was thereafter reached. The incidence increased with age from 92 (95% CI 77–109) cases per 100,000 person-years at 30–39 years of age to 238 (95% CI 216–262) cases per 100,000 person-years at 60–69 years of age (Fig. 2). When adjusting the incidence for the age distribution of Sweden, in its entirety, it decreases slightly to 172 cases per 100,000 person-years.

Men had a much more even distributional incidence throughout their lives than females, with only a dip between 30 and 39 years of age. Among females, the

Table 1 Characteristics on 1756 cases of ankle fracture. Number and proportion of the different classes as well as proportion of elderly patients, women and low energy trauma. 95% CI was calculated using Wilson method

AO class	Number, n (%)	> 65 years	Women	Low energy
A	347 (19.8)	35.2 (30.3–40.3)	60.2 (55.0–65.2)	58.8 (53.6–63.9)
A1	243 (13.8)	36.6 (30.8–42.9)	67.9 (61.8–73.5)	64.9 (58.7–70.6)
A12	136 (7.7)	36.8 (29.1–45.1)	66.9 (58.6–74.2)	62.5 (54.1–70.2)
A13	107 (6.1)	36.4 (27.9–45.9)	69.2 (59.9–77.1)	67.9 (58.5–76.1)
A2	91 (5.2)	31.9 (23.2–42.0)	40.0 (30.5–50.3)	43.3 (33.6–53.6)
A21	71 (4.0)	25.4 (16.7–36.6)	31.4 (21.8–43.0)	37.1 (26.8–48.9)
A22	11 (0.6)	63.6 (35.4–84.8)	72.7 (43.4–90.3)	54.5 (28.0–78.7)
A23	9 (0.5)	44.4 (18.9–73.3)	66.7 (35.4–87.9)	77.8 (45.3–93.7)
A3	13 (0.7)	30.8 (12.7–57.6)	61.5 (35.5–82.3)	53.8 (29.1–76.8)
A31	7 (0.4)	14.3 (2.6–51.3)	57.1 (25.1–84.2)	57.1 (25.1–84.2)
A32	2 (0.1)	50.0 (9.5–90.6)	50.0 (9.5–90.6)	100.0 (34.2–100.0)
A33	4 (0.2)	50.0 (15.0–85.0)	75.0 (30.7–95.4)	25.0 (4.6–69.9)
B	1162 (66.2)	36.7 (33.9–39.5)	60.1 (57.2–62.9)	72.0 (69.4–74.5)
B1	649 (37.0)	36.5 (32.9–40.3)	53.0 (49.2–56.8)	71.6 (68.1–75.0)
B11	484 (27.6)	34.7 (30.6–39.1)	53.9 (49.5–58.3)	71.1 (66.9–74.9)
B12	145 (8.3)	42.8 (35.0–50.9)	49.0 (41.0–57.0)	73.8 (66.1–80.3)
B13	20 (1.1)	35.0 (18.1–56.7)	60.0 (38.7–78.1)	70.0 (48.1–85.5)
B2	221 (12.6)	35.7 (29.7–42.3)	59.7 (53.2–66.0)	72.4 (66.1–77.9)
B21	96 (5.5)	26.0 (18.3–35.6)	46.9 (37.2–56.8)	74.0 (64.4–81.7)
B22	111 (6.3)	45.0 (36.1–54.3)	69.4 (60.3–77.2)	72.1 (63.1–79.6)
B23	14 (0.8)	28.6 (11.7–54.7)	71.4 (45.3–88.3)	64.3 (38.8–83.7)
B3	292 (16.6)	37.7 (32.3–43.3)	76.0 (70.8–82.4)	72.6 (67.2–77.4)
B31	100 (5.7)	32.0 (23.7–41.7)	65.0 (55.3–73.6)	72.0 (62.5–79.9)
B32	156 (8.9)	42.3 (34.8–50.2)	80.8 (73.9–86.2)	71.2 (63.6–77.7)
B33	36 (2.1)	33.3 (25.6–55.3)	86.1 (71.3–93.9)	80.6 (65.0–90.3)
C	189 (10.6)	25.4 (19.6–32.1)	48.7 (41.7–55.8)	62.4 (55.4–69.0)
C1	95 (5.4)	29.5 (21.3–39.3)	56.8 (46.8–66.3)	64.2 (54.2–73.1)
C11	61 (3.5)	29.5 (19.6–41,9)	54.1 (41.7–66.0)	70.5 (58.1–80.4)
C12	5 (0.3)	60.0 (23.1–88.2)	60.0 (23.1–88.2)	60.0 (23.1–88.2)
C13	29 (1.7)	24.1 (12.2–42.1)	62.1 (44.0–77.3)	51.7 (34.4–68.6)
C2	59 (3.4)	18.6 (10.7–30.4)	47.5 (35.3–60.0)	59.3 (46.6–70.9)
C21	22 (1.3)	9.1 (2.5–27.8)	31.8 (16.4–52.7)	59.1 (38.7–76.7)
C22	8 (0.5)	37.5 (13.7–69.4)	50.0 (21.5–78.5)	37.5 (13.7–69.4)
C23	29 (1.7)	20.7 (9.8–38.4)	58.6 (40.7–74.5)	65.5 (47.6–80.1)
C3	35 (2.0)	25.7 (14.1–42.1)	28.6 (16.5–45.1)	62.9 (16.3–76.8)
C31	18 (1.0)	27.8 (12.5–50.9)	22.2 (8.5–43.3)	61.1 (38.6–79.7)
C32	3 (0.2)	33.3 (6.15–79.2)	0.0 (0.0–56.2)	0.0 (0.0–56.2)
C33	14 (0.8)	21.4 (7.6–47.6)	42.9 (21.4–67.4)	78.6 (52.4–92.4)
Unclassified	58 (3.3)	20.7 (12.3–32.8)	43.6 (31.4–56.7)	67.3 (53.8–78.5)
Total	1756 (100.0)	34.6 (32.4–36.8)	58.4 (56.1–60.7)	68.2 (66.0–70.4)

incidence increased from 83 (95% CI 63–108) per 100,000 person-years at 30–39 to 319 (95% CI 283–359) at 60–69 years (Fig. 3).

The incidence of type B fractures increased substantially with age and had a similar pattern as ankle fractures. From 62 (95% CI 50–77) at 30–39 years to 158

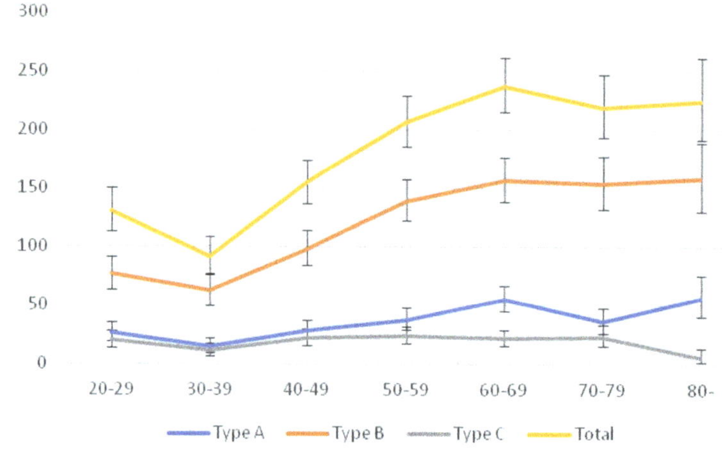

Fig. 2 Incidence per 100,000 person and year according to AO/OTA type and age. Ninety five percent CI was calculated using Mid-P exact test

(95% CI 131–190) at 80 years of age and older per 100,000 person-years. The incidence of type A fractures also increased similarly but not as markedly. From 14 (95% CI 9–22) at 30–39 to 56 (95% CI 45–68) per 100,000 person-years at 60–69 years. Type C fractures had a quite even incidence but with a significantly lower incidence at 30–39 and 80 years of age or older (Fig. 2).

Characteristics of ankle fractures

The mean age of patients in the study with an ankle fracture was 56.3 (range 20–101) years and 34.6% were 65 years of age or older. The percentage of female patients was 58.4 and 68.2% of the trauma leading to the fracture was defined as low-energy. In 1.5% of the cases the fracture was open.

There were more fractures of the right ankle, 53.3% compared to 46.7%. There was also a difference in the frequency of ankle fractures during the year, with three prominent peaks, in December, March and July, while the lowest incidence was in September (Fig. 4). More ankle fractures were observed during the weekend (Fig. 5).

Characteristics of subgroups

Type A, the infra-syndesmotic fractures, showed a smaller number of low-energy trauma than ankle fractures as a whole, but showed no difference in frequency for women or the elderly. Within the subgroups of type A fractures, a somewhat heterogeneous pattern is observed. The isolated medial malleolus fracture, A21, occurred significantly less frequently among females and after less low-energy trauma (Table 1).

The trans-syndesmotic type B fractures, which constituted two thirds of the total number of ankle fractures, had a slightly higher and significant number of low-energy fractures than type A and C fractures. The multi-malleolar type B fractures like B22, B32 and B33 has a somewhat higher frequency of females or/and elderly than unimalleolar B21fractures (Table 1).

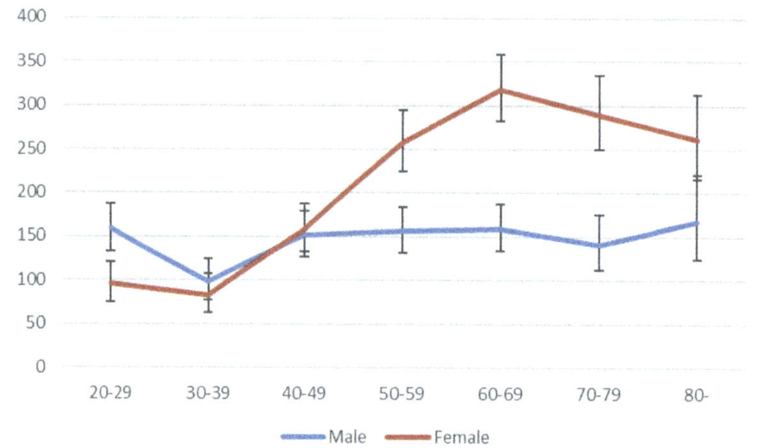

Fig. 3 Incidence per 100,000 persons and year according to gender and age. Ninety five percent CI was calculated using Mid-P exact test

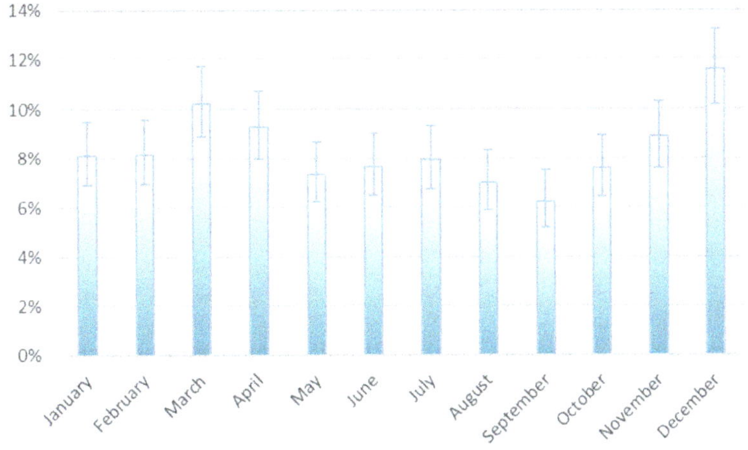

Fig. 4 Distribution of fractures throughout the year. Ninety five percent CI was calculated using Wilson method

Type C or the supra-syndesmotic fracture showed a significantly lower number in elderly and female patients than ankle fractures as a whole, and a lower amount of low-energy trauma than type B fractures (Table 1). Eight supra-syndesmotic fractures were included in the type C classification, even though they did not completely fulfil the conditions as they were equivalent to C13 and C23, but without a medial malleolus fracture.

Unclassified cases

Fifty-eight cases could not be classified according to the AO/OTA system. In 24 cases, pre-treatment X-rays were missing, often because the patients were surgically treated at hospitals outside Norrbotten County. In another 26 cases they only consisted of an isolated posterior malleolus fracture. Three of these cases were caused by axial force, five by dorsal flexion, 13 by twist and in five cases the injury could not be classified.

Discussion

This study shows an incidence of 179 ankle fractures per 100,000 person-years in the county. In comparison to both earlier and similar studies, this study shows a slightly higher incidence. The incidence of ankle fractures has been reported as between 71 and 187 per 100,000 person-years. [4–9]. We see a few reasons for this high incidence in Norrbotten County. Different presuppositions and methodology does, of course, make it difficult to make a completely identical comparison.

A major strength of this study is that we believe we have found almost every possible ankle fracture in the county during the period of study and validated them by examining and classifying every case. However, the strength of the study is also in a way its weakness. The population is relatively small, in a limited area in the far north of Sweden. One can question whether it is possible to generalize the results. Another weakness is that it is a quite low interobserver agreement of the subgroup level of the AO/OTA classification of ankle fracture that

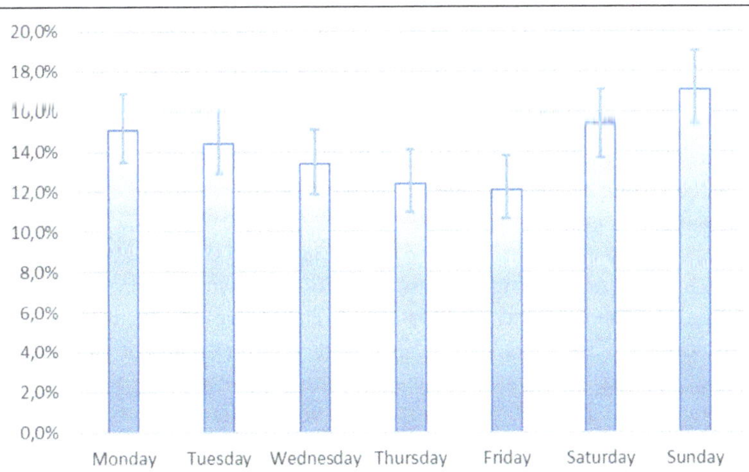

Fig. 5 Distribution of fractures throughout the week. Ninety five percent CI was calculated using Wilson method

can affect the results in the smaller subgroups (e.g. A32 and A33). Even though we have gone to great lengths to find all fractures there may be scenarios where cases have escaped our search. One would be if a patient injured outside the county and did not return within the period of the cast immobilisation.

Elsoe et al. recently published a study on ankle fracture epidemiology in Denmark, reporting an incidence of 169 per 100,000 person-years [8]. In Norrbotten County the mean age of the population is about 2.5 years higher than Sweden's general population [21]. Adjusted for this age difference, the incidence equates to 172 adult ankle fractures per 100,000 person-years. Our results are thereby very similar to those of Elsoe et al. and it seems that this is the true incidence for the period of the study and the region. We can expect similar countries to have a similar incidence.

There is general agreement that the incidence of ankle fractures increases with time, due to an ageing population [4–6, 8, 10]. We agree with this and believe it to be the main reason for the relatively high incidence in our population. The population in Norrbotten County is ageing relatively quickly, the mean age increasing from 40.5 years in 1998 to 43.7 years in 2015 [21]. Another factor that could explain a higher incidence is the long winter season in the county. The incidence increases markedly at the beginning and the end of the winter, when the average temperature is around zero degrees Celsius, resulting in icy and slippery roads and pavements. Our data shows an increase in incidence during the weekend, implying that a general increase in activity, as expected, is also a factor.

One third of the adult ankle fracture patients in the study were 65 years or older. We also observed an increase in incidence from the age of 30–39 to the age of 60–69 and this age group has the highest incidence. This rise in incidence is almost totally caused by the rise among females of nearly four times while men have a more even spread throughout their lives. Elsoe et al. show a similar pattern of incidence but report a decreasing trend among men [8]. We chose not to present the age span over 90 years of age separately, as this group is very small and hence the confidence interval is large.

There is controversy regarding ankle fractures. Should it be characterised as an osteoporotic fracture or not [2, 5, 8, 13, 14, 22–30]? Since a fracture is one of the strongest risk factors for another fracture this is still an important question [31]. A high frequency among women, low-energy trauma as a cause and the incidence increasing with age is seen in osteoporotic fractures. [23, 24]. The proportion of low-energy trauma, as a cause of fractures, was two-thirds in this study. Thur et al. report similar proportions, but in comparison to earlier studies it is slightly higher [4, 6, 9]. This is probably an additional result of an ageing population.

The increase of incidence with age is shown in a number of earlier studies where the highest incidence in females occurs after the age of 65 [4, 6, 8]. Furthermore, a study published recently show an association between lower bone mineral density and ankle fractures [30].

It is difficult to explain the pattern with the rising incidence among women both by age and time, without explaining it as being due to loss of strength in the bone. However, when using a definition of a fragile fracture due to low-energy trauma in an elderly person, they only constitute around one out of four fractures [8, 10]. With a prominent component of osteoporosis as cause of the fracture, this would contradict the plateau in incidence reached after 60 years of age.

We show some differences between the different classes of ankle fracture in the amount of low-energy trauma, gender and age. At one end of the spectrum are the multimalleolar trans-syndesmotic ankle fractures corresponding to B22–3 and B3 representing about every fifth ankle fracture. These occur in female patients in about three-quarters of cases and are caused by low-energy trauma in 70% of cases. It is difficult not to see bone fragility, at least partly, as a cause of this.

At the other end of the spectrum we found type A21 fractures and C fractures. A21 is equivalent to an isolated medial malleolus fracture and shows clear signs of being a non-osteoporotic fracture. It is the one subgroup in our population that stands out and has a low proportion of elderly people; caused in a majority of the cases by a non-low-energy trauma and the patients are mainly men. This is also in agreement with earlier studies [4, 6, 32].

The supra syndesmotic type C ankle fracture has been described as less of an osteoporotic fracture with a lower mean age and a lower frequency of low-energy trauma [6, 9]. Sakaki et al. demonstrate in their study in São Paulo of surgically-treated ankle fractures with a high amount of high-energy trauma that type C fractures compose about 37% of the fractures. More than half of them were high-energy traffic accidents [33]. Briet et al. show in a similar study that all Lauge-Hansen classes except supination external rotation fractures (SER) is, in a majority of the cases, caused by high energy trauma. [32]. In our population, type C fractures show a similar pattern with fewer elderly females and low-energy trauma. However, low-energy trauma is still the cause in over 60% of type C fractures and still one out of four patients are 65 years of age and older.

Court-Brown et al. present a theory where they give medial, lateral, bimalleolar, trimalleolar and supra-syndesmotic ankle fractures different incidence patterns [2]. Even though we do not see this somewhat simplified pattern, we noticed a tendency that supports the theory of an increase with age in lateral malleolus and bimalleolar and trimalleolär ankle fractures, but not in the same way in medial malleolar and supra-syndesmotic ankle fractures.

Compared with Thur et al., we see a lot of similarities in the incidence pattern, except for two differences. One is the decrease in incidence of bimalleolar and trimalleolar fractures after 70 years of age in their study. This can be due to the fact that type C is included in that category. The other difference is that the incidence of lateral malleolar fractures is very low. Our incidence of these is about 2–3 times higher, probably because of the limitation of only including inpatients [4].

Conclusion

This study shows an incidence of 179 adult ankle fractures annually per 100,000 persons. More than two thirds of the fractures were caused by a low-energy trauma and ankle fractures are more frequent among females. Females generally have an increased incidence during their life, mainly between the ages of 30 and 60. This is in contrast to men who have more of an even distribution throughout their life. Classification according to AO/OTA reveals some heterogeneity among the classes of ankle fractures in age and gender as well as the energy involved in the trauma.

Abbreviations

AO: Arbeitsgemeinschaft für osteosynthesefragen; ICD-10: International Statistical Classification of Diseases and Related Health Problems - Tenth Revision; OTA: American Orthopaedic Trauma Association; VAS: Vårdadministrativt System (Digital medical record and administrative system)

Acknowledgements

Appreciation goes to Robert Lundqvist, Research and Invention Department (FoI), Norrbotten County Council, for helping with the statistics. Regarding the extraction of X-rays and information about the fractures we would like to thank Patrik Brännberg and Agnes Bergström.

Funding

Financially the project was supported by grants from FoI Department, Norrbotten County Council.

Authors' contributions

HJ and PM designed the study. HJ and HN extracted X-rays and information from VAS. HJ, HN and PM classified the X-rays according to AO/OTA. HJ carried out the statistical analysis and wrote the first version of the manuscript but all authors took an active part in the revision of it. All authors read and approved the final manuscript.

Consent for publication

Not applicable.

Competing interests

The authors declare that they have no competing interests.

References

1. Möller M. Årsrapport 2013, Svenska Frakturregistret. 2014. (In Swedish) Available at: www.frakturregistret.se
2. Court-Brown CM, Caesar B. Epidemiology of adult fractures: a review. Injury. 2006;37:691–7.
3. Somersalo A, Paloneva J, Kautiainen H, Lönnroos E, Heinänen M, Kiviranta I. Incidence of fractures requiring inpatient care. Acta Orthop. 2014;85:525–30.
4. Thur C, Edgren G, Jansson K, Wretenberg P. Epidemiology of adult ankle fractures in Sweden between 1987 and 2004: a population-based study of 91,410 Swedish inpatients. Acta Orthop. 2012;83:276–81.
5. Bengnér U, Johnell O, Redlung-Johnell I. Epidemiology of ankle fracture 1950 and 1980. Increasing incidence in elderly women. Acta Orthop Scand. 1986;57:35–7.
6. Court-Brown CM, McBirnie J, Wilson G. Adult ankle fractures - an increasing problem? Acta Orthop Scand. 1998;69:43–7.
7. Daly PJ, Fitzgerald RH Jr, Melton LJ, Ilstrup DM. Epidemiology of ankle fractures in Rochester, Minnesota. Acta Orthop Scand. 1987;58:539–44.
8. Elsoe F, Ostgaard SE, Larsen P. Population-based epidemiology of 9767 ankle fractures. Foot and Ankle Surgery. 2017;24(1):34–9. https://doi.org/10.1016/j.fas.2016.11.002.
9. Jensen SL, Andresen BK, Mencke S, Nielsen PT. Epidemiology of ankle fractures. A prospective population-based study of 212 cases in Aalborg, Denmark. Acta Orthop Scand. 1998;69:48–50.
10. Kannus P, Palvanen M, Niemi S, Parkkari J, Järvinen M. Increasing number and incidence of low-trauma ankle fractures in elderly people: Finnish statistics during 1970-2000 and projections for the future. Bone. 2002;31:430–3.
11. Audigé L, Bhandari M, Kellam J. How reliable are reliability studies of fracture classifications? A systematic review of their methodologies. Acta Orthop Scand. 2004;75:184–94.
12. Barbosa P, Bonnaire F, Kojima K. AO surgery reference. 2006. Available at: https://www2.aofoundation.org/wps/portal/surgery?showPage=diagnosis&bone=Tibia&segment=Malleoli. Accessed 11/01, 2014.
13. Seeley DG, Browner WS, Nevitt MC, Genant HK, Scott JC, Cummings SR. Which fractures are associated with low appendicular bone mass in elderly women? The study of osteoporotic fractures research group. Ann Intern Med. 1991;115:837–42.
14. Hasselman CT, Vogt MT, Stone KL, Cauley JA, Conti SF. Foot and ankle fractures in elderly white women. Incidence and risk factors Journal of Bone and Joint SurgeryAmerican Volume (JBJS AM). 2003;85-A:820–4.
15. Baron JA, Barrett JA, Karagas MR. The epidemiology of peripheral fractures. Bone. 1996;18(3 Suppl):209S–13S.
16. Gunnes M, Mellström D, Johnell O. How well can a previous fracture indicate a new fracture? A questionnaire study of 29,802 postmenopausal women. Acta Orthop Scand. 1998;69:508–12.
17. Koval KJ, Lurie J, Zhou W, Sparks MB, Cantu RV, Sporer SM, et al. Ankle fractures in the elderly: what you get depends on where you live and who you see. J Orthop Trauma. 2005;19:635–9.
18. Beerekamp MSH, de Muinck Keizer RJO, Schep NWL, Ubbink DT, Panneman MJM, Goslings JC. Epidemiology of extremity fractures in the Netherlands. Injury. 2017;48:1355–62.
19. Singer BR, McLauchlan GJ, Robinson CM, Christie J. Epidemiology of fractures in 15,000 adults: the influence of age and gender. J Bone Joint Surg Br. 1998;80:243–8.
20. van Staa TP, Dennison EM, Leufkens HG, Cooper C. Epidemiology of fractures in England and Wales. Bone. 2001;29:517–22.
21. SCB – Statistict Sweden Online Databas. Available at: www.scb.se/en. Accessed 11/01, 2016.
22. Kanis JA, Oden A, Johnell O, Jonsson B, de Laet C, Dawson A. The burden of osteoporotic fractures: a method for setting intervention thresholds. Osteoporos Int. 2001;12:417–27.
23. Kannus P, Parkkari J, Niemi S, Palvanen M. Epidemiology of osteoporotic ankle fractures in elderly persons in Finland. Ann Intern Med. 1996;125:975–8.
24. Valtola A, Honkanen R, Kröger H, Tuppurainen M, Saarikoski S, Alhava E. Lifestyle and other factors predict ankle fractures in perimenopausal women: a population-based prospective cohort study. Bone. 2002;30:238–42.
25. Stone KL, Seeley DG, Lui LY, Cauley JA, Ensrud K, Browner WS, Nevitt MC, Cummings SR. BMD at multiple sites and risk of fracture of multiple types: long-term results from the study of osteoporotic fractures. J Bone Miner Res. 2003;18:1947–54.

26. Stein EM, Liu XS, Nickolas TL, Cohen A, Thomas V, McMahon DJ, Zhang C, Cosman F, Nieves J, Greisberg J, Guo XE, Shane E. Abnormal microarchitecture and stiffness in postmenopausal women with ankle fractures. J Clin Endocrinol Metab. 2011;96:2041–8. https://doi.org/10.1210/jc.2011-0309.
27. FitzGerald G, Boonen S, Compston JE, Pfeilschifter J, LaCroix AZ, Hosmer DW Jr, et al. Differing risk profiles for individual fracture sites: evidence from the global longitudinal study of osteoporosis in women (GLOW). J Bone Miner Res Off J Am Soc Bone Miner Res. 2012;27:1907–15.
28. Guggenbuhl P, Meadeb J, Chalès G. Osteoporotic fractures of the proximal humerus, pelvis, and ankle: epidemiology and diagnosis. Joint Bone Spine. 2005;72:372–5.
29. Lee KM, Chung CY, Kwon SS, Won SH, Lee SY, Chung MK, Park MS. Ankle fractures have features of an osteoporotic fracture. Osteoporos Int. 2013;24:2819–25. https://doi.org/10.1007/s00198-013-2394-6.
30. Biver E, Durosier C, Chevalley T, Herrmann FR, Ferrari S, Rizzoli R. Prior ankle fractures in postmenopausal women are associated with low areal bone mineral density and bone microstructure alterations. Osteoporos Int. 2015;26:2147–55. https://doi.org/10.1007/s00198-015-3119-9.
31. Johnell O, Kanis J. Epidemiology of osteoporotic fractures. Osteoporos Int. 2005;16(suppl 2):S3–7.
32. Briet JP, Houwert RM, Smeeing DPJ, Dijkgraaf MGW, Verleisdonk EJ, Leenen LPH, Hietbrink F. Differences in classification between mono- and polytrauma and low- and high-energy trauma patients with an ankle fracture: a retrospective cohort study. J Foot Ankle Surg. 2017;56:793–6.
33. Sakaki MH, Matsumura BA, Dotta Tde A, Pontin PA, Dos Santos AL, Fernandes TD. Epidemiologic study of ankle fractures in a tertiary hospital. Acta Ortop Bras. 2014;22:90–3. https://doi.org/10.1590/1413-78522014220200874.

17

Comparison of screening strategies for prevalent vertebral fractures in South Korea: vertebral fracture assessment vs. spine radiography

Sung-Hee Oh[1,2], Dam Kim[3], Young Eun Lee[1,4], Deog-Yoon Kim[5], Yu Kyung Lee[1], Joo-Hyun Lee[6], Sang-Cheol Bae[3], Yun Young Choi[7], Junhee Pyo[8], Jeonghoon Ahn[1,9*] and Yoon-Kyoung Sung[3*]

Abstract

Background: Vertebral Fracture Assessment (VFA) is a useful tool to detect the vertebral fracture (VF) with low cost and radiation exposure. We aimed to compare screening strategies including VFA and spine radiography (X-ray) for detecting VF in terms of clinical effectiveness, cost and radiation exposure.

Methods: Three screening strategies: 1) X-ray following VFA, 2) VFA only, and 3) X-ray only were compared using a Markov model based on administrative data from South Korea in a population aged ≥50 years. We compared the incidence of new VFs, cost-effectiveness of reducing new VFs and radiation exposure in each strategy.

Results: The incidence of new VFs was reduced in all screening strategies compared to no screening: 29.4% for women and 12.5% for men in both X-ray following the VFA and VFA only strategies and 35% for women and 17. 5% for men in the X-ray only strategy. The X-ray following VFA strategy had the lowest cost, followed by the X-ray only, and VFA only strategies. The radiation doses for X-ray only were 2,647–2,989 μSv and 3,253–3,398 μSv higher than in the X-ray following VFA and VFA only strategies. The new VF prevention effect was greater in women, and more prominent in older people (women ≥ 70, men ≥ 80) than people ≥ 50 years.

Conclusions: The X-ray following VFA strategy is a cost-effective option for screening prevalent VF to prevent new VF in people aged ≥50 years due to its high effectiveness, lowest cost, and least radiation exposure.

Keywords: Spinal fracture, Radiography, Diagnostic imaging, Cost effectiveness, Radiation

Background

Vertebral fracture (VF) is the most common sign of osteoporosis and indicates a higher risk of subsequent VFs [1, 2]. According to previous literature, only around one-fourth to one-third of prevalent VFs are recognized clinically [3–5]. However, detection of prevalent VFs is important because new VFs can be prevented by starting osteoporosis medication at the time of detection, even though bone mineral density (BMD) is not low [5–8]. In clinical practice, screening of VFs is rarely performed because of its cost, fear about radiation exposure, and inconvenience.

Spine radiography (X-ray) and vertebral fracture assessment (VFA) by dual energy X-ray absorptiometry (DXA) can readily detect prevalent VFs [9]. Until now, lateral thoracic and lumbar X-rays have been used as the gold standard for VF identification [6], because of the potential false negative rate of VF due to the poor image quality of the upper thoracic vertebrae in VFA [10, 11]. However, VFA has recently been considered as a practical and reliable diagnostic tool with a lower radiation dose of 2–50 μSv compared to 600 μSv for X-rays [12] and

* Correspondence: ahnjeonghoon@ewha.ac.kr; sungyk@hanyang.ac.kr
Sung-Hee Oh and Dam Kim contributed equally to this work and are joint first authors.
Jeonghoon Ahn and Yoon-Kyoung Sung contributed equally to this work and are joint corresponding authors.
[1]National Evidence-based Healthcare Collaborating Agency, Seoul, Republic of Korea
[3]Department of Rheumatology, Hanyang University Hospital for Rheumatic Diseases, 222-1 wangsimni-ro, Seoundong-gu, Seoul 133-792, Republic of Korea

provides greater convenience in assessing VFs at the same time as measurement of BMD [5].

Increasing evidence indicates that the sensitivity and specificity of VFA are as high as those of X-ray with lower cost and radiation exposure [13]. There has been one study of the cost-effectiveness of VFA versus X-ray in postmenopausal women with osteopenia [14] but none assessing the clinical benefits and disadvantages of X-ray and VFA as a screening tool in the general population. Therefore, in this study, we aimed to compare the clinical effectiveness, cost-effectiveness, and radiation exposures of VF screening strategies in adults aged 50 years and older using X-ray following VFA, VFA only and X-ray only as performed to detect prevalent VFs early and to prevent new VFs.

Methods

Model overview

A model structure comparing the screening strategies for prevalent VFs was developed from a review of the literature [15], clinical guidelines [9, 16], and expert opinion. A Markov model using a cohort simulation with each cohort of 1000 samples for women and men aged 50 years and older that compared screening strategies for identifying the presence of both asymptomatic and symptomatic VFs was created. We ran three Markov models simultaneously, one for each of the screening strategies for detecting prevalent VFs: 1) X-ray following VFA, which is screening of VFA followed by X-ray as confirmation test in patients who were suspicious of vertebral fracture, 2) VFA only, and 3) X-ray only. This index strategy of screening was compared to not doing any screening strategy before recognition of a new VF (No screening) (Fig. 1a).

The health states used in the Markov model were *No VF, Prevalent VF, Post VF, New VF,* and *VFA impossible. Prevalent VF* included radiographic VFs diagnosed by X-ray as well as symptomatic VFs. The subjects started at an initial state of *No VF* or *Prevalent VF*. We assumed that the patients with a VF could not move back to the *No VF* state. All patientswho tested positive for VF were assumed to receive anti-osteoporotic therapy for one year, and patients who tested negative for VF were

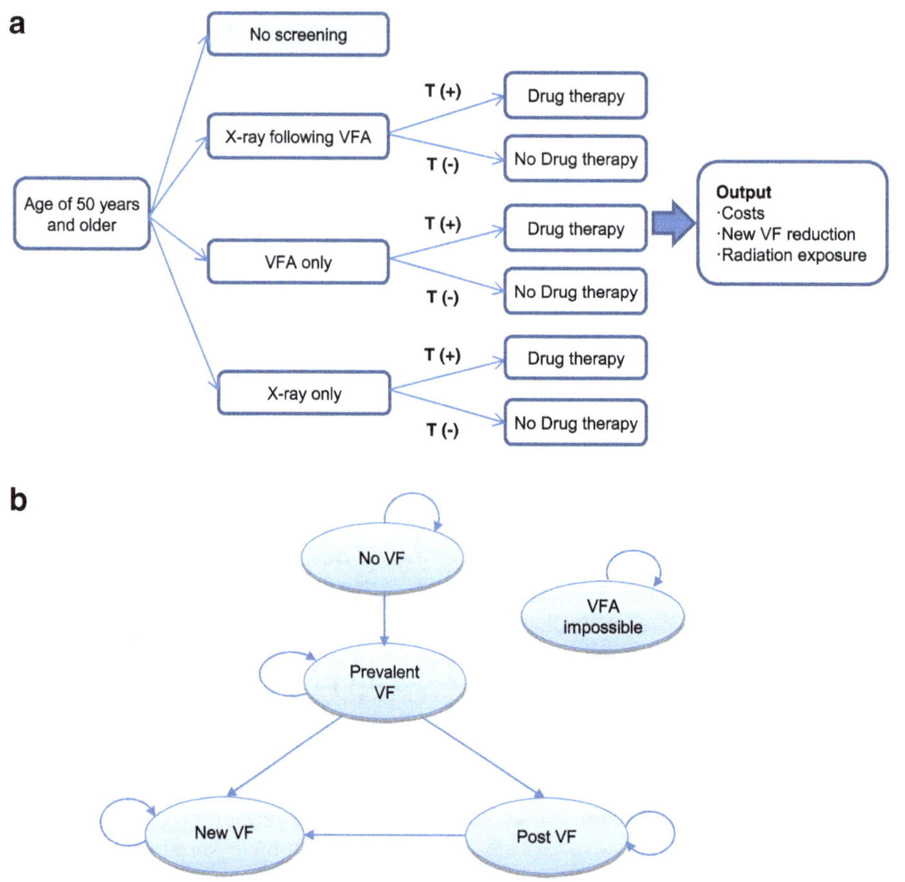

Fig. 1 Model structure for screening strategies to identify prevalent VF. T, test; VF, vertebral fracture; VFA, vertebral fracture assessment; (+), positive; (–), negative. **a** Simplified decision tree: Subjects who tested positive for prevalent VF were treated with anti-osteoporotic drugs, and the cycle length of the screening test was two years. b State transition diagram: the Markov model had five health states: No VF, Prevalent VF, Post VF, New VF, and VFA impossible. If the diagnosis of the new VF has been made once, patients with drug therapy are ruled out of the simulation targets

assumed not to receive anti-osteoporotic therapy. They could either remain in the present state or transit to *Post VF* or *New VF* in a subsequent cycle depending on the effect of drug therapy. Throughout the 10-year period, each subject was allowed to experience a new VF after the first VF. Once diagnosis of a new VF was made, a patient on drug therapy was excluded from the simulation. The model also considered *VFA impossible* as the absorbing state, which means that the VFA was unreadable as a result of poor image quality (Fig. 1b) [11].

Probability data and key assumptions

The prevalence of VFs in adults aged 50 years and older was obtained from a large-scale cohort study conducted in South Korea [17, 18]. The incidence of VFs was estimated based on the linked data between a hospital cohort and the National Health Insurance (NHI) claims database of South Korea [19]. Moreover, the adjusted value was multiplied by an asymptomatic to symptomatic VF ratio of 2.8, which was the weighted average calculated by the literature [4, 20, 21]. This was used because the incidence of VFs before adjustment only considers patients who are clinically diagnosed VFs (Table 1).

In regard to diagnostic accuracy of VFA, the sensitivity and specificity VFA per-patient were taken from a published systematic review and report [13, 22]. In addition, we calculated the unreadable vertebrae on the VFA as 0.03 (95% CI, 0.04–0.17) per patient and 0.05 (95% CI, 0.04–0.08) per vertebra using random-effect estimates [22]. We assumed that the X-ray has a sensitivity and specificity of 1.00 as the gold standard (Table 1).

The relative risk (RR) for new VFs was derived from five systematic review studies [19, 23–26]. The pooled RR was calculated by averaging the RRs weighted by the market share of the prescribed drug based on the 2012 claims database by health insurance review and assessment service (HIRA) (Table 1). We assumed that patients with diagnosed VFs will receive pharmacotherapy for a one year treatment period according to a previous trial [7] and expert opinions. However, the model did not consider the likelihood of adverse drug reaction

Table 1 Summary of the input parameters in the model for base case analysis and univariate sensitivity analysis

Parameter	Value[a]		Sources	Note
	Women	Men		
Probabilities				
VF prevalence	0.22 [0.08]	0.11 [0.03]	HIRA, [17, 18]	NHI database [Community-based cohort]
two-year VF incidence	0.12 [0.13]	0.05 [0.05]	HIRA, [32]	NHI database [Community-based cohort]
two-year new VF incidence	0.22 [0.23]	0.22 [0.23]	[19, 32]	Hospital cohort- NHI database linked data [Community-based cohort]
RR of new VF on drug therapy	0.58 [0.64]	0.38 [0.41]	[19, 23–26]	Meta-analysis literature review, pooled RR [decrease by 10%]
Diagnostic accuracy				
Sensitivity of X-ray	1.00	1.00		Gold standard
Specificity of X-ray	1.00	1.00		Gold standard
Sensitivity of VFA	0.82 [0.74]	0.82 [0.74]	[22]	SR [95% CI lower limit, conservative]
Specificity of VFA	0.93 [0.89]	0.93 [0.89]	[22]	SR [95% CI lower limit, conservative]
VFA impossible	0.03 [0.05]	0.03 [0.05]	[22]	SR, per patient [per vertebrae]
Costs (€)[b]				
VFA[c]	17 [40]	17 [40]	[27]	50% of X-ray test costs [Increase by 200% of X-ray costs, conservative]
X-ray[c]	24 [17]	24 [17]	HIRA	EDI code, thoracic and lumbar spine in the AP and lateral
VFs treatment	1526 [1249]	1707 [1336]	HIRA	NHI database, per patient [Mild VF relatively]
Physician visits	9	9	HIRA	NHI database, per visit
Drug therapy	180	194	HIRA	Drug weighted average charge, one-year administration
Procedure	809	934	HIRA	NHI database, only in symptomatic VF cases
Radiation doses (μSv)				
X-ray	600	600	[12]	
VFA	25 [2]	25 [2]	[12]	Average level of 2 to 50 μSv [lower limit]

VF vertebral fracture, *HIRA* Health Insurance Review and Assessment Service, *NHI* National Health Insurance, *RR* relative risk, *AP* anterior-posterior, *VFA* vertebral fracture assessment, *SR* systematic review

[a]Value in brackets, []: Inputs data for univariate sensitivity analysis

[b]Korean won converted to euros (€) using an exchange rate of 1€ = 1482 KRW (2013)

[c]VFA and X-ray costs included the test and a physician visit

from unnecessary treatment with a false-positive VFA image.

Cost and radiation exposure data

Cost data were collected from the NHI claims data from the HIRA in South Korea [22]. The unit costs for two categories, screening tests and VF treatment, are presented in Table 1. When estimating the costs of the index tests, X-ray was defined as using standard radiographic techniques for VF identification [6]. Since we do not have determined cost of VFA, we calculated that VFA imaging would cost half that of the X-ray, reflecting the U.S. relative cost [27]. The treatment cost of VFs included medical costs such as physician visits, drug therapy, or related procedures. A discount rate of 5% was applied to the future costs with half-cycle corrections according to the South Korean economic evaluation guidelines [28]. All costs were estimated in year 2013 euros using the health care component of the Consumer Price Index [29] and the exchange rate (1€ = 1482 KRW in 2013).

We applied the exposure to radiation at every cycle length of the test at 600 μSv for X-ray; 25 μSv— middle level of the reported range (2–50 μSv)—for VFA; and 625 μSv for X-ray following VFA, respectively [12]. The strategy of no screening was assumed to have no significant exposure to radiation.

Statistical analysis

In the base case analysis, we compared the clinical benefits and harm of doing the screening strategies (defined as Do screening, which presents the average expected values of the X-ray following VFA, VFA only, and X-ray only strategies) every two years and No screening. The outcome measures included incidence of new VFs (%), costs of tests and VFs treatment (€), and radiation exposure (μSv) of the three screening strategies compared to the No screening strategy. Consequently, the results were calculated as follows.

$$\text{Incremental effectiveness } (\Delta E) = \text{Effect}_{\text{index test}} - \text{Effect}_{\text{no screening}}\ (\%)$$

$$\text{Incremental costs } (\Delta C) = \text{Costs}_{\text{index test}} - \text{Costs}_{\text{no screening}}\ (€)$$

$$\text{Incremental radiation exposure } (\Delta RE) = \text{Radiation doses}_{\text{index test}} - \text{Radiation doses}_{\text{no screening}}\ (\mu Sv)$$

* Index test: X-ray following VFA, VFA only, and X-ray only as the Do screening.

Next, we performed univariate and multivariate sensitivity analyses to probe the validity of our model. In the univariate sensitivity analyses, the parameters of the prevalence and incidence of VFs, efficacy of drugs, diagnostic accuracy of VFA, costs of test and VFs treatment, and radiation doses of VFA were varied, using the various sources, range, and conservative approach (Table 1). Since there was no recommended test interval available in the guidelines [16], multivariate sensitivity analysis was conducted using a cycle length of one year.

Finally, the subgroup analysis of old age was conducted for women aged 70 years and older and all men aged 80 years and older since these age groups are recommended especially for VFA in the guidelines [16, 30], for which the input parameters are presented in Table 2.

All the statistical analyses were performed by SAS software version 9.2 (SAS Institute Inc., Cary, NC, USA).

Table 2 Summary of the input parameters in the model for multivariate sensitivity analysis and subgroup analysis

Parameters	Value[a]		Sources	Note
	Women	Men		
Cycle length one-year				
one-year VF incidence	0.06	0.02	HIRA	NHI database
one-year new VF incidence	0.11	0.11	[19]	Hospital cohort-NHI database linked data
VFs treatment cost[a] (€)	1458	1509	HIRA	NHI database
Women aged 70 and older, men aged 80 and older				
VF prevalence	0.43	0.46	[18]	Community-based cohort
two-year VF incidence	0.29	0.17	HIRA	NHI database
two-year new VF incidence	0.32	0.32	[19]	Hospital cohort-NHI database linked data
RR of new VF on drug therapy	0.60	0.60	[33]	Meta-analysis, pooled RR
Sensitivity of VFA	0.88	0.88	[34]	Diagnostic accuracy study for elderly adults
Specificity of VFA	0.99	0.99	[34]	Diagnostic accuracy study for elderly adults
VFs treatment cost[a] (€)	1513	1675	HIRA	NHI database

HIRA Health Insurance Review and Assessment Service, *NHI* National Health Insurance, *VF* vertebral fracture, *VFA* vertebral fracture assessment, *RR* relative risk
[a]Korean won converted to euros (€) using an exchange rate of 1€ = 1482 KRW (2013)

The model was estimated using TreeAge Pro 2013 (TreeAge Software, Williamstown, MA).

Results

Base case analysis

No screening versus do screening for prevalent VF

For women aged 50 and over for a 10-year time horizon, the new VF incidence was 54.6% for No screening, and 23.3% for Do screening with a two-year interval (calculated as the average incidence of X-ray following VFA, VFA only, and X-ray only strategies: 25.2%, 25.2%, and 19.6%, respectively). The expected costs were €967 higher for Do screening; and the radiation exposure was 1427 μSv per capita for Do screening. For men aged 50 and over it was also associated with lower new VF incidence (8.4% for Do screening vs. 22.5% for No screening) and higher costs (€658 for Do screening vs. €27 for No screening). Comparing Do screening to identify a prevalent VF to No screening, the new VF incidence decreased by 23.3% with increased costs of €810, and radiation exposure of 1422 μSv for both women and men aged 50 and over as the weighted average by the 2013 registration population by gender based on the South Korean Statistical Information Service statistics (Table 3) [29].

Three screening strategies for prevalent VF

Among the three screening strategies performed every two years (Table 3), the X-ray following VFA and VFA only strategies showed the same clinical effect of reducing the new VF incidence by as much as 29.4% for women, and 12.5% for men. The most effective strategy was the X-ray only strategy with a new VF incidence reduction of 35% for women and 17.5% for men over a 10-year period. With regard to the costs, X-ray following VFA strategy was less expensive than the others for both women and men. The second economic option was X-ray only strategy, then VFA only strategy (ΔC of €821, €938, and €1142 for women; €477, €515, and €899 for

Table 3 Results of the base case analysis and multivariate sensitivity analysis for the diagnostic strategies during a 10-year period

Category	Diagnostic strategies	Effectiveness (%)	ΔE[a] (%)	Costs (€)	ΔC[b] (€)	ΔRE[c] (μSv)
Women						
Base case	No screening	54.6		60		
	Do screening[e]	23.3	−31.3	1027	967	1427
	X-ray following VFA	25.2	−29.4	881	821	747
	VFA	25.2	−29.4	1202	1142	141
	X-ray	19.6	−35.0	998	938	3394
Multivariate sensitivity (CI = 1 year)	No screening	54.6		60		
	Do screening[e]	23.2	−31.4	1102	1042	2455
	X-ray following VFA	24.8	−29.7	862	802	996
	VFA	24.8	−29.7	1418	1358	254
	X-ray	19.9	−34.7	1025	966	6115
Men						
Base case	No screening	22.5		27		
	Do screening[e]	8.4	−14.2	658	630	1416
	X-ray following VFA	10.1	−12.5	504	477	556
	VFA	10.1	−12.5	927	899	147
	X-ray	5.0	−17.5	542	515	3545
Multivariate sensitivity (CI = 1 year)	No screening	34.0		60		
	Do screening[e]	8.3	−14.2	734	707	2526
	X-ray following VFA	10.1	−12.4	498	471	828
	VFA	10.1	−12.4	1143	1116	267
	X-ray	4.8	−17.7	560	533	6483
Total[d]	Do screening[e]	16.4	−23.3	854	810	1422

VFA vertebral fracture assessment, *CI* Cycle length

[a]ΔE (Incremental effectiveness, %) = $Effect_{index\ test}$−$Effect_{no\ screening}$ in new VFs incident

[b]ΔC (Incremental Costs, €) = $Costs_{index\ test}$−$Costs_{no\ screening}$ in the costs of test and VFs treatment

[c]ΔRE (Incremental radiation exposure, μSv) = Radiation $doses_{index\ test}$−Radiation $doses_{no\ screening}$; Radiation $doses_{no\ screening}$ was assumed to be '0 μSv'

[d]In the base case, the weighted average by the registration population by gender (female = 8,649,974 people; male = 7,590,057 people) based on Statistics

[e]Do screening presents the average expected values of X-ray following VFA, VFA only, and X-ray only

men per capita, respectively). Also, the 10-year radiation doses in the X-ray only strategy was from 2647 to 2989 μSv and 3253 to 3398 μSv higher than in the X-ray following VFA or VFA only strategies for both women and men.

Sensitivity analysis

The results of the univariate sensitivity analysis compared with the base case analysis are shown in Fig. 2. The input parameters of the sensitivity analysis are given in Table 1. The decrease of VF prevalence indicates that not only was the new VF incidence lower, by 1.7% to 6.9%, but the expected cost was reduced by €70 to €112 in all the screening strategies for both women and men. A similar pattern was found for VF incidence, as reduced effectiveness and cost resulted from an increase in VF incidence. Even though these parameters made great changes in effectiveness and cost, the relative rankings among the strategies did not change. In addition, when the sensitivity and specificity of VFA were reduced, the costs of the strategies that included VFA changed. However, the relative rankings of the strategies were maintained.

The multivariate sensitivity analysis examined the influence of a one-year cycle length compared to the base case analysis of a cycle length of two years during a 10-year period (Table 3). In particular, the X-ray following VFA strategy performed every year for women was beneficial as it was associated with an effect increase in terms of new VF incidence reduction, cost savings, and a slight increase in radiation dose, whereas the X-ray only produced the opposite effect of the X-ray following VFA strategy. The results of the X-ray following VFA strategy for men were similar regardless of the cycle length and the X-ray only strategy of every year increased the effectiveness, cost, and radiation dose. On average, the effectiveness of Do screening on the reduction of new VF incidence was almost identical between the one- and two -year screen intervals. However, the expected cost (about €80 in women and men) and the radiation exposure (about 1000–1100 μSv in women and men) were slightly increased in the one-year cycle length.

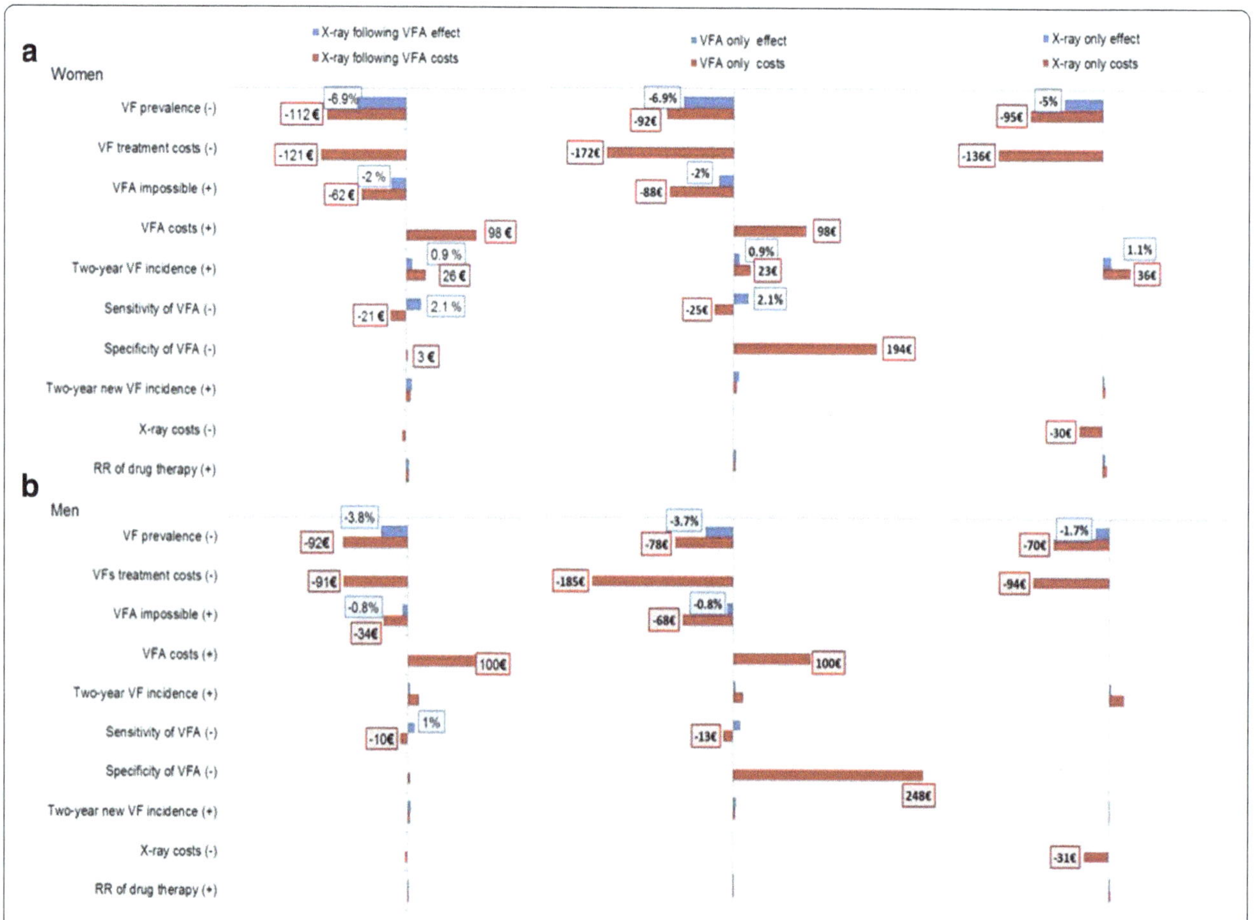

Fig. 2 VF, vertebral fracture; VFA, vertebral fracture assessment; RR, relative risk; (+), increase; (-), decrease (refer to Table 1). Effect and impact of parameter variation on new VF incidence compared with the base case analysis; Costs and impact of parameter variation on costs compared with the base case analysis. (**a**) represent for women and (**b**) for men

Subgroup analysis

Figure 3 shows the results from the subgroup analysis for old age people; women aged 70 and older and men aged 80 and older. The preventive effect of Do screening on new VFs was 41.0% for women and 32.8% for men compared with No screening. The expected costs were €1602 per woman aged 70 and over, and €1429 per man aged 80 and over. The radiation exposure for the old age women and men was comparable with the base case results. Among the three strategies, the overall expected cost of X-ray only strategy was the highest in the subgroup for old people whereas the cost of VFA only strategy was the highest in the base case analysis (Data not shown).

Discussion

This study demonstrated that doing screening strategies for prevalent VFs has a high preventive effect on reducing new VF incidence for women and men aged 50 years and older compared to a No screening strategy. A cost-effective option was X-ray following VFA strategy, considering that the radiation exposure in X-ray only strategy was much higher than the X-ray following VFA or VFA only strategies.

For a change of two years into the one-year screening interval, the average effects of the three screening strategies for prevalent VF on reducing new VF incidence were almost identical, but the X-ray following VFA strategy for women was especially beneficial resulting in a reduction of the incidence of new VFs, cost savings, and relatively low levels of radiation dose. On average, the clinical effect of incident VF reduction was more than two times in women than in men, more in old people aged 70 and over than in people aged 50 and over, and its effect on old people was increased more in men than in women.

In clinical practice, the X-ray, the gold standard tool for detecting VF, is not routinely performed in the clinical evaluation of people at risk of future fractures. In our study, considering the highest radiation exposure and the second highest cost, a routine X-ray screening strategy might be inferior to the X-ray following VFA. Given that the worldwide average effective dose from natural background radiation was reported to be 2.4 mSv per year [12], the potential risk to an individual might be small because the annual radiation doses of the X-ray strategy in our study had a much lower dose at 0.35 mSv. However, cyclical use could have a psychological impact on the compliance of people who are eligible for routine screening for VF.

On the other hand, VFA had the lowest radiation dose and a high preventive effect of new VFs. However, we should carefully consider whether to replace the X-ray with VFA because performing the VFA has a risk of misdiagnosis caused by false negative rates of about 20% [10]; the costs of VFA are increased with the additional costs of patients receiving unnecessary treatment with a false-positive result. Moreover, even if most osteoporotic VFs occur between T7 and L3, the poor image quality of the upper thoracic vertebrae superior to T7 is a major

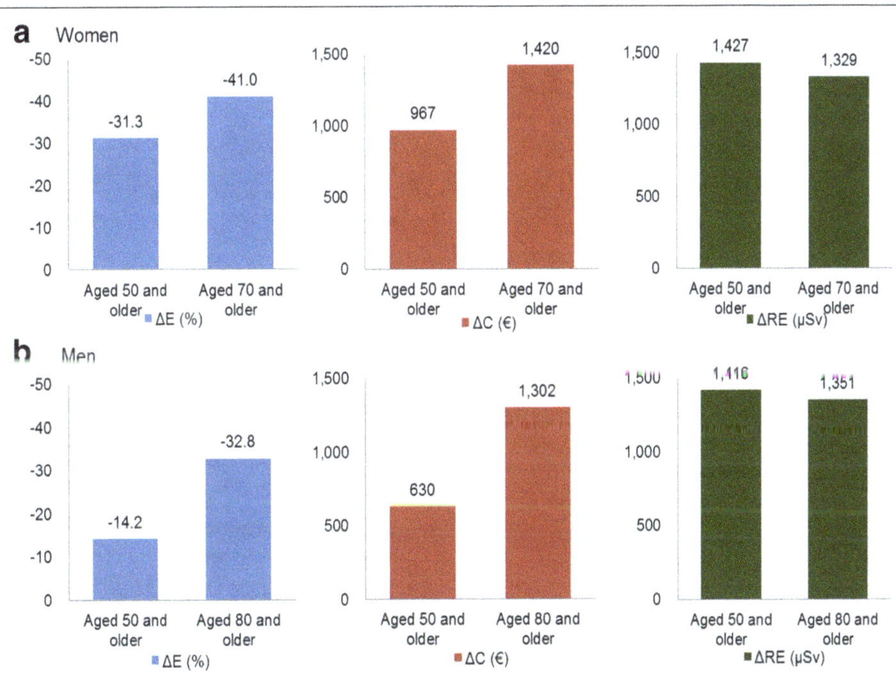

Fig. 3 Subgroup analysis by old age people who had received prevalent VF screening strategies compared to No screening in a 10-year time horizon. ΔE, new VFs incident reduction; ΔC, increased costs; ΔRE, radiation exposure. VF, vertebral fracture; VFA, vertebral fracture assessment. **a** and **b** represent the average values of the X-ray following VFA, VFA, and X-ray as a Do screening strategy

limitation of VFA [11]. Thus our model applied the unreadable probability of VFA, and additional confirmatory imaging (e.g. X-ray) should be considered.

The X-ray following VFA strategy can overcome these problems of VFA with the lowest cost, lower radiation dose than X-ray, and high effect of reducing the new VF. In addition, it can assess VFs at the same time as BMD assessment in contrast to X-ray, which may need referral to another facility [8].

Our study has some limitations. First, since there were no reliable data about adherence to screening and osteoporosis medication, we assumed 100% adherence for screening as well as medication use. Therefore, this assumption probably overstates the clinical effectiveness of this study. In addition, the use of anti-osteoporotic agents based on BMD values was not considered, since it would be equally applicable to all the patients. Modeling that included information on BMD values in the subject population would be very complex, but it would be possible to perform such additional modeling if real world data from observational studies were included. Second, as we assume that the costs of the VFA test would be half of the X-ray as in the U.S., it should be updated for costs after pricing in each countries. Third, our analysis did not consider patient outcome or health-related quality of life (HRQoL). However, this study has great strength that it revealed the benefits and harm of X-ray following VFA, VFA only, and X- ray only strategies, as a population screening tool. Moreover, we used accurate data on prevalence, incidence and cost using real world data from the NHI claims database to obtain a more accurate result. Although the new DXA devices such as iDXA are not widely used in the clinical field, the results of this study would be different if we used such a device because of its high sensitivity and specificity [31].

Conclusion

We suggest that routine screening for VF every one to two years is justified in all populations aged 50 years and older. In particular, an X-ray following VFA strategy can be a relevant option for prevalent VF detection and new VF prevention. Further studies of both HRQoL and cost-utility analysis are needed to promote informed decision making.

Abbreviations

BMD: Bone mineral density; DXA: Dual energy X-ray absorptiometry; HIRA: Health insurance review and assessment service; HRQoL: Health-related quality of life; NHI: National Health Insurance; RR: Relative risk; VF: Vertebral fracture; VFA: Vertebral fracture assessment; X-ray: Spine radiography

Acknowledgments

None.

Funding

This study was completed as part of the health technology assessment project (no. NA-2013-007) funded by the National Evidence-based Healthcare Collaborating Agency in South Korea.

Authors' contributions

SHO, YEL, and YKL performed data correction and analysis. SHO, DK, YEL, DYK, YKL, JHL, SCB, YYC, JP, JA, and YKS contributed to the conception and design of the study. SHO, DK, JA, and YKS involved in drafting the manuscript and revising it critically for important intellectual content. All authors read and approved the final manuscript.

Consent for publication

Not applicable.

Competing interests

YKS reports grants from Pfizer and Eisai. SHO, DK, YEL, DYK, YKL, JHL, SCB, YYC, JHP, JA declare that they have no competing interests.

Author details

[1]National Evidence-based Healthcare Collaborating Agency, Seoul, Republic of Korea. [2]Social and Administrative Pharmacy, College of Pharmacy, Yonsei University, Incheon, Republic of Korea. [3]Department of Rheumatology, Hanyang University Hospital for Rheumatic Diseases, 222-1 wangsimni-ro, Seoundong-gu, Seoul 133-792, Republic of Korea. [4]Department of Biostatistics and Epidemiology, Graduate School of Public Health, Seoul National University, Seoul, Republic of Korea. [5]Department of Nuclear Medicine, Kyung Hee University Hospital, Seoul, Republic of Korea. [6]Department of Rheumatology, Inje University Ilsan Paik Hospital, Goyang, Republic of Korea. [7]Department of Nuclear Medicine, Hanyang University Hospital, Seoul, Republic of Korea. [8]WHO Collaborating Centre for Pharmaceutical Policy and Regulation, Department of Pharmaceutical Science, Utrecht University, Utrecht, Netherlands. [9]Department of Health Convergence, Ewha Womans University, 52 Ewhayeodae-gil, Seodaemun-gu, Seoul 03760, Republic of Korea.

References

1. Kanis JA, Johnell O, De Laet C, et al. A meta-analysis of previous fracture and subsequent fracture risk. Bone. 2004;35:375–82.
2. Black DM, Arden NK, Palermo L, Pearson J, Cummings SR. Prevalent vertebral deformities predict hip fractures and new vertebral deformities but not wrist fractures. Study of osteoporotic fractures research group. J Bone Miner Res. 1999;14:821–8.
3. Jang S, Park C, Jang S, et al. Medical service utilization with osteoporosis. Endocrinol Metab DE. 2010;25:326–39.
4. Fink HA, Milavetz DL, Palermo L, et al. What proportion of incident radiographic vertebral deformities is clinically diagnosed and vice versa? J Bone Miner Res. 2005;20:1216–22.
5. Ensrud KE, Schousboe JT. Clinical practice. Vertebral fractures. N Engl J Med. 2011;364:1634–42.
6. Genant HK, Li J, Wu CY, Shepherd JA. Vertebral fractures in osteoporosis: a new method for clinical assessment. J Clin Densitom. 2000;3:281–90.
7. Lindsay R, Silverman SL, Cooper C, et al. Risk of new vertebral fracture in the year following a fracture. JAMA. 2001;285:320–3.
8. Lewiecki EM, Laster AJ. Clinical review: clinical applications of vertebral fracture assessment by dual-energy x-ray absorptiometry. J Clin Endocrinol Metab. 2006;91:4215–22.
9. Schousboe JT, Vokes T, Broy SB, et al. Vertebral fracture assessment: the 2007 ISCD official positions. J Clin Densitom. 2008;11:92–108.
10. Cosman F, de Beur SJ, LeBoff MS, et al. Clinician's guide to prevention and treatment of osteoporosis. Osteoporos Int. 2014;25:2359–81.
11. Duboeuf F, Bauer DC, Chapurlat RD, Dinten JM, Delmas P. Assessment of vertebral fracture using densitometric morphometry. J Clin Densitom. 2005;8:362–8.

12. Damilakis J, Adams JE, Guglielmi G, Link TM. Radiation exposure in X-ray-based imaging techniques used in osteoporosis. Eur Radiol. 2010;20:2707–14.
13. Lee JH, Lee YK, Oh SH, et al. A systematic review of diagnostic accuracy of vertebral fracture assessment (VFA) in postmenopausal women and elderly men. Osteoporos Int. 2016;27:1691–9.
14. Schousboe JT, Ensrud KE, Nyman JA, Kane RL, Melton LJ 3rd. Cost-effectiveness of vertebral fracture assessment to detect prevalent vertebral deformity and select postmenopausal women with a femoral neck T-score>−2.5 for alendronate therapy: a modeling study. J Clin Densitom. 2006;9:133–43.
15. Gray A. Applied methods of cost-effectiveness analysis in health care. vi ed. New York: Oxford University Press; 2011.
16. Watts NB, Lewiecki EM, Miller PD, Baim S. National Osteoporosis Foundation 2008 Clinician's guide to prevention and treatment of osteoporosis and the World Health Organization fracture risk assessment tool (FRAX): what they mean to the bone densitometrist and bone technologist. J Clin Densitom. 2008;11:473–7.
17. Shin CS, Kim MJ, Shim SM, et al. The prevalence and risk factors of vertebral fractures in Korea. J Bone Miner Metab. 2012;30:183–92.
18. Kweon SS, Shin MH, Jeong SK, et al. Cohort profile: the Namwon study and the dong-gu study. Int J Epidemiol. 2014;43:558–67.
19. Ahn J, Hyun MK, Kim Y, et al. A study on the evaluation standards of osteoporosis in Korea. Seoul: National Evidence-based Healthcare Collaborating Agency; 2011.
20. Lee JH, Cho SK, Han M, et al. Validity and role of vertebral fracture assessment in detecting prevalent vertebral fracture in patients with rheumatoid arthritis. Joint Bone Spine. 2014;81:149–53.
21. Kanis JA, Johnell O, Black DM, et al. Effect of raloxifene on the risk of new vertebral fracture in postmenopausal women with osteopenia or osteoporosis: a reanalysis of the multiple outcomes of Raloxifene evaluation trial. Bone. 2003;33:293–300.
22. Sung YK, Ahn J, Oh SH, et al. Diagnostic accuracy of vertebral fracture assessment using DXA and comparison of diagnostic strategy of vertebral fracture. Seoul: National Evidence-based Healthcare Collaborating Agency; 2014.
23. Freemantle N, Cooper C, Diez-Perez A, et al. Results of indirect and mixed treatment comparison of fracture efficacy for osteoporosis treatments: a meta-analysis. Osteoporos Int. 2013;24:209–17.
24. Avenell A, Gillespie WJ, Gillespie LD, O'connell D. Vitamin D and vitamin D analogues for preventing fractures associated with involutional and post-menopausal osteoporosis. Cochrane Database Syst Rev. 2005;3:CD000227.
25. Sawka AM, Papaioannou A, Adachi JD, et al. Does alendronate reduce the risk of fracture in men? A meta-analysis incorporating prior knowledge of anti-fracture efficacy in women. BMC Musculoskelet Disord. 2005;6:39.
26. Zhong ZM, Chen JT. Anti-fracture efficacy of risedronic acid in men: a meta-analysis of randomized controlled trials. Clin Drug Investig. 2009;29:349–57.
27. Laster AJ, Lewiecki EM. Vertebral fracture assessment by dual-energy X-ray absorptiometry: insurance coverage issues in the United States. A white paper of the International Society for Clinical Densitometry. J Clin Densitom. 2007;10:227–38.
28. HIRA. A study on economic evaluation guideline. Seoul: Health Insurance Review and Assessment Service; 2012.
29. Statistics. Korean statistical information service (KOSIS). In: Consumer price index in healthcare; 2011.
30. Schousboe JT, Shepherd JA, Bilezikian JP, Baim S. Executive summary of the 2013 International Society for Clinical Densitometry Position Development Conference on bone densitometry. J Clin Densitom. 2013;16:455–66.
31. Hind K, Cooper W, Oldroyd B, Davies A, Rhodes L. A cross-calibration study of the GE-lunar iDXA and prodigy for the assessment of lumbar spine and total hip bone parameters via three statistical methods. J Clin Densitom. 2015;18:86–92.
32. Shin C, Jo N, Kim Y, et al. Study of an osteoporosis management program in Korea. Seoul: Seoul National Univeristy; 2007.
33. Inderjeeth CA, Foo AC, Lai MM, Glendenning P. Efficacy and safety of pharmacological agents in managing osteoporosis in the old old: review of the evidence. Bone. 2009;44:744–51.
34. Schousboe JT, Debold CR. Reliability and accuracy of vertebral fracture assessment with densitometry compared to radiography in clinical practice. Osteoporos Int. 2006;17:281–9.

18

Pre-operative radiographic findings predicting concomitant posterior malleolar fractures in tibial shaft fractures

Zhipeng Huang[1†], Yuan Liu[2†], Wenjun Xie[1], Xiang Li[1], Xiaodong Qin[1*] and Jun Hu[1*]

Abstract

Background: A concomitant tibial shaft and posterior malleolar fracture is a type of regular compound fracture. The associated posterior malleolar fractures are mostly occult fractures, which often do not show a fracture line on ordinary films, and thus lead to a high rate of misdiagnosis. The aim of the present study was to investigate factors helpful for the pre-operative detection of concomitant posterior ankle fractures using the ipsilateral radiographic tibia and fibula shaft fracture characteristics.

Methods: One hundred eleven adult patients with tibial shaft fractures were selected using inclusion and exclusion criteria. Pre-operative ankle radiographs and computed tomography (CT) scans were obtained for all patients, and clinical data, including age and gender, were collected. Patients were divided into two groups (posterior malleolar fracture and no posterior malleolar fracture groups). Fracture height, fracture length, fracture shape, and Haraguchi type of posterior malleolar fracture were measured on radiographs and CT images, and were compared between the two groups. Multiple logistic regression analysis was performed to identify the factors that significantly contributed to concomitant posterior malleolar fractures. Receiver operating characteristic curves were calculated, and cut-off values were used to predict posterior malleolar fractures on pre-operative imaging measurements.

Results: Of the 111 patients with tibial shaft fractures, 42 (37.8%) had a concurrent posterior malleolar fracture. Age, gender and affected side were not significantly different, but tibial fracture location, fracture length, and fibular and tibial fracture shape were significantly different between the two groups. In the multiple logistic analysis, tibial fracture location, fracture length, and tibial fracture shape were shown to be significant factors contributing to posterior malleolar fractures. Receiver operating characteristic curves showed that the status of tibial shaft fractures is closely related to the associated posterior malleolar fracture.

Conclusion: Ipsilateral posterior ankle fractures are commonly associated with tibial shaft fractures, especially spiral-type injuries. An analysis of the imaging features of such fractures and evaluation of the diagnostic value of various methods can provide imaging basics for the development of accurate and appropriate treatment options.

Keywords: Tibial shaft fracture, Spiral, Posterior malleolar fracture, Radiograph

* Correspondence: infection118@163.com; junhu89@vip.sina.com
†Equal contributors
[1]Department of Orthopedics, The First Affiliated Hospital of Nanjing Medical University, Nanjing 210029, China
Full list of author information is available at the end of the article

Background

Posterior malleolus fractures are a common type of ankle fracture with variations ranging from small posterior malleolus avulsion fractures to large displaced fractures. The integrity of the posterior malleolus and the posterior tibiofibular ligaments play an important role in load transfer of ankle joints, the stability of the back talus, and the stability of ankle joint rotation [1]. Posterior malleolus fractures account for 7%–44% of ankle fractures, and most of the posterior malleolus fractures occur in post-rotatory extorsion fractures [1]. Tibial shaft fractures with ankle fractures have recently attracted increasing attention in clinical practice. In this type of fracture, posterior malleolus fractures mostly manifest as crack fractures and non-obvious displacement, which are challenging to detect on X-ray films. Indeed, the misdiagnosis rate on x-ray films is 67.9% – 91.2% [2]. Therefore, how to optimize the imaging examination method to reduce the misdiagnosis rate is an important clinical problem.

The aim of this study was to determine factors helpful for the pre-operative detection of concomitant posterior ankle fractures using the ipsilateral radiographic tibia and fibula shaft fracture characteristics. It was hypothesized that the morphologic features of tibial shaft fractures contribute to posterior malleolus fractures.

Methods

This study was approved by the clinical research ethics committee of the First Affiliated Hospital of Nanjing Medical University. All patients with tibial shaft fractures underwent CT examinations between 2012 and 2017; the obtained data was retrospectively analyzed. The exclusion criteria were as follows: fractures primarily involving the knee joint (tibial plateau fractures); fractures primarily involving the ankle joint (uni-, bi-, and trimalleolar ankle fractures); old fractures or fractures due to unhealed fractures; congenital dysplasia; neuromuscular disorders; infections; bone tumors and other diseases possibly altering the normal anatomy of skeletal muscle; bilateral comminuted tibial shaft fractures; and fractures without ipsilateral ankle CT images or fractures with X-ray filming excluding the full length of the tibia and fibula [3].

Demographic data, including age and gender, were recorded. As part of our institution's standard pre-operative evaluation, all tibial shaft fracture patients have orthogonal tibia radiographs with supplemental radiographic views of the ankle and knee. A CT scan without iodinated contrast of the entire tibia that included the ankle was also obtained to assess for concomitant injuries. All CT scans were performed on a 64-slice scanner utilizing 1.25-mm axial slices (Siemens SOMATOM Definition AS 64-slice spiral CT machine [detector dimension, 64 * 1.25 mm, pitch, 0.8, tube voltage, 130 kV, 80 ~ 520 mAs]; Shanghai, China).

Pre-operative radiographs were independently reviewed by three orthopedic surgeons. X-ray films were preliminarily analyzed according to the location of the tibia and fibula fractures. Tibial shaft fractures were divided into four types (transverse, oblique, spiral, and complex). Fibular and tibial fracture location was defined as the midpoint of the fracture line, and the point was calculated as the percentage between the ankle and knee joint lines, where the ankle joint line was 0% and the knee joint line was 100%. Similarly, fibular fracture location was calculated as the percentage between the distal and proximal tips of the fibula. Fracture length was defined as the vertical height between the lowest and highest points of the fracture line of the tibial shaft [3].

Three-dimensional evaluation of posterior malleolus fractures with tibial shaft fractures was performed in cross-sectional, sagittal, and coronal surfaces. If the posterior malleolus fracture involves > 25% of the articular surface or fracture displacement is > 2 mm, fixation of the posterior ankle injury (distal tibial articular surface) by surgery is necessary [4].

A technique of mapping fracture lines for a given bone, which has been previously described, was used for this study [5–7]. A brief description follows. The CT axial cut located 3 mm above the distal tibial subchondral surface from each of the 42 patients was selected for analysis and fracture "mapping." Each image was obtained digitally, and subsequently enlarged to fit a grid to standardize the size of the images, which were then uploaded into a graphics design program (Macromedia Fireworks MX software; Macromedia, Inc., San Francisco, CA, USA). To identify the common fracture patterns, all 42 images were divided into 2 sides and were superimposed to create a "heat map" of the plafond. These superimposed images resulted in a frequency diagram based on the density of the fracture lines.

The inter-observer reliability of the three orthopedic surgeons was evaluated using intra-class correlation coefficients (ICCs). The surgeons measured the radiologic indices independently without having access to the patients' clinical information and the measurement results of other surgeons. One of the orthopedic surgeons repeated the measurements of the radiologic indices 3 weeks after the observer reliability test to assess the reliability of the intra-observer. Inter- and intra-observer reliability testing was performed on 111 patients. After the reliability test, all flat sheet measurements were done by one of the authors who performed intra-observer reliability testing.

Descriptive statistics, including the mean, standard deviation, and proportions, were determined. A Kolmogorov-Smirnov test verified the normality of the distribution of continuous variables. Comparisons between the patients with and without concomitant posterior malleolar fractures were performed using a t-test or Mann-Whitney U test and a chi-square test according to the data characteristics. To combine the factors that significantly contributed to predict posterior ankle fractures, multiple logistic regression with the stepwise selection method was used. The sensitivity and specificity of the receiver operating characteristic curve were calculated for each radiographic measurement. All statistics were two-tailed, and a p value < 0.05 was considered significant [8].

Results

In this study, a total of 111 patients with tibial shaft fractures met the inclusion and exclusion criteria. Of these patients, 72 were males and 39 were females, with an average age of 46.6 ± 16.1 years. Of the 111 patients with tibial fractures, 42 (37.8%) had ipsilateral posterior ankle fractures. Of 42 ankle joint injuries, 30 were isolated posterior malleolus fractures, 11 were posterior malleolus fractures combined with lateral malleolus fractures, and 1 was a posterior malleolus fractures combined with lateral and medial malleolus fractures. In 42 patients with posterior malleolus fractures, 19 underwent surgical treatment and 23 underwent conservative treatment (Fig. 1).

After critically reviewing all of these images, consistent fracture lines were identified and deemed major fracture lines. We identified two major fracture lines, as follows: 1) larger posterolateral-oblique type fragments (Haraguchi type I); and 2) small posterolateral avulsion type fragments (Haraguchi type III; Fig. 2).

Radiographic measurements showed satisfactory inter- and intra-observer reliabilities (Table 1). A comparison between the groups with and without posterior malleolar fractures, univariate logistic regression analysis indicated that there were no significant differences in age, gender, mechanism of injury, fibular fracture location, and fibular fracture shape, but there were significant differences in the location of tibial fractures, fracture length, and tibial fracture shape ($p < 0.05$; Table 2).

We then further analyzed age, gender, mechanism of injury, tibial and fibular fracture location, fracture length, and tibial and fibular fracture shape using multiple logistic regression model, and the results showed that tibial fracture location, fracture length, and tibial fracture shape were significant contributing factors to posterior malleolar fracture injuries in tibial fractures (Table 3).

The receiver operating characteristic curves for tibial fracture location and fracture length on radiographs of posterior ankle fractures were also calculated. The cut-off value for tibial fracture location was 40.0%, with a sensitivity of 92.9% and a specificity of 44.9% (Fig. 3a). The cut-off value for fracture length was 11.4%, with a sensitivity of 85.7% and a specificity of 52.2% (Fig. 3b). In addition, we analyzed the combination between tibial fracture location and fracture length. And we analyzed the combination between the shape of the tibial shaft fractures (transverse, oblique, spiral, and complex) and the shape of fibular fractures (intact, proximal, middle, distal, and complex). We found that the area under the curve for the combination of tibial fracture location and fracture length was 0.7208, with a sensitivity of 40.5% and a specificity of 78.3% (Fig. 3c). The area under the

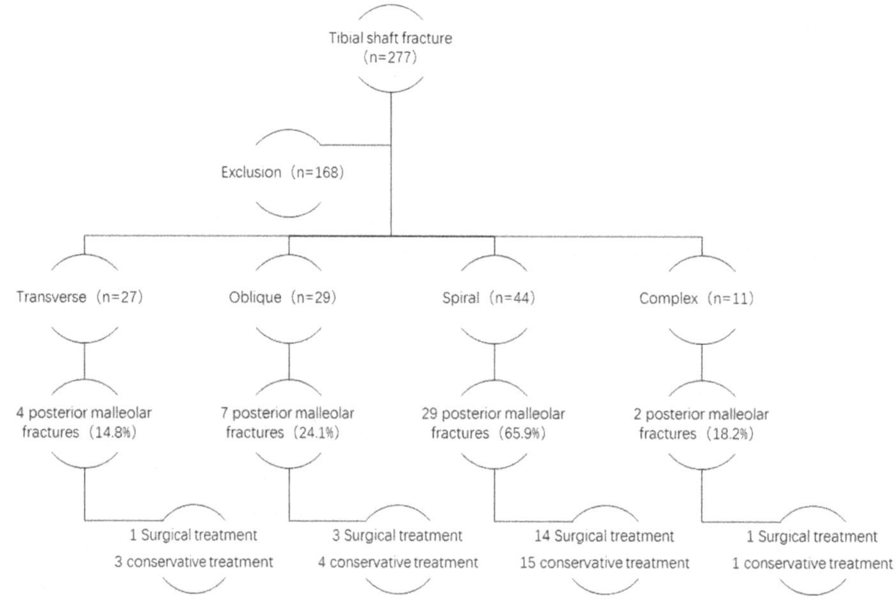

Fig. 1 According to tibial fracture shape, our study consisted of 27 transverse, 29 oblique, 44 spiral, and 11 complex fractures

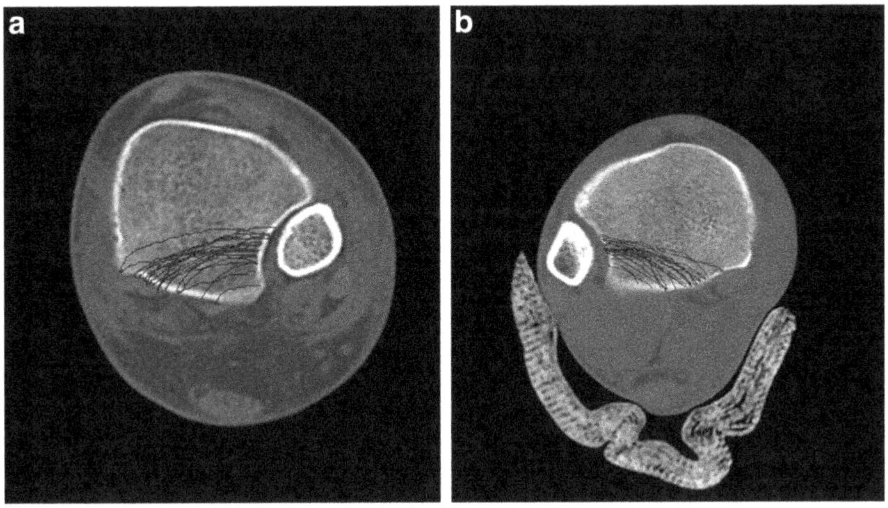

Fig. 2 Axial CT (**a** right side, **b** left side) scans demonstrating the posterior malleolus fracture pattern. The Posterior Malleolar Map revealed a fracture pattern and morphology consistent with the fracture lines, as originally described by Haraguchi

curve for the combination of tibial and fibula fracture shapes was 0.8094, with a sensitivity of 66.7% and a specificity of 81.2% (Fig. 3d).

Discussion

The present study investigated the factors that could be used to detect posterior malleolar fractures concurrent with tibial shaft fractures pre-operatively and to provide cut-off values based on pre-operative radiographic measurements. Tibial fracture location, fracture length, and tibial fracture shape were significant pre-operative factors that were associated with posterior malleolar fractures. When the tibial fracture location is ≤40% or the fracture length is > 11.4% on a radiograph, posterior malleolar fractures should be suspected, appropriately evaluated, and managed at the time of tibial shaft fracture surgery.

The incidence of tibial shaft fractures combined with posterior malleolus fractures in each region show remarkable differences. Kempegowda [9] identified 1113 cases of tibial shaft fractures, 96 of which were associated with ankle fractures, thus accounting for 8.6% of all cases. Schottel and others [10] studied 71 cases of tibial shaft fractures, 35 of which showed combined ankle fractures, thus accounting for 49.3% of all cases. Stuermer et al. [11] reported that 43 (20.1%) of 214 patients with a tibial fracture were found to have an associated injury of the ankle joint. Hou Z et al. [12] found that 288 cases of tibial shaft fractures, 28 of which showed combined posterior malleolar fractures, thus accounting for 9.7% of all cases. Based on the previous studies, the incidence of tibial shaft fractures and concomitant ankle injuries had relatively large differences. We showed that the incidence of tibial shaft fractures combined with posterior malleolus fractures was 37.8% in our study.

The misdiagnosis of tibial shaft fractures combined with ankle fractures reflects the methods of examination. The lack of understanding of this concomitant injury is also an important reason resulting in misdiagnosis. At the time of initial consultation, most orthopedic surgeons only noticed a significant shift in the tibial shaft fracture, but often did not take into account the possible concomitant ankle fracture. When X-ray films were obtained, the ankle joint was not included, and the ankle fracture was therefore missed. Even if most X-ray examinations include the distal tibia, shooting angle and clarity also largely affect the diagnosis of fractures. It is challenging to visualize tibial ankle fractures from frontal films, and it is even more challenging to view the fractures from lateral radiographs due to the overlap with the fibula, especially when the fracture is combined with

Table 1 Intra- and inter-observer reliabilities of measurements

Measurements	Intra-observer Reliability		Inter-observer Reliability	
	ICC	95% CI	ICC	95% CI
Tibial fracture location, %	0.989	0.978 to 0.997	0.917	0.856 to 0.958
Fibular fracture location, %	0.949	0.876 to 0.981	0.926	0.836 to 0.961
Fracture length, %	0.891	0.808 to 0.949	0.808	0.701 to 0.912

Abbreviations: *ICC* Intraclass correlation coefficient, *CI* Confidence interval

Table 2 Comparison between groups with and without posterior malleolar fractures

	With posterior malleolar fracture	Without posterior malleolar fracture	*P* Value
Patients	42	69	
Age, y[a]	46.79 ± 14.06	46.49 ± 17.33	0.93
Gender			0.92
Male	27	45	
Female	15	24	
Side			0.96
Right	19	31	
Left	23	37	
Bilateral	0	1	
Fracture location, %[a]			
Tibial	27.52 ± 10.08	37.59 ± 18.08	< 0.01
Fibular	38.94 ± 34.53	38.68 ± 27.94	0.97
Fracture length, %[a]	15.11 ± 6.08	11.31 ± 9.52	< 0.05
Fibular fracture shape			< 0.01
Intact	5	10	
Proximal level	13	11	
Middle level	2	24	
Distal level	20	21	
Complex	2	3	
Tibial fracture shape			< 0.01
Transverse	4	23	
Oblique	7	22	
Spiral	29	15	
Complex	2	9	
Haraguchi Type			
Type I	41		
Type II	0		
Type III	1		

[a]The values are given as the mean and the standard deviation

distal fibula fractures. In addition, most ankle fractures of this type are occult fractures, and it is difficult to diagnose these fractures through X-ray examinations. In these cases, non-displaced distal ankle fractures are often misdiagnosed [10].

Tibial shaft fractures combined with posterior malleolus fractures are a regular combined injury, and the cause of injury, mechanism of injury, and epidemiologic characteristics are different from ankle fractures. It has been shown that the incidence of posterior malleolus fractures in tibial shaft fractures combined with ankle joint injuries is significantly higher than in patients with ankle fractures only [13] .Ankle fractures are most commonly found in Lauge-Hansen classification degree III or above post-rotatory extorsion fractures and degree IV pronation-external rotation fractures. The typical posterior ankle coronal fractures often occur in rotational injuries. When the foot is in the pronation or posterior

Table 3 Logistic regression analysis (Stepwise selection method)

Variable	Estimate	Standard Error	Odds Ratio	95% CI	*P* Value
Tibial fracture location, %	−0.05	0.02	0.96	0.93 to 0.99	< 0.01
Fracture length, %	0.05	0.03	1.05	1.00 to 1.11	< 0.05
Tibial fracture shape					
Spiral	2.32	0.70	10.22	2.57 to 40.56	< 0.01

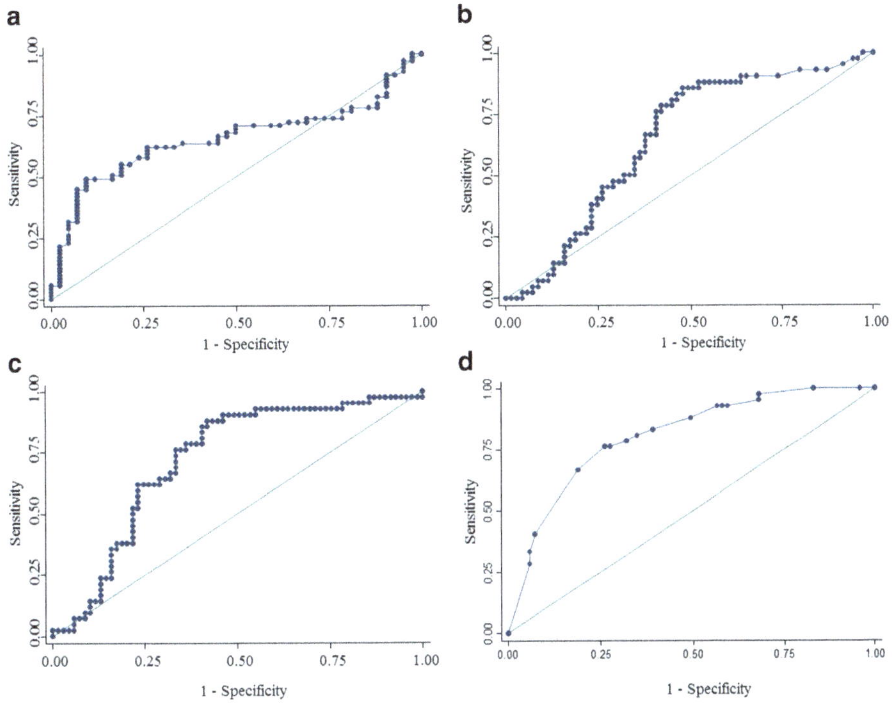

Fig. 3 The receiver operating characteristic curve of the pre-operative radiographic measurements on the anteroposterior tibia and fibula view between the with posterior malleolar fracture group and without posterior malleolar fracture group. **a** the tibial fracture location; (**b**) fracture length; (**c**) combination between tibial fracture location and fracture length; (**d**) combination between shape of the tibial shaft fractures and fibular shaft fractures

rotation position, the lower tibiofibular ligament injury may be injured upon external force on the talus due to rotation or valgus. One side of this ligament is attached to the distal posterior margin of the tibia, which is the posterior ankle. Posterior malleolus fractures are caused by avulsion of the lower tibiofibular ligament. At present, the mechanism of tibial shaft fractures combined with posterior malleolus injuries is still controversial. Some researchers believe that the fracture is mostly caused by indirect low-energy torsional forces. The mechanism of injury is due to rotation to the outside during forward movement because of inertia when the ankle is fixed, resulting in a spiral fracture in the weak parts involving one-third of the distal tibia. The fracture line goes from the inside lower aspect to the outside upper aspect, the ankle fracture is due to the talus shear during the movement upon sudden fixation of the foot or due to avulsion fractures caused by traction between the ankle and lower tibiofibular posterior ligament [14] .There are still some other types of tibial shaft fractures that cannot be included in the situation we discussed herein. Some scholars have stated that when tibial shaft fractures occur, the lateral leg muscles contract, resulting in excessive plantar flexion of the ankle joint, extrusion of the tibial fossa trailing edge by the talus, and thus ankle fractures [15]. Nevertheless, the mechanism leading to damage needs to be verified by further biomechanical studies.

Among the 42 posterior malleolus fractures in this study, 19 patients underwent surgical treatment and 23 patients were conservatively treated. Surgical fixation is necessary if the posterior ankle fracture is > 25% of the tibial articular surface or the fracture displacement is > 2 mm [4]. Fitzpatrick et al. [16] found that the mean and peak contact stress did not increase significantly, even in the cases in which posterior malleolar fracture involve > 50% of the articular surface. The results of the Fitzpatrick et al. [16] study showed that in a posterior malleolus fracture model, contact stress of the ankle joint is redistributed to the anterior medial side during movement of the ankle joint. This stress concentration may lead to changes in the weight load of the cartilage within the contact interface, resulting in the final induction of post-traumatic arthritis. Drijfhout van Hooff et al. [17] showed that the fixation should be implemented when the posterior malleolus fracture block is > 5%; an articular surface step > 1 mm will lead to the development of osteoarthritis.

The limitations of the current study include those inherent to the retrospective design. Secondly, intra-observer reliability is better to be calculated from the data of the 3 orthopedics. In addition, in our study all tibia shaft fracture surgery was used an intramedullary nail fixation, but because posterior malleolar fractures were performed by different surgeons and different surgical approaches were adopted, including hollow screws and buttress plates, we cannot discuss the choice of surgical methods, and we cannot evaluate functional outcomes after fixation of posterior malleolus fractures with a tibial shaft fracture. Boraiah et al. [18] reported on a series of 24 patients of posterior malleolar fractures associated with tibia fractures, where the malleolus was fixed before intramedullary nailing of the tibia, and there were no complications during the post-operative follow-up. Kempegowda et al. [9] strongly suggests that malleolar fractures should be fixed before nailing of the tibia to reduce the risk of intra-operative displacement and poor reduction. The Kempegowda et al. [9] study was based on a small number of patients, bringing into question the power of the results. Sufficiently powered, good-quality, randomized trials are warranted.

Conclusions

Our clinical experience shows that it is necessary to have pre-operative regular radiography, including frontal and lateral X-ray films of ankle joints and carefully check the films, which are critical the diagnosis. For the suspected cases, it is important to perform a CT examination to determine whether or not an ankle fracture is present. In the current study, we performed CT examinations for all diagnosed and suspected tibial shaft fractures with ankle fractures. For the regions that lack medical resources or with high medical costs, diagnosis according to the pre-operative films can save a substantial amount of medical costs. For combined ankle fractures with tibial shaft fractures in busy trauma centers, if ipsilateral ankle joint CT films are not obtained, surgeons can also determine concomitant ankle fracture according to analysis of characteristics in flat films, which can help intra-operative restoration and avoid misdiagnosis.

Abbreviations

CT: Computed tomography; ICCs: Intra-class correlation coefficients

Acknowledgements

Not applicable.

Funding

This study was supported by grants from the National Natural Science Foundation of China (Nos. 81672218 and 81603092).

Authors' contributions

1. Study conception and design: XQ, JH 2. Acquisition, analysis and/or interpretation of data: ZH, YL, WX, XL, JH 3. Drafting/revision of the work for intellectual content and context: ZH, YL, JH 4. Final approval and overall responsibility for the published work: XQ, JH.
2. All authors read and approved the final manuscript.

Consent for publication

Not applicable.

Competing interests

The authors declare that they have no competing interests.

Author details

[1]Department of Orthopedics, The First Affiliated Hospital of Nanjing Medical University, Nanjing 210029, China. [2]Department of Infectious Diseases, The First Affiliated Hospital of Nanjing Medical University, Nanjing 210029, China.

References

1. Irwin TA, Lien J, Kadakia AR. Posterior malleolus fracture. J Am Acad Orthop Surg. 2013;21(1):32–40.
2. Kukkonen J, Heikkilä JT, Kyyrönen T, Mattila K, Gullichsen E. Posterior malleolar fracture is often associated with spiral tibial diaphyseal fracture: a retrospective study. J Trauma. 2006;60(5):1058–60.
3. Jung KJ, Chung CY, Park MS, et al. Concomitant ankle injuries associated with Tibial shaft fractures. Foot Ankle Int. 2015;36(10):1209–14.
4. Ruokun H, Ming X, Zhihong X, et al. Postoperative radiographic and clinical assessment of the treatment of posterior tibial plafond fractures using a posterior lateral incisional approach. J Foot Ankle Surg. 2014;53(6):678–82.
5. Cole PA, Mehrle RK, Bhandari M, Zlowodzki M. The pilon map: fracture lines and comminution zones in OTA/AO type 43C3 pilon fractures. J Orthop Trauma. 2013;27(7):e152–6.
6. Mangnus L, Meijer DT, Stufkens SA, et al. Posterior malleolar fracture patterns. J Orthop Trauma. 2015;29(9):428–35.
7. Armitage BM, Wijdicks CA, Tarkin IS, et al. Mapping of scapular fractures with three-dimensional computed tomography. J Bone Joint Surg Am. 2009;91(9):2222–8.
8. Choi Y, Kwon SS, Chung CY, Park MS, Lee SY, Lee KM. Preoperative radiographic and CT findings predicting syndesmotic injuries in supination-external rotation-type ankle fractures. J Bone Joint Surg Am. 2014;96(14): 1161–7.
9. Kempegowda H, Maniar HH, Richard R, et al. Posterior malleolar fractures associated with Tibial shaft fractures and sequence of fixation. J Orthop Trauma. 2016;30(10):568–71.
10. Schottel PC, Berkes MB, Little MT, et al. Predictive radiographic markers for concomitant ipsilateral ankle injuries in tibial shaft fractures. J Orthop Trauma. 2014;28(2):103–7.
11. Stuermer EK, Stuermer KM. Tibial shaft fracture and ankle joint injury. J Orthop Trauma. 2008;22(2):107–12.
12. Hou Z, Zhang Q, Zhang Y, Li S, Pan J, Wu H. A occult and regular combination injury: the posterior malleolar fracture associated with spiral tibial shaft fracture. J Trauma. 2009;66(5):1385–90.
13. Wu HT, Hou ZY. Zhang Q, et al. [comparison of two kinds of fractures involving posterior malleolar fracture]. Zhonghua Yi Xue Za Zhi. 2008; 88(39):2775–8.
14. Robinson CM, McLauchlan GJ, McLean IP, Court-Brown CM. Distal metaphyseal fractures of the tibia with minimal involvement of the ankle. Classification and treatment by locked intramedullary nailing. J Bone Joint Surg Br. 1995;77(5):781–7.
15. Colville MR, Colville JM, Manoli A. Posteromedial dislocation of the ankle without fracture. J Bone Joint Surg Am. 1987;69(5):706–11.
16. Fitzpatrick DC, Otto JK, McKinley TO, Marsh JL, Brown TD. Kinematic and contact stress analysis of posterior malleolus fractures of the ankle. J Orthop Trauma. 2004;18(5):271–8.

19

Posterior pedicle screw fixation to treat lower cervical fractures associated with ankylosing spondylitis: a retrospective study of 35 cases

Liang Yan[1†], Zhenguo Luo[2†], Baorong He[1*], Jijun Liu[1] and Dingjun Hao[1*]

Abstract

Background: The most common site of fractures in patients with ankylosing spondylitis (AS) is the cervical spine, especially the lower cervical spine and cervicothoracic junction. The optimal treatment for cervical spine fractures secondary to AS is controversial. This study aimed to explore the effects of posterior pedicle screw fixation alone on fractures of the lower cervical spine in patients with AS.

Methods: From January 2006 to January 2013, a total of 35 patients with AS and a lower cervical spine fracture were treated using only posterior cervical/thoracic pedicle screw fixation. In this retrospective study, we reviewed the patients' charts to assess their case histories, operations, neurological outcomes, and complications. We also evaluated their postoperative radiographs to determine the time of bone fusion.

Results: Altogether, 32 (91.4%) of the 35 fractures resulted from an acute injury and 3 (8.6%) from a chronic injury. In 25 cases, the fracture resulted from a low-energy spinal injury and in 8 cases from a high-energy injury. Posterior pedicle screw fixation was successful in all patients, with radiographic fusion confirmed by computed tomography. The average time of bone fusion was 3.6 months (range 3 – 6 months). The surgery improved the American Spinal Injury Association grade in 15 (42.9%) patients. No intraoperative complications occurred. None of the corrections resulted in neurological decompensation. The average postoperative correction was 18°.

Conclusions: Pedicle screw fixation and autologous bone grafting through a single posterior approach to lower cervical spine fractures in AS patients could stabilize the spine, correct kyphosis, and relieve pressure. It is thus reasonable to recommend this surgical strategy for AS-associated fractures of the lower cervical spine.

Keywords: Ankylosing spondylitis, Cervical, Fracture, Pedicle screw, Posterior

Background

Ankylosing spondylitis (AS) is a seronegative, progressive, systemic, inflammatory, rheumatic spondyloarthropathy that mainly affects the spine and sacroiliac joints [1]. The condition is associated with progressive ossification of the spinal ligaments and ankylosis of the facet joints, eventually leading to a completely stiff spine. Calcification of the longitudinal ligaments eventually results in the classic radiographic "bamboo spine" appearance. AS affects 0.5% of the global population. The creation of a rigid spinal column, with associated osteoporosis as the disease progresses, results in a brittle, rigid structure that is poorly suited to withstand stress. Thus, even minor trauma can result in a fracture [2–5].

Globally, the relative risk of traumatic vertebral fractures has been estimated to be three times higher in patients with AS than in the general population [4]. The cervical spine, especially the lower cervical spine and cervicothoracic junction, is the most common site of

* Correspondence: hebr888@sina.com; haodingjunspine@sina.com
[†]Equal contributors
[1]Department of Spinal Surgery, Hong Hui Hospital, Xi'an Jiaotong University College of Medicine, 555 Friendship East Road, Xi'an 710054, Shaanxi, China

fractures in these patients. The diagnosis is difficult and thus may be delayed. The delay is partly attributed to the lack of pain associated with these fractures because (1) the patients are undergoing corticosteroid therapy for AS and (2) the preexisting spinal alterations. Plain radiography is inadequate for fully evaluating the shearing fractures due to osteoporosis and to the position of the shoulders [3, 6–9].

AS-related fractures are frequently more severe than cervical spinal fractures in an otherwise healthy population because of their specific features. For instance, AS fractures are highly unstable because of the anterior and the posterior elements that are involved. Moreover, the broken "bamboo spine," resembling long-lever arms, is extremely unstable with a high risk of neurological deterioration. In addition, the kyphotic deformation does not provide the most appropriate sagittal balance for primary stability. Despite these considerations, these bones display a good propensity to fuse [8, 10].

Surgical treatment is controversial, with several reports having described an array of surgical techniques to treat these fractures and their resulting deformities [3, 5–8, 11]. The aim of this study was to show the surgical experience of treating lower cervical spine fractures in patients with AS using posterior pedicle screw fixation alone.

Methods

Patient population

The study is based on data from patients with AS and lower cervical spine fractures who underwent posterior cervical/thoracic pedicle screw fixation between 2006 and 2013. The study design is a retrospective chart review with radiological follow-up. The study group consisted of 35 patients (34 men, 1 woman; mean age 57 years, range 37 – 68 years). On average, AS had been diagnosed 21 years previously. The mechanism of the injury was of low energy in 25 cases, violent in 8 cases, and unknown in 2 cases (Table 1). On inspection, the patients had obvious preexisting thoracolumbar and cervicothoracic kyphosis, with markedly forward head positioning.

Table 1 Summary of patient's demographic data

Variables	
Sex (F/M)	1/34
Age (mean, yrs)	57
Mechanism of injury	
Low-energy	25
High-energy	8
Unknown	2
Level of fracture	
C5–6	11
C6	5
C6–7	16
C7	3

All patients were evaluated with plain radiography, computed tomography (CT), and magnetic resonance imaging (MRI). CT scans were used to elucidate the bone detail of the fracture, deformity, and tissues surrounding the fixation site. MRI was used to differentiate the various causes of cord compression and to identify cord contusion. Two experienced spinal surgeons performed all of the radiological studies. The fracture levels were C5-6 in 11 patients, C6 in 5 patients, C6-7 in 16 patients, and C7 in 3 patients.

The neurological injury was evaluated based on the American Spinal Injury Association (ASIA) impairment scale. At admission, there was a high incidence of neurological deficit after the fracture. Among the 33 cases with neurological deficit, the deficit was reported as grade A in 5 cases, grade B in 4 cases, grade C in 12 cases, and grade D in 12 cases.

Treatment and surgical techniques

Management was based on the presence or absence of spinal instability and neurological symptoms. In the presence of both instability and neurological deficit, surgery was performed to achieve stabilization and decompression. All 35 of our patients underwent posterior surgery alone. Posterior stabilization was achieved using pedicle screw fixation between C4 and T2.

Decompression of spinal stenosis may be performed during the same operative session. Patients with AS are at increased risk for posture deterioration and iatrogenic fractures of the spine during the surgical procedure, especially while under sedation/anesthesia. A possible detrimental consequence is worsening of the neurological impairment. To avoid further motion of the cervical spine in AS patients, an awake nasoendotracheal intubation should be performed blindly using a laryngeal mask to guide the tube.

Cervical pedicle screws are the most reliable—although the most challenging—type of fixation. A modified Abumi technique was used to place these screws. Using a lateral C-arm view and anatomical landmarks, a large hole was created in the lamina at the pedicle entrance, and the pedicle was gently probed before screw insertion. A definitive tapered rod, which tapered from 3.2 to 5.5 mm, was applied from the immobilized lower cervical vertebrae to T2. A pre-bending rod and distraction can be performed to increase the chin-to-chest distance gradually and restore the former lordosis. The rhythm and amount of correction must be performed under neurophysiological monitoring. Usually, postoperative immobilization is mandatory because of the specificities of those patients (i.e., residual kyphosis and sagittal imbalance, poor bone quality, highly unstable lesions). A custom-made cervicothoracic orthosis could be sufficient.

Follow-up

Patients were monitored for neurological outcome, radiographic fusion, and complications. Complications were categorized as general (e.g., infection, dysphagia, death) or surgical (e.g., instrumentation failure) subtypes. Postoperative follow-up examinations were performed at intervals of 4 weeks, 3 months, 6 months, and annually thereafter, with radiographic evaluations including CT scans and sagittal reconstruction obtained immediately postoperatively and again at the 3-, 6-, and 12-month follow-up examinations. Fusion was considered complete when trabecular bone was visible and spanned the fracture site. Cervical deformation and correction of the pre-fracture kyphosis were evaluated by comparing the regional deformation immediately preoperatively, postoperatively, and/or at the last follow-up.

Results

In our series, 32 (91.4%) of the 35 fractures were due to acute injuries, and 3 (8.6%) were chronic in nature. A single spinal segment was involved in each patient. The C6-7 level was the most frequently injured site (16 cases, 45.7%). A low-energy injury of the spine occurred in 25 cases and a high-energy injury in 8 cases. The mechanisms of the fractures were hyperextension in 19 patients, flexion in 12 patients, and compression in 2 patients. All 35 patients were treated successfully using posterior pedicle screw fixation (Fig. 1). Posterior decompression was performed in the patients with a neurological deficit.

The mean duration of the operation was 4.4 h (range 3.2 – 6.4 h). The average estimated blood loss was 740 ml (600 – 1200 ml). Instrumentation spanned four vertebrae: two cephalad and two caudal to the fracture. Altogether, 280 pedicle screws were placed: 32 in C4 pedicles, 70 in C5 pedicles, 38 in C6 pedicles, 70 in T1 pedicles, and 70 in T2 pedicles.

Two cervical pedicle screws were misplaced superiorly, and two were misplaced laterally in the pedicles. Three thoracic pedicle screws were misplaced slightly medially. Although all of the misplaced pedicle screws were evaluated using postoperative CT to determine their positions, none of the seven displaced screws induced any symptoms, and they did not require surgical extraction. In summary, 4 of the 140 cervical pedicle screws (2.9%)

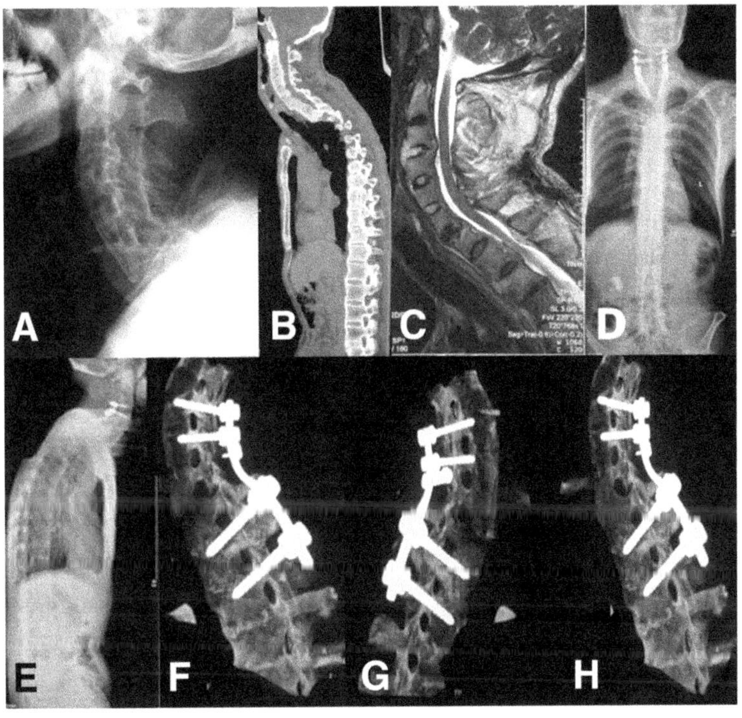

Fig. 1 A 53-year-old man with ankylosing spondylitis and a complete fracture of C7 and partial dislocation. **a** Preoperative plain radiograph showing a displaced fracture together with an obvious gap in the anterior column at C7 because the rigid elevation of the shoulders prevents adequate imaging at the cervico-thoracic junction and so called bamboo spine resulting from ankylosing spondylitis; (**b**) and (**c**) CT with sagittal reconstruction and MR imaging showing an obvious fracture of C7. **d** and (**e**) Immediate antero-posterior and lateral radiographs showing posterior stabilization using pedicle screw fixation between C4 and T2. **f** and (**g**) Postoperative CT with sagittal reconstruction showing good screws placement in the cervical and thoracic pedicles, the cervicothoracic pre-existing kyphosis has been corrected. **h** Bone fusion has been confirmed by sagittal reconstruction CT after 6 months postoperatively

and 3 of the 140 thoracic pedicle screws (2.1%) were misplaced.

An average of 5.6 segments were instrumented in each case, with harvesting of iliac crest bone graft material in 10 patients (28.6%). All of the others received autogenous local bone graft obtained from the spinous processes and lamina.

Four patients died from unrelated causes during the postoperative follow-up period. Death was due to pneumonia in two of the patients, at 6 and 13 months, respectively. Intestinal obstruction occurred in one patient at 13 months postoperatively, and one patient suffered a heart attack at 4 months. The other 31 patients had a mean follow-up time of 26 months (range 11 – 48 months).

All patients achieved radiographic fusion, which was confirmed by CT. The average bone fusion time was 3.6 months (range 3 – 6 months). There was no hardware failure (e.g., broken screws, pullout, migration) during the follow-up period.

Before the operation, two (5.7%) patients were neurologically intact, and five (14.3%) patients had a complete cord injury. In all, 28 (80%) patients sustained an incomplete cord injury, with four (11.4%) patients at ASIA grade B, 12 (34.3%) at ASIA grade C, and 12 (34.3%) at ASIA grade D. Although the number of patients was limited, the patients' neurological status, when influenced, had improved. Postoperatively, 15 (42.9%) patients had improved ASIA grades: two (5.7%) from grade B to grade C; eight (22.9%) from C to D; and five (14.3%) from D to E (Table 2).

There were no intraoperative complications. One patient experienced a superficial wound infection, which was managed with daily wound changes and the use of local and systematic antibiotics. A cervical esophageal fistula occurred 3 days postoperatively in one patient. Reoperation was undertaken, and the fistula was repaired with a pedicled fascial patch. Follow-up included fasting and gastrointestinal nutrition. The patient recovered 2 weeks later.

Preexisting cervicothoracic kyphosis was corrected during the posterior fixation procedure. The average postoperative correction was 18° (range 12° – 32°). The correction did not result in neurological decompensation.

Table 2 Patients' neurological status before and after the operation according to American Spinal Injury Association (ASIA) impairment scale

Preoperatively		Neurological status	Postoperatively	
5	14.3%	ASIA A	5	14.3%
4	11.4%	ASIA B	2	5.7%
12	34.3%	ASIA C	6	17.1%
12	34.3%	ASIA D	15	42.9%
2	5.7%	ASIA E	7	20.0%

Discussion

Clinical characteristics of lower cervical spine fracture with AS

Patients with AS are at higher risk of vertebral fractures than the rest of the global population. A recent retrospective cohort study of more than 230,000 patients reported a 3.3 times greater risk of vertebral fractures in patients with AS than in healthy persons [4, 10]. This higher risk of fracture is related to: (1) the spinal rigidity in AS due to progressive bone bridges that ultimately incorporate posterior facet joints, ligaments, and intervertebral discs; (2) kyphotic deformation, leading to trauma during hyperflexion – hyperextension and reduction of the visual field; and (3) association of AS with osteoporosis (25% – 50% of patients with AS present with associated osteoporosis) [9, 12–15].

AS-related cervical spine fractures are frequently more severe, with specific features, than the corresponding fractures in the healthy population. First, osteoporosis and deformity lead to increased weakness of the spine. As a consequence, even minor trauma can cause fractures because of the spine's poor elasticity. A recent review of the literature showed that 65% of 345 patients with a cervical spine fracture in a context of AS presented after minor trauma. In our series, minor trauma was responsible for the fracture in 25 patients. Two patients presented with a fracture unrelated to trauma.

AS-associated fractures are highly unstable because the anterior and posterior elements exhibit a transverse or short oblique pattern that does not follow the classic three-column criterion for stability, as is seen in normal spines. Moreover, the broken "bamboo spine" behaves somewhat like a long bone with a diaphyseal fracture. That is, the long-lever arms are extremely unstable, with an associated higher risk of neurological deterioration. In addition, the kyphotic deformation does not provide the most appropriate sagittal balance for primary stability, and the hemorrhagic trend produces a supplementary risk of neurological complications because of the increased possibility of a compressive epidural hematoma.

In our series, all fractures occurred in the lower cervical spine and were accompanied by dislocation [13, 16]. Overall, 26 patients had neurological signs at admission, and 7 patients presented with neurological deterioration prior to surgical treatment. In addition, there was a high incidence of respiratory complications. A previous study reported a mortality rate of 20% – 57%, which was twice as high as that for a cervical spine fracture in the general population [17]. One explanation may be that it is associated with a systemic disease, AS, which can result in pulmonary fibrosis and reduced lung capacity. Finally, the diagnosis is difficult and may be delayed. The delay could be partly attributed to (1) the lack of pain associated with these fractures as the patients are undergoing corticosteroid therapy, and (2) the preexisting spinal alterations. Standard radiography is inadequate for fully evaluating shearing fractures due to osteoporosis and the position of the shoulders. Some authors have advocated MRI for detecting traumatic lesions specifically at the cervicothoracic junction, which is poorly documented radiologically. At the very least, a CT scan is necessary to show the fracture line, which usually runs transversely or is shortly oblique and complete from the anterior to the posterior side, similar to the classic Chance fracture at the thoracolumbar spine [2, 10, 18].

Treatment of the AS-associated lower cervical spine fracture

The definitive treatment for cervical spine fractures in AS patients remains controversial, with various treatment modalities and outcomes reported in the literature [4, 6, 12, 16, 19]. Conservative treatment has long been the gold standard. It typically involves bed rest, skull traction, and/or wearing a halo vest or a head - cervical chest cast. Bed rest, however, is not appropriate for these patients as they are susceptible to pulmonary and decubitus complications. Skull traction cannot satisfactorily reduce or stabilize the cervical spine because of its stiffness and the irreducible surrounding soft tissues. Neurological deterioration had been reported as a result of distraction at the fracture site while applying traction. Simple external fixation cannot eliminate movement between the fracture sites, leading to pseudoarthroses. Non-union, loss of reduction, and neurological deterioration have been reported after non-operative treatment, often leading to a second operation. According to recent publications and in our own experience, such treatment strategies are not to be recommended because of the associated long-term immobilization and to complications related to bed rest and skull traction.

The primary aim of surgical treatment is to maintain the fracture's realignment with adequate stabilization measures until the bone has healed completely. Spinal stenosis may be decompressed during the same operative session. It may be achieved through a single anterior, single posterior, or combined one-time or staged posteroanterior or anteroposterior approach. The anterior approach has the benefit of short operative times, lower neurological deterioration due to positional changes, restoration of cervical alignment, and direct decompression. However, the poor results and high complication rate (cervical esophageal fistula, internal fixation failure) cannot be ignored. In AS patients, the esophageal mucosa is prone to injury due to ossification of the anterior longitudinal ligament and fracture displacement. Moreover, the anterior approach to the cervicothoracic junction is extremely difficult because of the great inclination and the kyphosis that exist in this region. The esophageal mucosa is prone to iatrogenic injury during the operation and to repeated friction by the anterior plate postoperatively. In our series, although not an anterior operation, a cervical esophageal fistula occurred within 3 days postoperatively in one case (Fig. 2). A possible cause was that the esophageal mucosa experienced gradual, repeated friction caused by progressive ossification of the anterior longitudinal ligament. After injury, the esophageal fistula was due to a shift of the sharp fracture end. The failure rate of anterior internal fixation is 50% because anterior implants are unstable and do not resist or absorb the tension from the posterior spinal column after three-column spinal injuries and because of the presence of severe osteoporosis. According to recent publications and in our own experience, anterior-only stabilization is rarely performed because of the aforementioned conditions.

Most authors have indicated that posterior fixation alone seems stable enough, provided that the number of fixations is sufficient (at least two above and two below the fracture). Cervical pedicle screws are reported to be the most reliable—but most challenging—type of fixation. The pull-out strength of various screw placement techniques in the cervical spine has been analyzed. Pedicle screws have been demonstrated to offer the best pull-out resistance of all available posterior fixation techniques, with an 88% increase in pull-out strength, compared with lateral mass screws [5, 13]. Given the anatomical bone distortion secondary to the underlying disease process, the typical landmarks are often obscured, making hardware placement a unique challenge

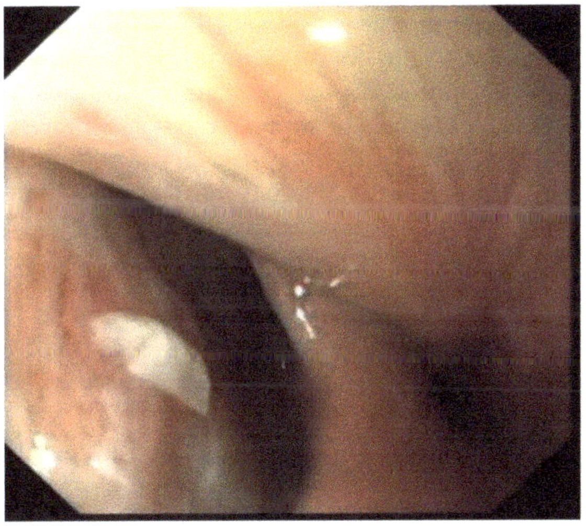

Fig. 2 Gastroscopy performed three days postoperatively showing 1.5 cm × 1.5 cm circular fistula located at esophageal entrance posterior wall

in patients with AS. Detailed knowledge and familiarity with the lateral mass and pedicle anatomy are essential for extrapolation of limited recognizable landmarks during hardware placement and trajectory infiltration [18]. In our series, posterior pedicle screw fixation was completed successfully in all 35 patients, who had satisfactory clinical outcomes.

Because the cervical spine is kyphotic, the occurrence of the fracture could be an opportunity to increase lordosis at the site of the fracture. Most published series, however, have aimed only at restoring the former kyphosis [15, 17, 20]. In our experience, the pre-bending rod and distraction can be used to increase the chin-to-chest distance gradually and restore the former lordosis. This procedure did not increase the surgical duration. It is clear that the risk of translation and overdistraction is high during the lordosis maneuvers because of the instability. The anterior opening must be limited, specifically above C6, to avoid any additional cerebral risk of stretching the vertebral arteries. In our study, the correction did not result in neurological decompensation, and the average postoperative correction was 18°. All of the patients were satisfied with the results as their field of vision had improved.

There are several limitations in this study. First, the enrollment in this study was relatively small. As more cases are performed using this technique, however, its safety and efficiency can be more thoroughly evaluated. Second, we did not have controls to prove the outcomes. Prospective, controlled studies are currently being performed to meet this objective.

Conclusions

Pedicle screw fixation and autologous bone graft through a single posterior approach for treating lower cervical spine fractures in AS patients can stabilize the spine, correct kyphosis, and relieve pressure. It is reasonable, therefore, to recommend this surgical strategy in patients with AS who have a fracture of the lower cervical spine.

Abbreviations

3D-CT: Three-dimensional computed tomography; AS: Ankylosing Spondylitis; ASIA: American Spinal Injury Association; CT: Computed tomography; ICBG: Iliac Crest Bone Graft; MRI: Magnetic resonance imaging

Acknowledgements

Dr Liang Yan and Dr Zhenguo Luo contributed equally to this work and should be considered as co-first authors. Dr Dingjun Hao and Dr Baorong He contributed equally to this work and should be considered as co-corresponding authors. The authors wish to thank the National Natural Science Foundation of China (81401843) and China Postdoctoral Science Foundation (2016M590965). The funders had no role in the study design, data collection and analysis, decision to publish, or preparation of the manuscript.

Funding

This research was supported by a grant from the National Natural Science Foundation of China (81401843) and China Postdoctoral Science Foundation (2016M590965).

Authors' contributions

DJH conceived of the study, performed all operations. LY, ZGL and BRH performed all operations and drafted the manuscript. JJL carried out the follow-up for the patients and collected the patients' data. All authors read and approved the final manuscript.

Competing interests

The authors declare that they have no competing interests.

Consent for publication

Not applicable.

Author details

[1]Department of Spinal Surgery, Hong Hui Hospital, Xi'an Jiaotong University College of Medicine, 555 Friendship East Road, Xi'an 710054, Shaanxi, China. [2]Department of Anesthesiology, Hong Hui Hospital, Xi'an Jiaotong University College of Medicine, 555 Friendship East Road, Xi'an 710054, Shaanxi, China.

References

1. Feldtkeller E, Vosse D, Geusens P, van der Linden S. Prevalence and annual incidence of vertebral fractures in patients with ankylosing spondylitis. Rheumatol Int. 2006;26:234–9.
2. Etame AB, Than KD, Wang AC, La Marca F, Park P. Surgical management of symptomatic cervical or cervicothoracic kyphosis due to ankylosing spondylitis. Spine (Phila Pa 1976). 2008;33:E559–64.
3. Cornefjord M, Alemany M, Olerud C. Posterior fixation of subaxial cervical spine fractures in patients with ankylosing spondylitis. Eur Spine J. 2005;14:401–8.
4. El Masry MA, Badawy WS, Chan D. Combined anterior and posterior stabilisation for treating an unstable cervical spine fracture in a patient with long standing ankylosing spondylitis. Injury. 2004;35:1064–7.
5. Mountney J, Murphy AJ, Fowler JL. Lessons learned from cervical pseudoarthrosis in ankylosing spondylitis. Eur Spine J. 2005;14:689–93.
6. Shen FH, Samartzis D. Surgical management of lower cervical spine fracture in ankylosing spondylitis. J Trauma. 2006;61:1005–9.
7. Mundwiler M, Siddique K, Dym J, Perri B, Johnson JP, Weisman MH. Complications of the spine in ankylosing spondylitis with a focus on deformity correction. Neurosurg Focus. 2008;24:1–9.
8. Kouyoumdjian P, Guerin P, Schaelderle C, Asencio G, Gille O. Fracture of the lower cervical spine in patients with Ankylosing Spondylitis: Retrospective study of 19 cases. Orthop Traumatol Surg Res. 2012;98:543–51.
9. Anwar F, Al-Khayer A, Fraser M, Allan DB. Concomitant cervical and thoracic spinal fractures in ankylosing spondylitis: a case report and review of literature. Injury Extra. 2009;40:242–5.
10. Anwar F, Al-Khayer A, Joseph G, Fraser MH, Jigajinni MV, Allan DB. Delayed presentation and diagnosis of cervical spine injuries in long-standing ankylosing spondylitis. Eur Spine J. 2011;20:403–7.
11. Payer M. Surgical management of cervical fractures in ankylosing spondylitis using a combined posterior-anterior approach. J Clin Neurosci. 2006;13:73–7.
12. Braun J, Sieper J. Ankylosing spondylitis. Lancet. 2007;369:1379–90.
13. Caron T, Bransford R, Nguyen Q, Agel J, Chapman J, Bellabarba C. Spine fractures in patients with ankylosing spinal disorders. Spine (Phila Pa 1976). 2010;35:E458–64.
14. Dean LE, Jones GT, MacDonald AG, Downham C, Sturrock RD, Macfarlane GJ. Global prevalence of ankylosing spondylitis. Rheumatology (Oxford). 2014;53:650–7.

15. Einsiedel T, Schmelz A, Arand M, Wilke HJ, Gebhard F, Hartwig E, et al. Injuries of the cervical spine in patients with ankylosing spondylitis: experience at two trauma centers. J Neurosurg Spine. 2006;5:33–45.
16. Westerveld LA, van Bemmel JC, Dhert WJ, Oner FC, Verlaan JJ. Clinical outcome after traumatic spinal fractures in patients with ankylosing spinal disorders compared with control patients. Spine J. 2014;14:729–40.
17. Westerveld LA, Verlaan JJ, Oner FC. Spinal fractures in patients with ankylosing spinal disorders : a systematic review of the literature on treat-ment, neurological status and complications. Eur Spine J. 2009;18:145–56.
18. Kanter AS, Wang MY, Mummaneni PV. A treatment algorithm for the management of cervical spine fractures and deformity in patients with ankylosing spondylitis. Neurosurg Focus. 2008;24:E11.
19. Klingberg E, Lorentzon M, Mellström D, Geijer M, Göthlin J, Hilme E, et al. Osteoporosis in Ankylosing Spondylitis-prevalence, risk factors and methods of assessment. Arthritis Res Ther. 2002;14:R108.
20. Sambrook N, Geusens P. The epidemiology of osteoporosis and fractures in Ankylosing Spondylitis. Ther Adv Musculoskelet Dis. 1998;4:287–92.

20

Increased fragility fracture risk in Korean women who snore: a 10-year population-based prospective cohort study

Soo Beom Choi[1,2], Il Suk Lyu[3], Wanhyung Lee[4] and Deok Won Kim[1,2*]

Abstract

Background: Snoring is frequently associated with obstructive sleep apnea (OSA). Previous studies have shown that bone mineral density was significantly lower in patients with OSA than in controls; however, these studies did not focus on fractures. Fragility fractures can lead to long-term disabilities and a decrease in quality of life. The present study aimed to investigate the association between snoring and fragility fractures.

Methods: This study included 2969 men and 3220 women aged 40 years and older from the Ansung and Ansan cohort studies in Korea. During a 10-year follow-up period, 129 and 273 fracture cases were reported in men and women, respectively.

Results: Severe snoring (6–7 nights per week or sleep disturbance by snoring in the next room) was a statistically significant risk factor for fracture ($p = 0.006$, hazard ratio 1.68, 95% confidence interval 1.16–2.43) after adjusting for covariates related to fragility fracture in women. However, both snoring and severe snoring groups did not show significant associations with the fracture risk in men.

Conclusions: Thus, information on the frequency of snoring in women may improve the accuracy of fragility fracture risk prediction, which can help in deciding whether intervention or treatment is necessary.

Keywords: Cohort study, Snoring, Fracture, Osteoporosis, Pre-screening

Background

Fragility fractures are a major and increasingly common cause of morbidity, and they pose a considerable burden on healthcare systems [1]. Moreover, most osteoporosis-related fractures can lead to significant long-term disabilities and a decrease in the quality of life [2, 3]. Screening for low bone mineral density (BMD) using dual-energy X-ray absorptiometry (DXA) is an accepted strategy to identify people with an elevated risk of fragility fracture. However, mass screening with DXA in the general population, without pre-screening for high-risk individuals, is generally not recommended [4]. Moreover, people who have not experienced fractures may not recognize the necessity of having their BMD measured; therefore, people with osteoporosis may not realize that their BMD is low before fragility fractures actually occur. Thus, it is important to identify risk factors for fragility fractures that can be easily assessed without special examination.

Obstructive sleep apnea (OSA) syndrome is a common disorder characterized by recurring episodes of apnea or hypopnea due to total or partial pharyngeal collapse during sleep [5]. Previous studies have reported on the risk of osteoporosis in patients with OSA. A previous retrospective study of 66 chronic obstructive pulmonary disease (COPD) patients found that lumbar spine BMD was significantly lower in COPD patients with OSA than in COPD patients without OSA [6]. Additionally, a 6-year retrospective cohort study of 1377 OSA patients and 20,655 matched controls found that the risk of osteoporosis was 2.52-fold higher in the OSA patients than in the matched controls [7]. Moreover, a 10-year retrospective cohort study of 846 OSA patients and a

* Correspondence: kdw@yuhs.ac
[1]Department of Medical Engineering, Yonsei University College of Medicine, CPO Box 8044, Seoul, Korea
[2]Graduate Program in Biomedical Engineering, Yonsei University, Seoul, Korea

control group of 89,380 people with no sleep disorders found that OSA patients had an adjusted hazard ratio of 2.98 for osteoporosis when compared with the control group [8]. Furthermore, a cross-sectional study of 26 male OSA patients and 21 male participants without OSA showed that the spine and femoral neck BMDs were significantly lower in the OSA patients than in the participants without OSA [9].

Snoring is frequently associated with OSA, and patients who initially have only primary snoring may be at risk for the future development of OSA with increasing age or weight gain [10]. However, the above-mentioned previous studies focused on BMD and not fragility fractures. Moreover, studies on the association between snoring and fragility fracture risk are rare. Therefore, the objective of the present study was to investigate the association between snoring and fragility fractures in elderly people using data obtained in a cohort study performed in Korea.

Methods

Study population

Two communities were selected for the Korean Health and Genome Study (KHGS) in 2001; the Ansung and Ansan cohorts represented rural and urban communities, respectively. This is an ongoing prospective study involving a biennial examination. Detailed information on the study design and procedures has been published previously [11]. At each visit, informed written consent was obtained from all participants. Initial data were obtained from the 10,030 subjects who participated in the Ansung and Ansan cohort studies. The fifth and sixth follow-up examinations (2009–12) collected data related to fractures. Among the 10,030 subjects, 2982 did not participate in the fifth and sixth follow-up examinations and were thus excluded. Among the remaining 7048 subjects, 859 subject had missing data. These subjects were excluded from this study. Therefore, 2969 men and 3220 women were finally included in this study (Fig. 1). The institutional review board of the Yonsei University Health System approved the protocol of this study (No. 4-2016-0572).

Selection of fracture events

Fracture events were recorded using a standardized self-administered questionnaire. In this study, we only included fracture events that occurred when the participants fell while walking or while performing activities of daily living. Fractures clearly caused by high-trauma events, such as motor vehicle accidents, violence, and falls from more than the standing height of the individual, were excluded [12]. In addition, we considered fracture events from all sites.

Clinical risk factors

Information on the presence of snoring was obtained using a questionnaire administered face to face. One of the questions asked was "Have you ever been told that you snored? If so, how many nights per week? The response options were "rarely," "1–3 times a week," "4–5 times a week," and "6–7 times a week." Another question asked was "Have you ever been told that your snoring disturbed a person's sleep in next room?" The incidences of fractures in women were 7.4% ($n = 103$) among those who did not snore, 8.4% ($n = 108$) among those who rarely snored, 9.5% ($n = 15$) among those who snored 1–3 times a week, 8.6% ($n = 8$) among those who snored 4–5 times a week, and 13.7% ($n = 39$) among those who snored 6–7 times a week. Based on the statistical analysis for optimal criterion of snoring frequency, snoring frequency was classified into the following 3 groups: non-snoring, snoring (1–5 nights per week), and severe snoring (6–7 nights per week or sleep disturbance by snoring in the next room). In this study, the covariates for fracture included age, weight, height, body mass index, waist circumference, hip circumference, regular exercise, alcohol consumption, lifetime smoker, history of previous fracture, family history of osteoporosis or fracture, degenerative arthritis, rheumatoid arthritis, hypertension, diabetes mellitus, medications for osteoporosis, years since menopause, estrogen therapy, and BMD. Regular exercise was defined as engaging in any of a variety of activities for the purpose of exercise at least once per week. The smoking and alcohol consumption variables were smoking status (never, former, or current) and alcohol consumption status (never, former, or current), respectively. The number of years since menopause was defined as "0" for premenopausal subjects and was the actual value for postmenopausal subjects.

Quantitative ultrasound (qUS) measurements of BMD at the radius and tibia were performed using the Omnisense 7000 device (Sunlight Medical, Ltd., Rehovot, Israel) with a handheld probe specifically designed for the measurement of the axial speed of sound (SoS, m/s) along the surface of bone [12]. In addition, T and Z scores were calculated in both the radius and tibia.

Statistical analysis

The characteristics of the study participants are reported as mean ± standard deviation (SD) for continuous variables and as number (%) for categorical variables. In order to evaluate the association between each of these variables and the fragility fracture risk, analysis of variance (ANOVA) was performed for each continuous variable and the chi-square test was performed for each categorical variable.

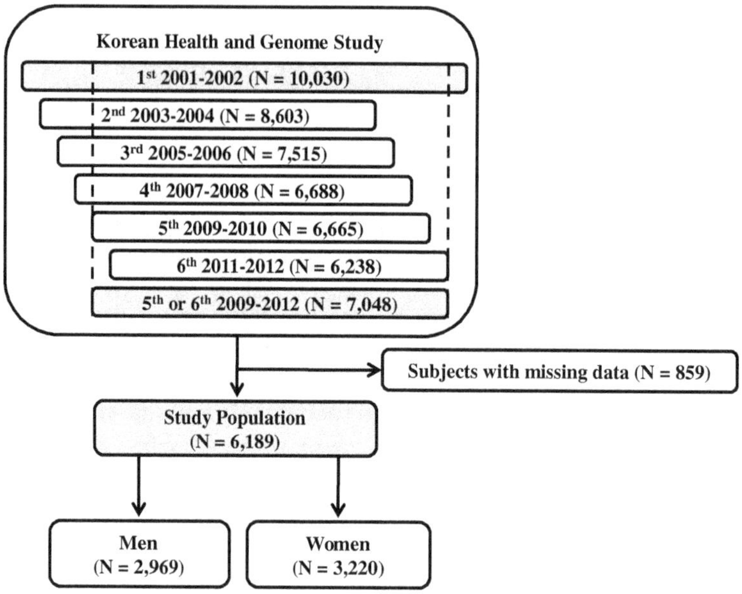

Fig. 1 Flow chart of participants for the Ansung and Ansan cohort studies with subject exclusion

Cox regression was performed to investigate whether snoring was associated with an increase in the risk of fragility fractures. Among the Cox regression analysis results, hazard ratios and 95% confidence intervals were reported. The survival time was defined as the time interval between the first examinations (2001) and the first fragility fracture since the first examinations. Non-fracture cases were censored at the time of the sixth follow-up examinations (2011). First, crude univariate Cox regression was performed without controlling for any covariate. Second, Cox regression analysis was performed after controlling for age, weight, height, waist circumference, hip circumference, regular exercise, alcohol consumption, lifetime smoker, history of previous fracture, family history of osteoporosis or fracture, degenerative arthritis, rheumatoid arthritis, hypertension, diabetes mellitus, years since menopause, estrogen therapy, and qUS measurements at the radius and tibia. Third, a Cox regression model with backward stepwise elimination was used to restrict adjustment for confounding factors with a threshold of $p = 0.1$. The Cox regression model proportionality of hazard assumption was verified using the log-minus-log method (LML) and time-dependent coefficients.

Finally, Kaplan-Meier analysis was performed in the non-snoring, snoring, and severe snoring groups, and the log-rank test was performed to check for statistically significant differences among these 3 groups. All statistical analyses were two-sided and were performed using SPSS 23.0 (IBM Corp., Armonk, NY). A p-value <0.05 was considered statistically significant.

Results

Clinical characteristics of fractures

The mean (SD) survival time of the study population was 9.5 (1.3) years for women. During the follow-up period, 273 women (8.5% of all women) experienced fractures. Among these 273 fracture cases, 52 (19.0% of all fracture cases) involved the hip, 14 (5.1%) vertebrae, 33 (12.1%) wrist, 3 (1.1%) coccyx, 16 (5.9%) humerus, 17 (6.2%) forearm, 25 (9.2%) rib, 80 (29.3%) lower limb, 1 (0.4%) clavicle, and 32 (11.7%) other locations. The mean (SD) survival time of the fracture cases was 6.6 (2.4) years. The mean (SD) survival time of the study population was 9.6 (1.1) years for men. During the follow-up period, 129 men (4.3% of all men) experienced fractures (Additional file 1: Table S1).

The results of ANOVA and the chi-square test suggested that age, weight, height, body mass index, waist circumference, hip circumference, degenerative arthritis, rheumatoid arthritis, hypertension, diabetes mellitus, years since menopause, SoS at the radius, T and Z scores of the radius, SoS at the tibia, and T and Z scores of the tibia were significantly different between the non-snoring, snoring, and severe snoring groups in women (Table 1).

Hazard ratios for fracture

When the non-snoring group was used as the reference group, the snoring and severe snoring groups in women had hazard ratios of 1.14 and 1.97, respectively, in the crude Cox regression model (Table 2). After adjusting for all covariates, the fracture risk was 1.68-fold higher in the severe snoring group than in the non-snoring

Table 1 Demographic and clinical characteristics of the female participants in the snoring groups ($n = 3220$)

	Non-snoring ($n = 1398$)	Snoring (1–5 nights/week) ($n = 1493$)	Severe snoring (6–7 nights/week) ($n = 329$)	p-value
Survival time (years)	9.6 ± 1.1	9.5 ± 1.4	9.3 ± 1.6	0.003*
Age (years)	51.3 ± 8.9	52.6 ± 8.6	55.7 ± 8.2	<0.001*
Weight (kg)	57.1 ± 7.8	59.8 ± 8.2	62.5 ± 8.6	<0.001*
Height (cm)	153.9 ± 5.6	154.1 ± 5.5	153.5 ± 5.5	<0.001*
Body mass index (kg/m^2)	24.1 ± 3.0	25.2 ± 3.1	26.5 ± 3.2	<0.001*
Waist circumference (cm)	79.8 ± 9.2	82.3 ± 9.5	86.6 ± 9.2	<0.001*
Hip circumference (cm)	92.4 ± 5.7	93.9 ± 5.8	96.2 ± 6.2	<0.001*
Regular exercise, n (%)	325 (23.3)	366 (24.5)	69 (21.0)	0.359
Alcohol consumption, n (%)				0.314
Never	1012 (72.4)	1052 (70.5)	221 (67.2)	
Past	32 (2.3)	40 (2.7)	12 (3.7)	
Current	354 (25.3)	401 (26.9)	96 (29.2)	
Lifetime smoker, n (%)				0.814
Never	1342 (96.0)	1438 (96.3)	312 (94.8)	
Past	29 (2.1)	29 (1.9)	9 (2.7)	
Current	27 (1.9)	26 (1.7)	8 (2.4)	
History of previous fracture, n (%)	31 (2.2)	42 (2.8)	15 (4.6)	0.062
Family history of osteoporosis or fracture, n (%)	78 (5.6)	79 (5.3)	18 (5.5)	0.943
Degenerative arthritis, n (%)	187 (13.4)	279 (18.7)	94 (28.6)	<0.001*
Rheumatoid arthritis, n (%)	98 (7.0)	118 (7.9)	37 (11.3)	0.037*
Hypertension, n (%)	172 (12.3)	289 (19.4)	89 (27.1)	<0.001*
Diabetes mellitus, n (%)	60 (4.3)	86 (5.8)	35 (10.6)	<0.001*
Medications for osteoporosis, n (%)	62 (4.4)	87 (5.8)	17 (5.2)	0.239
Years since menopause (years)	6.5 ± 8.5	7.2 ± 8.5	9.7 ± 8.8	<0.001*
Current estrogen therapy, n (%)	55 (3.9)	45 (3.0)	15 (4.6)	0.245
Speed of sound of radius (m/s)	4212.2 ± 185.5	4187.6 ± 186.1	4136.6 ± 187.4	<0.001*
T-score of radius	0.3 ± 1.6	0.1 ± 1.6	−0.3 ± 1.6	<0.001*
Z-score of radius	1.1 ± 1.4	0.9 ± 1.4	0.8 ± 1.4	<0.001*
Speed of sound of tibia (m/s)	3867.6 ± 164.3	3854.3 ± 161.9	3822.2 ± 171.3	<0.001*
T-score of tibia	−0.8 ± 1.5	−0.9 ± 1.5	−1.2 ± 1.6	<0.001*
Z-score of tibia	−0.1 ± 1.3	−0.1 ± 1.3	−0.2 ± 1.5	<0.001*
Fracture, n (%)	103 (7.4)	124 (8.3)	46 (14.0)	0.001*

Data are presented as mean ± standard deviation or number of participants (%)
The p-values of continuous and binary variables were calculated using analysis of variance (ANOVA) and the chi-square test, respectively
*$p < 0.05$

group (model 2). Moreover, the Cox regression model (model 3) with backward stepwise elimination showed that the fracture risk was 1.68-fold higher in the severe snoring group than in the non-snoring group. However, the snoring group did not show a significant association with the fracture risk in all the models. In both models 2 and 3, severe snoring, height, waist circumference, hip circumference, family history of osteoporosis or fracture, rheumatoid arthritis, and medications for osteoporosis were selected as risk factors for fractures in women. However, both the snoring and severe snoring groups did not show significant associations with the fracture risk in men (Additional file 1: Table S2).

Kaplan-Meier survival analysis and log-rank test

We performed Kaplan-Meier analyses and log-rank tests to evaluate the association between snoring and fracture risk in women (Fig. 2). The log-rank test results indicated

Table 2 Crude and adjusted hazard ratios with 95% confidence intervals for fractures among the female participants in Cox regression analyses

	Fracture		Model 1		Model 2		Model 3	
	No ($n = 2947$)	Yes ($n = 273$)	*p*-value	HR (95% CI)	*p*-value	HR (95% CI)	*p*-value	HR (95% CI)
Survival time (years)	9.8 ± 0.6	6.6 ± 2.4						
Snoring, *n* (%)								
Non-snoring	1295 (43.9)	103 (37.7)	Reference		Reference		Reference	
Snoring	1369 (46.5)	124 (45.4)	0.320	1.142 (0.879–1.483)	0.495	1.097 (0.841–1.432)	0.506	1.094 (0.840–1.424)
Severe snoring	283 (9.6)	46 (16.9)	<0.001*	1.969 (1.391–2.787)	0.006*	1.682 (1.164–2.430)	0.005*	1.680 (1.168–2.416)
Age (years)	52.2 ± 8.8	54.0 ± 8.5			0.178	1.019 (0.991–1.048)	0.007*	1.023 (1.006–1.039)
Weight (kg)	58.9 ± 8.2	59.1 ± 8.3			0.956	0.999 (0.964–1.035)		
Height (cm)	154.0 ± 5.5	153.1 ± 5.5			0.014*	0.966 (0.939–0.993)	0.004*	0.965 (0.941–0.988)
Body mass index (kg/m^2)	24.8 ± 3.2	25.2 ± 3.2						
Waist circumference (cm)	81.6 ± 9.6	82.1 ± 9.5			0.039*	0.978 (0.957–0.999)	0.006*	0.977 (0.960–0.993)
Hip circumference (cm)	93.4 ± 5.9	94.2 ± 5.7			0.014*	1.047 (1.009–1.086)	<0.001*	1.048 (1.022–1.076)
Regular exercise, *n* (%)	693 (23.5)	67 (24.5)			0.776	1.043 (0.780–1.394)		
Alcohol consumption, *n* (%)								
Never	2088 (70.9)	197 (72.2)			Reference			
Former	74 (2.5)	10 (3.7)			0.375	1.336 (0.704–2.536)		
Current	785 (26.6)	66 (24.2)			0.615	0.929 (0.697–1.238)		
Lifetime smoker, *n* (%)								
Never	2832 (96.1)	260 (95.2)			Reference			
Former	61 (2.1)	6 (2.2)			0.995	0.998 (0.441–2.256)		
Current	54 (1.8)	7 (2.6)			0.423	1.365 (0.638–2.921)		
History of previous fracture, *n* (%)	80 (2.7)	8 (2.9)			0.803	0.913 (0.448–1.862)		
Family history of osteoporosis or fracture, *n* (%)	154 (5.2)	21 (7.7)			0.029*	1.658 (1.052–2.612)	0.028*	1.658 (1.055–2.605)
Degenerative arthritis, *n* (%)	504 (17.1)	56 (20.5)			0.764	0.953 (0.694–1.308)		
Rheumatoid arthritis, *n* (%)	219 (7.4)	34 (12.5)			0.020*	1.563 (1.073–2.278)	0.019*	1.552 (1.076–2.238)
Hypertension, *n* (%)	499 (16.9)	51 (18.7)			0.847	0.968 (0.698–1.342)		
Diabetes mellitus, *n* (%)	165 (5.6)	16 (5.9)			0.860	0.955 (0.569–1.601)		
Medications for osteoporosis, *n* (%)	141 (4.8)	25 (9.2)			0.004*	1.877 (1.225–2.876)	0.004*	1.856 (1.221–2.819)
Years since menopause (years)	7.0 ± 8.6	8.4 ± 8.7			0.821	0.997 (0.973–1.022)		
Estrogen therapy, *n* (%)	104 (3.5)	11 (4.0)			0.771	0.912 (0.492–1.690)		
Speed of sound in radius (m/s)	4195.9 ± 187.3	4162.4 ± 184.5			0.318	1.000 (0.999–1.000)		
Speed of sound in tibia (m/s)	3859.1 ± 164.6	3832.1 ± 160.9			0.627	1.000 (0.999–1.001)		

Data are presented as mean ± standard deviation or number of participants (%)
Crude univariate Cox regression model 1 did not control for any covariate
Cox regression model 2 controlled for age, weight, height, waist circumference, hip circumference, regular exercise, alcohol consumption, lifetime smoker, history of fracture, family history of osteoporosis or fracture, degenerative arthritis, rheumatoid arthritis, hypertension, diabetes mellitus, years since menopause, estrogen therapy, and quantitative ultrasound measurements at the radius and tibia
Cox regression model 3 with backward stepwise elimination involved a threshold of $p = 0.1$
Abbreviations: *HR* hazard ratio, *CI* confidence interval
*$p < 0.05$

that the fracture risk was significantly higher in the severe snoring group than in the non-snoring group ($p < 0.001$).

Discussion

In this study, female participants with severe snoring had a statistically significant increase in the fracture risk, even after adjusting for covariates. To the best of our knowledge, the present study is the first to investigate the association between snoring and fragility fractures using data from a 10-year cohort study. Information about snoring can easily be obtained with history taking, and it does not require medical examinations, such as DXA. Thus, we expect that collecting information about snoring may be an inexpensive and simple approach to help increase the accuracy of the prediction of fragility fracture events. Furthermore, if future studies identify

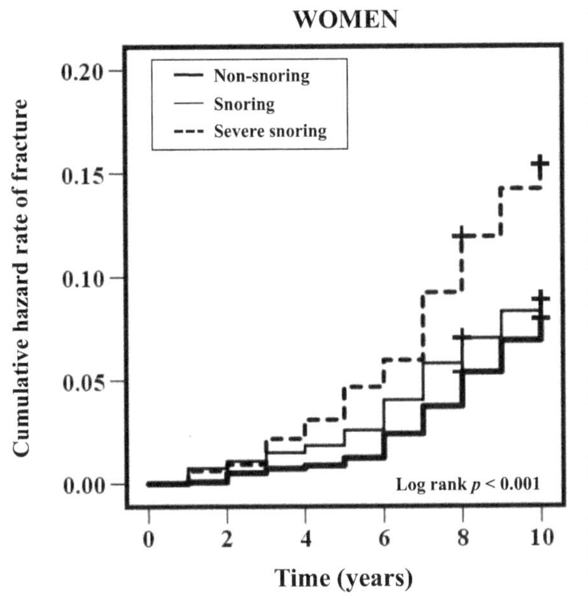

No. at risk

	0	2	4	6	8	10
Non-snoring	1398	1397	1388	1381	1347	1169
Snoring	1493	1482	1471	1455	1409	1238
Severe snoring	329	327	322	314	300	259

Fig. 2 The cumulative hazard rates of fractures and the log rank values for the non-snoring, snoring, and severe snoring groups in women

the exact mechanism by which snoring increases the fragility fracture risk, treatment of snoring may become an accepted approach to reduce the fragility fracture risk.

This study showed that snoring was significantly associated with fragility fractures in women aged 40 years and older. Although few if any previous studies have specifically investigated the association between snoring and fragility fractures, several previous studies have analyzed the osteoporosis risk in OSA patients [6–9]. Snoring has been reported to be frequently associated with OSA [10]. Moreover, Jennum et al. demonstrated that snoring was associated with the respiratory distress index, which was calculated as the number of apnea and hypopnea episodes lasting longer than 10 s per hour [13]. However, the authors mentioned that self-reported snoring alone was not sensitive enough to identify individuals with sleep apnea [13]. The repetitive hypoxia and subsequent reoxygenation that occur in OSA may lead to oxidative stress, which may result in acidosis because of insufficient vascular perfusion [7]. Furthermore, hypoxia may inhibit the proliferation of osteoblasts and promote proliferation of osteoclasts, resulting in osteoporosis [7, 14]. A decrease in BMD caused by the above-mentioned mechanisms may increase the fragility fracture risk in the elderly.

Suzuki et al. investigated the association between sleep disturbance and hip fracture risk, which may provide more insights into the association between snoring and an increase in the fracture risk [15]. In that study, the authors followed participants for 6 months and reported that there was a significant association between sleep disturbance and hip fracture risk (odds ratio 2.60, 95% confidence interval 1.31–5.17) [15]. Sleep disturbance may increase the fracture risk in the elderly by decreasing the alertness level during the daytime and thus increasing the risk of falling [15]. However, further studies are needed to investigate the exact association between snoring and fragility fracture risk.

Zhang et al. demonstrated the associations between insomnia and falls using cross-sectional data (954 subjects) in Boston, Massachusetts [16]. Adults with insomnia had a 32% increased likelihood of falls after adjustment for multiple covariates, but insomnia was not associated with recurrent falls or fractures. The authors also assessed snoring and falls; however, there was no significant difference. The study for insomnia and falls involved only 2 years of follow-up data. A longer follow-up duration is required for fractures. Moreover, Upala et al. performed a systematic review and meta-analysis of 9 articles to evaluate the association between OSA and the risk of osteoporosis [17]. Their analysis did not find a significant association between osteoporosis and OSA or a difference in bone loss between the groups.

The present study has 4 limitations. First, we did not investigate the OSA of subjects using polysomnography; therefore, the definition of severe snoring in this study was not experimentally verified. However, information about snoring, which can easily be obtained with simple questions, could be useful in pre-screening for fragility fractures. Second, BMD was not measured with DXA. However, qUS has been shown to be a fairly accurate method for measuring BMD [18], and therefore, qUS is being used in the clinical setting along with DXA. Third, fracture history was not obtained from official medical records maintained by physicians but was obtained from survey results, which relied on the memory of the respondents. Moreover, the memory of the respondents about fractures was retrospective up to a 10-year lag, and fracture time was asked by the year. Fourth, this cohort study was designed to investigate the genome-wide association and associated risk factors of chronic disease in urban and rural Koreans; therefore, it might be difficult to extend our findings to the general population. Moreover, there were unmeasured confounders for snoring and fractures, such as mental status, insomnia disorders, dairy product consumption, and pregnancy information.

Conclusions

This study showed that snoring is significantly associated with fragility fracture risk in women aged 40 years and older. Snoring may be associated with a decrease in

BMD and a decrease in the alertness level during the daytime. These 2 health problems are in turn probably associated with an increase in the fracture risk. Information about snoring can easily be obtained with history taking, and treatment options for snoring are available. Thus, information on the frequency of snoring in women may improve the accuracy of fragility fracture risk prediction, which can help in deciding whether intervention or treatment is necessary.

Abbreviations
BMD: Bone mineral density; COPD: Chronic obstructive pulmonary disease; KHGS: Korean health and genome study; OSA: Obstructive sleep apnea; qUS: Quantitative ultrasound; SoS: Speed of sound

Acknowledgments
This data set was provided by the National Genome Research Institute, Korean Center for Disease Control and Prevention (2001-2003-348-6111-221, 2004-347-6111-213, and 2005-347-2400-2440-215).

Funding
We did not receive any funding or support.

Authors' contributions
SBC and DWK contributed to the concept and design of the study. SBC and WL contributed to data acquisition, analysis, and interpretation. SBC and ISL contributed to the drafting of the manuscript. ISL also contributed to the statistical analysis of data. DWK takes full responsibility for the integrity of the data analysis. All authors read and approved the final manuscript.

Competing interests
The authors have no competing interests.

Consent for publication
Not applicable.

Author details
[1]Department of Medical Engineering, Yonsei University College of Medicine, CPO Box 8044, Seoul, Korea. [2]Graduate Program in Biomedical Engineering, Yonsei University, Seoul, Korea. [3]Department of Medicine, Yonsei University College of Medicine, Seoul, Korea. [4]Graduate School of Public Health, Yonsei University College of Medicine, Seoul, Korea.

References
1. Johnell O, Kanis JA, Odén A, Sernbo I, Redlund-Johnell I, Petterson C, et al. Mortality after osteoporotic fractures. Osteoporos Int. 2004;15(1):38–42.
2. Adachi JD, Ioannidis G, Berger C, Joseph L, Papaioannou A, Pickard L, et al. The influence of osteoporotic fractures on health-related quality of life in community-dwelling men and women across Canada. Osteoporos Int. 2001; 12(11):903–8.
3. Hallberg I, Rosenqvist AM, Kartous L, Löfman O, Wahlström O, Toss G. Health-related quality of life after osteoporotic fractures. Osteoporos Int. 2004;15:834–41.
4. Maghraoui AE, Habbassi A, Ghazi M, Achemlal L, Mounach A, Nouijai A, et al. Validation and comparative evaluation of four osteoporosis risk indexes in Moroccan menopausal women. Arch Osteoporos. 2006;1:1–6.
5. Mannarino MR, Di Filippo F, Pirro M. Obstructive sleep apnea syndrome. Eur J Intern Med. 2012;23(7):586–93.
6. Wang TY, Lo YL, Chou PC, Chung FT, Lin SM, Lin TY, et al. Associated bone mineral density and obstructive sleep apnea in chronic obstructive pulmonary disease. Int J Chron Obstruct Pulmon Dis. 2015;10:231–7.
7. Chen YL, Weng SF, Shen YC, Chou CW, Yang CY, Wang JJ, et al. Obstructive sleep apnea and risk of osteoporosis: a population-based cohort study in Taiwan. J Clin Endocrinol Metab. 2014;99(7):2441–7.
8. Yen CM, Kuo CL, Lin MC, Lee CF, Lin KY, Lin CL, et al. Sleep disorders increase the risk of osteoporosis: a nationwide population-based cohort study. Sleep Med. 2014;15(11):1339–44.
9. Uzkeser H, Yildirim K, Aktan B, Karatay S, Kaynar H, Araz O, et al. Bone mineral density in patients with obstructive sleep apnea syndrome. Sleep Breath. 2013;17(1):339–42.
10. American Academy of Sleep Medicine. International classification of sleep disorders: diagnostic and coding manual. 2nd ed. Westchester: American Academy of Sleep Medicine; 2005.
11. Shin C, Abbott RD, Lee H, Kim J, Kimm K. Prevalence and correlates of orthostatic hypotension in middle-aged men and women in Korea: the Korean Health and Genome Study. J Hum Hypertens. 2004;18(10):717–23.
12. Lee SH, Khang YH, Lim KH, Kim BJ, Koh JM, Kim GS, et al. Clinical risk factors for osteoporotic fracture: a population-based prospective cohort study in Korea. J Bone Miner Res. 2010;25(2):369–78.
13. Jennum P, Sjøl A. Epidemiology of snoring and obstructive sleep apnoea in a Danish population, age 30–60. J Sleep Res. 1992;1(4):240–4.
14. Chakhtoura M, Nasrallah M, Chami H. Bone loss in obesity and obstructive sleep apnea: a review of literature. J Clin Sleep Med. 2015;11(5):575–80.
15. Suzuki T, Yoshida H, Hashimoto T, Yoshimura N, Fujiwara S, Fukunaga M, et al. Case-control study of risk factors for hip fractures in the Japanese elderly by a Mediterranean Osteoporosis Study (MEDOS) questionnaire. Bone. 1997;21(5):461–7.
16. Zhang Y, Cifuentes M, Gao X, Amaral G, Tucker KL. Age- and gender-specific associations between insomnia and falls in Boston Puerto Rican adults. Qual Life Res. 2017;26(1):25–34.
17. Upala S, Sanguankeo A, Congrete S. Obstructive Sleep Apnea is Not Associated with an Increased Risk of Osteoporosis: a Systematic Review and Meta-Analysis. J Clin Sleep Med. 2015;11(9):1069–70.
18. Tao B, Liu JM, Li XY, Wang JG, Wang WQ, Ning G. An assessment of the use of quantitative ultrasound and the Osteoporosis Self-Assessment Tool for Asians in determining the risk of nonvertebral fracture in postmenopausal Chinese women. J Bone Miner Metab. 2008;26(1):60–5.

21

Clinical and radiographic predictors of acute compartment syndrome in the treatment of tibial plateau fractures

Axel Gamulin[1*], Anne Lübbeke[1], Patrick Belinga[1], Pierre Hoffmeyer[1], Thomas V. Perneger[2], Matthieu Zingg[1] and Gregory Cunningham[1]

Abstract

Background: The aim of the study was to evaluate the relation between demographic, injury-related, clinical and radiological factors of patients with tibial plateau fractures and the development of acute compartment syndrome.

Methods: All consecutive adult patients with intra-articular tibial plateau fractures admitted in our urban academic medical centre between January 2005 and December 2009 were included in this retrospective cohort study. The main outcome measurement was the development of acute compartment syndrome.

Results: The charts of 265 patients (mean age 48.6 years) sustaining 269 intra-articular tibial plateau fractures were retrospectively reviewed. Acute compartment syndrome occurred in 28 fractures (10.4%). Four patients presented bilateral tibial plateau fractures; of them, 2 had unilateral, but none had bilateral acute compartment syndrome. Non-contiguous tibia fracture or knee dislocation and higher AO/OTA classification (type 41-C) were statistically significantly associated with the development of acute compartment syndrome in multivariable regression analysis, while younger age (<45 years), male sex, higher Schatzker grade (IV-V-VI), higher tibial widening ratio (≥1.05) and higher femoral displacement ratio (≥0.08) were significantly associated in the analysis adjusted for age and sex.

Conclusions: Two parameters related to the occurrence of ACS in tibial plateau fractures were highlighted in this study: the presence of a non-contiguous tibia fracture or knee dislocation, and higher AO/OTA classification. They may be especially useful when clinical findings are difficult to assess (doubtful clinical signs, obtunded, sedated or intubated patients), and should rise the suspicion level of the treating surgeon. In these cases, regular clinical examinations and/or intra-compartmental pressure measurements should be performed before and after surgery, even if acute compartment syndrome seemed unlikely during initial assessment. However, larger studies are mandatory to confirm and refine both factors in predicting the occurrence of acute compartment syndrome.

Keywords: Tibial plateau fracture, Proximal tibia fracture, Acute compartment syndrome, Fasciotomy, Risk factors

* Correspondence: axel.gamulin@hcuge.ch
[1]Department of Surgery, Division of Orthopaedic and Trauma Surgery, University Hospitals of Geneva, 4 Rue Gabrielle-Perret-Gentil, CH-1211 Geneva 14, Switzerland
Full list of author information is available at the end of the article

Background

Tibial plateau fractures account for approximately 1% of all fractures [1]. Schatzker and AO/OTA classifications are widely used for their description [2, 3]. Tibial plateau fractures represent a broad range of injury pattern, from low-energy mainly undisplaced, isolated lateral plateau fractures, to high-energy displaced, medial plateau, bicondylar or epiphyso-metaphyso-diaphyseal fractures [4–6]. The amount of energy released in the bone and soft-tissues during trauma may determine associated soft-tissue lesions such as skin lacerations (open fracture) and acute compartment syndrome (ACS) [4–7]. Occurrence of ACS may be as high as 12% in overall tibial plateau fractures [8–11], and as high as 53% in higher-energy fracture subgroups (Schatzker IV, V and VI) [8, 11–15].

Trauma patients, especially those involved in high-energy polytrauma, may be intubated and/or sedated and/or obtunded at time of assessment by the orthopaedic surgeon. In such conditions, usual valuable clinical signs for diagnosing ACS (pain out of proportion with the findings on physical examination and exacerbated by passive stretch of the muscles in the area of the injury) may be impossible to evaluate [16, 17]. In addition to intra-compartmental pressure (ICP) measurement, alternative predictors of impending ACS need to be determined.

The literature regarding risk factors for the occurrence of ACS after tibial plateau fractures is scarce. Radiographic determinants have been recently reported, such as higher Schatzker and AO/OTA grades, increased tibial widening ratio (TWR), increased femoral displacement ratio (FDR), increased fracture length and associated fibular fracture [8, 11–15]. Identified risk factors for ACS following tibial shaft fractures include young age, male sex, mechanism of injury, high-energy trauma and open fracture [9, 16–19]. However, the presence of a concomitant non-contiguous tibia fracture or knee dislocation may be an additional valuable indicator for high-energy trauma associated with extended musculoskeletal damage, and may hence also be a predictive factor for development of ACS. To the authors' knowledge, no study has to date evaluated these potential risk factors simultaneously.

The objective of this study was therefore to evaluate the relation between key demographic, injury-related, clinical and radiographic factors in patients with tibial plateau fractures and the subsequent development of ACS.

Methods

Ethics statement

Approval from the local institutional research ethics board was obtained prior to initiation of the study.

Study participants

This retrospective cohort study was conducted in a 1900-bed urban academic medical centre providing primary and tertiary care for 500,000 inhabitants. All patients admitted for a proximal tibia fracture were identified using the institutional hospitalization diagnoses database, which lists all patients diagnoses upon hospitalization. Inclusion criteria were: 1) a proximal tibia fracture as defined by the AO/OTA classification code 41 [1]; 2) trauma as a cause of fracture; 3) presentation to our institution between January 2005 and December 2009; and 4) age > 16 years old at the time of injury. At this point, 319 fractures were eligible. Exclusion criteria were: 1) extra-articular fractures (AO/OTA type 41-A), as these are commonly excluded from studies about tibial plateau fractures (18 fractures); 2) open growth plates at the time of initial presentation (one fracture); 3) presentation to our institution more than 24 h after initial trauma (patient-based late presentation or referral from another institution; 27 fractures); 4) pathological (primary neoplasm, metastasis) or spontaneous fracture (preceding and as cause of the fall) (one fracture); 5) periprosthetic or peri-implant fracture (two fractures); 6) available radiographic workup inadequate for intra-articular involvement evidence and Schatzker and AO/OTA classifications; 7) above or below knee amputation within the first 24 h after the trauma; and 8) death within the first 24 h after the trauma (one fracture). Finally, 265 patients with 269 fractures were included in the analysis.

Outcome

The outcome was presence of ACS leading to fasciotomy. Standard clinical evaluation was performed on every patient, at admission in the emergency room and during every preoperative and postoperative visit. The attending orthopaedic surgeon established the diagnosis, with or without the use of ICP measurements [20, 21]. ICP monitoring was not used routinely but only in selected patients: those with equivocal clinical signs and those intubated, sedated or obtunded [20, 21]. When indicated, ICP was measured in each of the four leg compartments using an Intra-Compartmental Pressure Monitor (Stryker Osteosynthesis AG, Biberist, Switzerland). Patients with clinical signs of ACS and/or with pathological ICP values (a difference of less than 30 mmHg between diastolic blood pressure and ICP) were taken to the operative room for four compartments fasciotomy, and the presence or absence of muscle bulging at the time of fasciotomy was reported in the operative notes. For the purpose of this study, ACS was defined as pathological ICP values before fasciotomy, and/or by the presence of muscle bulging at the time of fasciotomy. When ICP was not measured (alert and collaborative patients with unequivocal clinical signs), muscle bulging had to be reported in the operative notes to confirm ACS. If the muscle aspect was not described in the operative notes, the diagnosis of ACS was based on ICP measurements. The diagnosis of ACS was not confirmed if fasciotomy was performed without prior ICP measurements, and if there was no muscle bulging at the time of surgery.

Variables of interest

Patient-related (age, sex) and fracture-related (mechanism of injury, closed vs. open fracture and Gustilo classification [22, 23] in case of open fracture) variables were extracted from the patients' charts. According to the mechanism of injury, trauma was further classified as either "fall from own height" or "other" (falls from more than one meter high, sports injuries, road traffic accidents, crushes, construction site accidents, farming accidents) in an attempt to differentiate between low and high-energy trauma. For statistical analysis, fractures were considered in two ways: 1) either closed or open; and 2) in three categories (closed, Gustilo type 1 and 2, and Gustilo type 3).

Based on the initial set of radiographs, Schatzker and AO/OTA classifications were determined, as well as the presence or absence of a non-contiguous tibial shaft or pilon fracture, or knee dislocation. Schatzker classification was divided in two groups: Schatzker I to III (exclusively lateral plateau fractures, involving less resistant bone than the medial plateau which is more sclerotic due to the physiologically slightly varus mechanical axis), and Schatzker IV to VI (involving either the medial plateau or a complete metaphyseal disruption, thus probably representing a higher energy pattern) [4–6]. Only the first level of the AO/OTA classification (41-B vs. 41-C) was used for the statistical analysis. Radiographic analysis of all cases was performed by a single trauma-fellowship trained orthopaedic surgeon, who was blinded to the outcome. Moreover, since intra- and interobserver reliability of Schatzker and AO/OTA classifications has been shown to be poor (moderate to substantial) in a recent study [24], a new reliability assessment of these both classifications was performed: an Internet based random integer generator (http://www.random.com) was used to randomly select 30 cases among the 269 fractures. As cases were picked independently from each other, duplicates may occur that were excluded from the reliability assessment. The trauma-fellowship trained orthopaedic surgeon performed new Schatzker and AO/OTA classifications on the randomly picked radiographs a second time, 6 months after the first analyse (intraobserver reliability). An orthopaedic chief resident also performed the above-mentioned classifications on the selected series (interobserver reliability). Non-contiguous tibial shaft or pilon fractures were defined as a second fracture complex separated from the tibial plateau fracture and located distal to the metaphyso-diaphyseal junction, thus representing a different pattern from Schatzker VI fractures [3]. Knee dislocation was defined as dislocation on both medial and lateral femoro-tibial joint lines (Fig. 1). This injury pattern has not yet been described in the literature to the best of our knowledge and must thus be very rare. It possibly represents a specific injury mechanism, with energy dissipated on one hand in the bone (producing the tibial plateau fracture) and on the other hand in the soft tissue structures supporting the joint (tearing the ligaments and producing a complete knee dislocation). This differs from the more common knee fracture-dislocation described by Moore, where only one (medial or lateral) joint line is dislocated, while the other stays reduced [25]; the tear in the supporting ligament of the dislocated compartment is possibly a direct consequence of displacement of the fracture fragment, without additional energy dissipated in the soft tissue structures supporting the joint. In this sense, tibial plateau fracture associated with complete knee dislocation might be a specific injury pattern comparable to segmental fractures, and we therefore included associated non-contiguous tibia fractures and knee dislocation in the same group. In order to control the radiographic evaluation of complete knee dislocation, both cases showing this condition were inserted in the group of cases randomly picked for reliability assessment of Schatzker and AO/OTA classifications, and were reviewed by the trauma-fellowship trained orthopaedic surgeon and the orthopaedic chief resident. Specific radiographic measurements (Figs. 2 & 3) were taken from the initial antero-posterior plain radiograph of the knee after the limb was grossly aligned, as described by Ziran et al. [11]. The following measurements were obtained using a dedicated open-source PACS workstation DICOM viewer (OsiriX, Pixmeo Sàrl, Bernex, Switzerland): 1) the width of the tibial plateau at its widest point; 2) the width of the femoral condyles at their widest point; 3) TWR (width of the tibial plateau at its widest point/width of the femoral condyles at their widest point); 4) anatomical axis displacement (absolute value of the displacement of the tibial anatomic axis to the femoral anatomic axis, measured at the best estimate of the joint line which is 1.5 cm proximal to the fibular head); 5) FDR (anatomical axis displacement/width of the femoral condyles at their widest point); and 6) anatomical axis displacement direction (neutral, lateral or medial). The rationale for and specific steps in obtaining these measurements have been extensively discussed by Ziran et al. [11]. However, intra- and interobserver reliability of TWR and FDR have never been assessed to the best of our knowledge. To estimate it, the same method previously

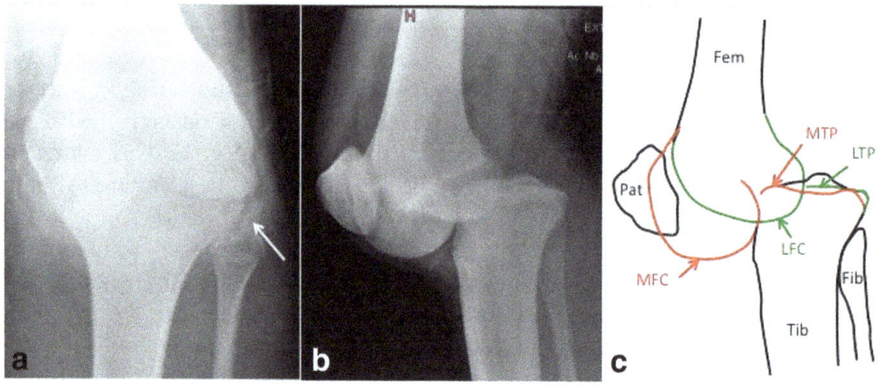

Fig. 1 Plain antero-posterior (**a**) and lateral (**b**) radiographs of the left knee of a 17 year old male with a complete dislocation of the knee and a lateral tibial plateau fracture (Schatzker II, AO/OTA 41-B3.1). The white arrow shows the lateral plateau fragment on the antero-posterior view. Schematic diagram (**c**) of the lateral radiograph showing dislocation on both medial (red drawing) and lateral (green drawing) femoro-tibial joint lines. The line representing the lateral tibial plateau is interrupted due to the fracture of the anterior part of the lateral plateau. *Fem*: femur; *Fib*: fibula; *LFC*: lateral femoral condyle; *LTP*: lateral tibial plateau; *MFC*: medial femoral condyle; *MTP*: medial tibial plateau; *Pat*: patella; *Tib*: tibia

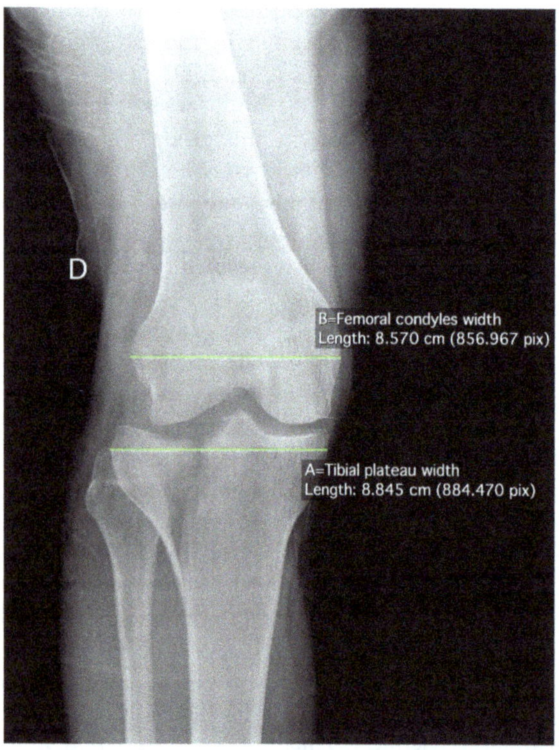

Fig. 2 Plain antero-posterior radiograph of a right knee with a Schatzker II, AO/OTA 41-B3.1 fracture. Line A represents the tibial plateau width (the width of the tibial plateau at its widest point). Line B represents the femoral condyles width (the width of the femoral condyles at their widest point). To compensate for any magnification error, a unitless ratio was calculated in order to depict tibial widening: Tibial Widening Ratio (TWR) = Line A/Line B. In the case illustrated, TWR was 8.85/8.57 = 1.03

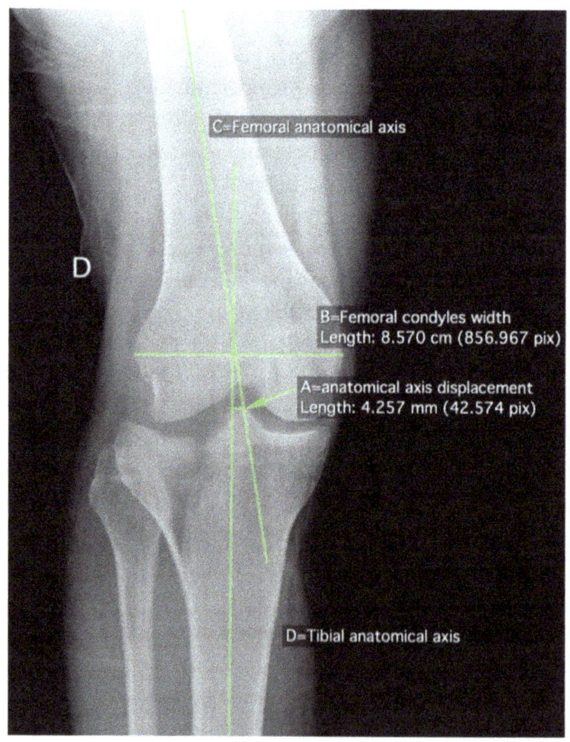

Fig. 3 Plain antero-posterior radiograph of a right knee with a Schatzker II, AO/OTA 41-B3.1 fracture. Line A represents the displacement of the tibial anatomical axis (Line D) to the femoral anatomical axis (Line C), measured at the best estimate of the joint line which is 1.5 cm proximal to the fibular head. Line B represents the femoral condyles width (the width of the femoral condyles at their widest point). To compensate for any magnification error, a unitless ratio was calculated in order to depict femoral displacement: Femoral Displacement Ratio (FDR) = Line A/Line B. In the case illustrated, FDR was 0.43/8.57 = 0.05

described for Schatzker and AO/OTA classifications reliability assessment was used.

Statistical analysis

Clinical characteristics of patients and fractures with and without ACS were compared using frequency distributions for discrete variables and means and ranges for continuous variables. Univariate odds ratios (OR) and 95% confidence intervals (95% CI) for ACS were obtained for each clinical characteristic. For this analysis, we dichotomized continuous variables at approximate midpoints (age < 45 years, TWR ≥1.05, FDR ≥0.08).

The chi-square test for linear trend was used to evaluate ACS occurrence according to soft tissue injury classified in three categories (closed fractures, open fractures Gustilo type 1 and 2, and open fractures Gustilo type 3).

Because the risk of ACS may be related to the energy dissipated in the impact, and because men and younger patients may be more likely to sustain high-energy impacts, we adjusted the other clinical variables for age and sex, using logistic regression.

Finally, we constructed a multivariable logistic regression model, starting with the most statistically significant clinical predictors, and obtained OR and 95% CIs. Two variables remained significantly related to the occurrence of ACS (see results): risks of ACS for the four subgroups of patients defined by their status on both these variables were calculated.

Intraclass correlation coefficients (ICC two-way-random) were calculated to quantify intra- and interobserver reliability in assessing Schatzker and AO/OTA classifications, TWR and FDR. The ICC is a special case of the weighted kappa and has been considered equivalent [26]. We interpreted the results following the Landis and Koch guidelines: κ <0 = poor agreement, κ 0.0–0.20 = slight agreement, κ 0.21–0.40 = fair agreement, κ 0.41–0.60 = moderate agreement, κ 0.61–0.80 = substantial or good agreement, κ 0.81–1.00 = almost perfect agreement [27].

IBM® SPSS® Statistics version 19.0.0 software (IBM SPSS, Chicago, IL) was used for statistical analysis. Statistical significance was defined as $p < 0.05$.

Results

All 269 fractures in 265 patients had complete epidemiological and clinical data extracted from their charts, as well as complete radiographic measurements available for analysis, except for one case where radiographs were of insufficiently good quality to measure TWR, FDR, and anatomical axis displacement direction; in this case's available radiographs, both tibial proximal metaphysis and femoral distal metaphysis were never seen together on the same antero-posterior view, making every measurement that necessitated comparison of anatomical landmarks located on both tibia and femur impossible. However, Schatzker and AO/OTA classifications could be determined for this case, as well as the presence or absence of a non-contiguous tibial shaft or pilon fracture, or knee dislocation.

Overall, ACS occurred in 28 (10.4%) of 269 tibial plateau fractures. ACS was confirmed 20 times by ICP measurements, and diagnosed eight times solely on clinical findings (muscle bulging at the time of surgery). There was no false positive ACS diagnosis, meaning that every patient who underwent fasciotomy had pathological ICP values before fasciotomy, and/or presented muscle bulging at the time of fasciotomy (Fig. 4). Four patients presented bilateral tibial plateau fractures; of them, 2 had unilateral ACS, but none had bilateral ACS. Timing of ACS occurrence is showed in Table 1. None of the patients with ACS was on therapeutic anticoagulation before the injury or during hospital stay.

Table 2 shows demographics, injury characteristics and clinical and radiographic factors of the study patients. Younger age (<45 years), male sex, open fracture, non-contiguous tibia fracture or knee dislocation, higher Schatzker grade (IV-V-VI), higher AO/OTA classification (type 41-C), higher TWR (≥1.05) and higher FDR (≥0.08) were associated with an increased rate of ACS in univariate analysis (Table 3). There was a significant linear association (p = 0.002) between occurrence of ACS and severity of soft tissue injury: ACS occurred in 22 of 246 (8.9%) closed fractures, two of 13 (15.4%) open fractures Gustilo type 1 and 2, and four of 10 (40%) open fractures Gustilo type 3. Mechanism of injury and anatomical axis displacement direction were not significantly associated with ACS. Separate adjustment of each variable according to age and sex resulted in small changes in significance levels, except for open fracture, which lost its statistical significance (Table 3).

In the multivariable regression model, only non-contiguous tibia fracture or knee dislocation (OR 50.0, 95% CI 6.4–391.0, p < 0.001) and higher AO/OTA classification (OR 12.8, 95% CI 4.3–38.7, p < 0.001) remained statistically significantly associated with the development of ACS. Table 4 shows the relation between both these risk factors and ACS occurrence: the risk of ACS was very high in high AO/OTA grade fractures associated with another fracture or dislocation, and very low when both risk factors were absent.

Intra- and interobserver reliability showed almost perfect agreement for all measurements (Table 5). Of note, one duplicate was excluded from the 30 randomly picked cases, leaving 29 cases (10.8% of 269 cases) for the final analysis. The trauma-fellowship trained orthopaedic surgeon and the orthopaedic chief resident both identified the same cases with associated knee dislocation. There were no false positive or false negative results.

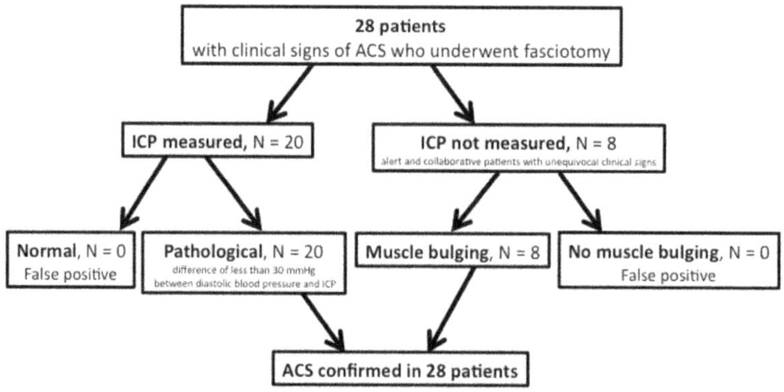

Fig. 4 Flowchart depicting how the diagnosis of ACS was confirmed in the 28 patients with clinical signs of ACS who underwent fasciotomy. ICP monitoring was used only in patients with equivocal clinical signs and those intubated, sedated or obtunded. ACS was defined as pathological ICP values before fasciotomy, and/or by the presence of muscle bulging at the time of fasciotomy. When ICP was not measured (alert and collaborative patients with unequivocal clinical signs), muscle bulging had to be reported in the operative notes to confirm ACS. If muscle aspect was not described in the operative notes, the diagnosis of ACS was based on ICP measurements. The diagnosis of ACS was not confirmed if fasciotomy was performed without prior ICP measurements, and if there was no muscle bulging at the time of surgery. There was no false positive ACS diagnosis, meaning that every patient who underwent fasciotomy had pathological ICP values before fasciotomy, and/or presented muscle bulging at the time of fasciotomy. *ACS*: acute compartment syndrome; *ICP*: intra-compartmental pressure

Discussion

We found a risk of 10.4% for ACS occurring after tibial plateau fracture. Multivariable regression analysis individually confirmed non-contiguous tibia fracture or knee dislocation, and higher AO/OTA classification as significantly associated with ACS.

Reported incidence of ACS following tibial plateau fracture ranges from 0.7 to 12% [8–11, 28]. This incidence may even be as high as 53% in higher-energy fracture subgroups (Schatzker IV-V-VI) [8, 11–15]. This incidence seems to have increased over the past decades, possibly due to an increase in high-energy trauma as a causative injury associated with improved survival rates among severe polytrauma patients [29, 30]. In this perspective, the 212 fractures in our study (78.8%) sustained during trauma other than a fall from one's own height, the 126 (46.8%) classified as Schatzker IV, V and VI, and the 91 (33.8%) as AO/OTA 41-C, represent a rather "modern" cohort of high-energy trauma patients and closely match the most recently reported incidence rates. Indeed, the incidence of ACS found in this study among high-energy pattern fracture types was 22 out of 126 (17.5%) Schatzker IV, V and VI fractures and 22 out of 91 (24.2%) AO/OTA 41-C fractures. Even though some ACS occurred during or after fixation (external or definitive internal fixation) and may be partly attributable to the surgery, we believe that the primary factor for developing ACS is the initial fracture with soft tissue injury, and that surgery only represents a decompensating factor. Traumatized soft tissues may indeed be vulnerable to further surgical aggression for a certain time after the initial injury. Surgical timing and protocol might therefore influence the development of ACS in the treatment of high-energy plateau tibial fractures. Common practice favors staged protocol with spanning fixators [13, 31]. A recent retrospective cohort study reporting the results of early definitive fixation (within 72 h of injury) of bicondylar tibial plateau fractures (AO/OTA 41-C) showed a favorable 2.9% incidence rate of ACS [32]. However, this study might have been biased by the fact that the choice of timing and protocol was left at the discretion of the attending surgeon, potentially leading to lower Injury Severity Score (ISS) in the early definitive fixation group (11 vs. 17, $p = 0.024$) and to a strong trend for patients with open fractures to sustain a staged

Table 1 Timing of occurrence of acute compartment syndrome

	ACS occurence *N* = 28	Remarks
Before external fixation[a]	18	
During external fixation[a]	4	
After external fixation[a]	3	–2 cases within 24 h after surgery –1 case 10 days after plateau tibial EF and 1 day after ORIF of an associated ipsilateral pilon fracture
After definitive ORIF	3[b]	–1 single approach 2 days after injury, without transitory EF –1 double approach 7 days after injury, without transitory EF –1 double approach 18 days after injury, after transitory EF

[a] External fixation was performed in all cases within 24 h after injury
[b] All 3 cases occurred within 24 h after ORIF
ACS acute compartment syndrome, *ORIF* open reduction and internal fixation, *EF* external fixation

Table 2 Demographics, injury characteristics and clinical and radiographic factors of the 265 study patients with 269 tibial plateau fractures

	ACS absent, *N* = 241 (89.6%)	ACS present, *N* = 28 (10.4%)
Age (years)	49.6 ± 18.2 (16.8–92.2)	40.9 ± 15.5 (17.7–75.9)
Male sex	134 (55.6%)	23 (82.1%)
Mechanism other than fall from own height	186 (77.2%)	26 (92.9%)
Open fracture[a]	17 (7.1%)	6 (21.4%)
Associated skeletal lesion		
non-contiguous tibia fracture	1 (0.4%)	3 (10.7%)
knee dislocation	1 (0.4%)	1 (3.6%)
Schatzker classification		
type I	21 (8.7%)	2 (7.1%)
type II	76 (31.5%)	4 (14.3%)
type III	40 (16.6%)	0
type IV	35 (14.5%)	0
type V	44 (18.3%)	9 (32.1%)
type VI	25 (10.4%)	13 (46.4%)
AO/OTA classification		
41-B1	42 (17.4%)	2 (7.1%)
41-B2	41 (17.0%)	0
41-B3	89 (36.9%)	4 (14.3%)
41-C1	19 (7.9%)	3 (13.6%)
41-C2	8 (3.3%)	6 (21.4%)
41-C3	42 (17.4%)	13 (46.4%)
TWR	0.99 ± 0.06 (0.89–1.47)	1.01 ± 0.07 (0.9–1.19)
FDR	0.07 ± 0.05 (0–0.32)	0.09 ± 0.05 (0–0.2)
Medial anatomical axis displacement	19 (7.9%)	5 (17.9%)

[a] Fractures were classified as either open or closed, without subgroup classification for the open ones
Values are expressed as mean ± SD (range) for age, TWR and FDR, and N (%) for other variables
ACS acute compartment syndrome, *TWR* tibial widening ratio, *FDR* femoral displacement ratio

Table 3 Association between variables of interest (demographics, injury characteristics and clinical and radiographic factors) and the occurrence of acute compartment syndrome

	Univariate analysis		Each variable adjusted for age and sex	
	OR (95% CI)	*P* value	OR (95% CI)	*P* value
Age < 45 years	2.93 (1.24–6.91)	0.014	-	
Male sex	3.67 (1.35–9.98)	0.011	-	-
Mechanism other than fall from own height	3.84 (0.88–16.71)	0.072	2.55 (0.57–11.45)	0.22
Open fracture	3.59 (1.28–10.05)	0.015	2.64 (0.90–7.70)	0.076
Associated skeletal lesion	19.92 (3.47–114.44)	0.001	11.68 (1.95–69.93)	0.007
Schatzker type IV-V-VI	4.83 (1.89–12.34)	0.001	4.11 (1.58–10.66)	0.004
AO/OTA type 41-C	9.14 (3.55–23.51)	<0.001	8.08 (3.09–21.13)	<0.001
TWR ≥1.05	3.66 (1.50–8.89)	0.004	3.85 (1.52–9.74)	0.004
FDR ≥0.08	2.74 (1.22–6.15)	0.015	3.46 (1.47–8.18)	0.005
Medial axis displacement	2.66 (0.90–7.80)	0.076	2.64 (0.86–8.13)	0.090

OR odds ratio, *95% CI* 95% confidence interval, *Associated skeletal lesion* non-contiguous tibia fracture or knee dislocation, *TWR* tibial widening ratio, *FDR* femoral displacement ratio

Table 4 Relation between variables identified by the multivariate analysis (presence of a non-contiguous tibia fracture or knee dislocation, and higher AO/OTA fracture classification) and acute compartment syndrome

	Total number of patients[a] N	Patients with ACS[b] N (%)
AO/OTA 41-B, no associated non-contiguous tibia fracture or knee dislocation	174	4 (2.3)
AO/OTA 41-C, no associated non-contiguous tibia fracture or knee dislocation	89	20 (22.5)
AO/OTA 41-B and associated non-contiguous tibia fracture or knee dislocation	4	2 (50.0)
AO/OTA 41-C and associated non-contiguous tibia fracture or knee dislocation	2	2 (100.0)

[a] Number of patients, with or without ACS, presenting the variables as described in the first column
[b] Number of patients with ACS presenting the variables as described in the first column; the percentage is calculated relative to the total number of patients presenting the same variables
ACS acute compartment syndrome

protocol (28,6% open fractures in the staged protocol group vs. 5.0% in the early definitive fixation population, $p = 0.012$). Patients theoretically more at risk to develop ACS due to a higher energy trauma (higher ISS, open fracture) were also more prone to be excluded from the early total care protocol. Another retrospective study compared early external fixation (within 12 h of injury) to delayed external fixation (after 12 h) in the treatment of high-energy plateau tibial fractures [33]. Once again, the choice of timing was left to the surgeon's discretion, and open fractures were more prone to be treated in the first 12 h than beyond (19% vs. 4% open fractures respectively, $p = 0.045$; 14% vs. 7% ACS incidence rate respectively, $p = 0.304$); this represents a potential source of bias. Thus, definitive conclusions about best practice in terms of timing and type of surgery to decrease ACS incidence rate cannot be drawn from both these studies.

All the ACS predictors highlighted by our univariate analysis are linked to the initial energy dissipated in the bone and soft tissue envelope at time of injury, possibly causing higher skeletal lesions (higher Schatzker and AO/OTA grades, higher TWR, higher FDR, non-contiguous tibia fracture or knee dislocation) and increased soft tissue envelope damage (open fracture) [4–7]. Younger age and male sex probably represent a propensity to sustain high-energy trauma, in a specific population more prone to engage in high-risk behaviour. It is noteworthy that in the past, there was a widespread wrongly reassuring theory assuming that an open fracture would relieve the pressure inside the muscle compartments and protect from the occurrence of ACS. Some reports showed that this was incorrect and that ACS could occur following an open fracture [9–11]. This parameter was even recognized as positively associated with the occurrence of ACS in tibial shaft fractures, with an incidence of ACS directly proportional to the severity of the open fracture [18, 19]. Our univariate analysis found a linear association between occurrence of ACS and severity of soft tissue injury, possibly linked with an increasing amount of fascial and muscle injury. Interestingly, none of the fractures classified as Schatzker IV evolved towards ACS in the present study. Reported incidence rates of ACS in Schatzker IV fractures vary from 0% to 53% [8, 11, 13–15]. There is possibly a subgroup of Schatzker IV fractures more prone to evolve towards ACS, but its identification is not clear and may involve specific factors that are not yet recognized.

Table 5 Intraobserver and interobserver reliability assessment of Schatzker and AO/OTA classifications, tibial widening ratio and femoral displacement ratio

	Intraobserver reliability ICC (95% CI)	Interobserver reliability ICC (95% CI)
Schatzker	0.972 (0.940–0.987)	0.917 (0.830–0.960)
AO/OTA	0.975 (0.948–0.988)	0.868 (0.738–0.936)
TWR	0.986 (0.970–0.993)	0.953 (0.902–0.978)
FDR	0.929 (0.854–0.966)	0.930 (0.857–0.967)

ICC intraclass correlation coefficient; values <0 represent poor agreement, values between 0.0 and 0.20 slight agreement, values between 0.21 and 0.40 fair agreement, values between 0.41 and 0.60 moderate agreement, values between 0.61 and 0.80 substantial or good agreement, and values between 0.81 and 1.00 almost perfect agreement. *95% CI* 95% confidence interval, *Schatzker* Schatzker classification, *AO/OTA* AO/OTA classification, *TWR* tibial widening ratio, *FDR* femoral displacement ratio

However, this study was unable to point out an association between mechanism of injury and development of ACS, despite a trend towards statistical significance. Retrospective trauma classification into "fall from own height" or "other" (in an attempt to differentiate between low and high-energy trauma) was based on chart review and may not provide a good representation of the energy released at the time of injury. For instance, not all road traffic accidents and sports injuries are high-energy trauma, and their retrospective assessments may be inaccurate as all the details of the injury (vehicle speed, type of sports injury, etc.) may be difficult to retrieve from patients' charts. This makes any conclusions about mechanism or energy of the injury weak.

In the multivariable regression model built for this study, non-contiguous tibia fracture or knee dislocation and higher AO/OTA classification remained independently highly associated with the development of ACS. Both these factors are hence red flags representing a high amount of energy transmitted to the injured limb, causing increased skeletal lesions (higher AO/OTA grade, non-contiguous tibia fracture or knee dislocation) and extensive soft tissue damage leading to the development of ACS.

Despite being the largest series to date to analyze the association between patient-related, fracture-related and radiological parameters in patients with tibial plateau fractures and the development of ACS, this study has several limitations: 1) its retrospective design with an attempt to differentiate between low and high-energy trauma based on chart review makes it prone to energy level misclassification, and weakens any conclusions about mechanism or energy of the injury; 2) ICP measurements were not performed on all patients presenting with tibial plateau fractures, which would have been the gold standard to diagnose or exclude ACS; this was not possible in the retrospective design of this study but could be performed in a future prospective study. This implies that there is a theoretical possibility of false negative diagnosis; however, we did not find any clinical records suspect of late ACS sequellae in the charts of patients that were not diagnosed with ACS; 3) in some occurrences, ACS was diagnosed clinically, without the use of ICP measurements, thus introducing the possibility of false positive diagnoses; however, common orthopaedic practice recognizes standard clinical examination as a valuable confirmation of ACS [20, 21]; 4) radiographs of the complete series of cases were analyzed by a single surgeon on one occasion, thus not addressing the possible issue of intra- and interobserver errors; however, intra- and interobserver reliability assessment performed on 10.8% of the cases showed almost perfect agreement for Schatzker and AO/OTA classifications, TWR and FDR; furthermore, the control of the radiographic evaluation of knee dislocation showed no false positive or false negative results; 5) Schatzker and AO/OTA classification systems may not adequately characterize some specific fracture patterns such as coronal plane fractures; new fracture classification systems analyzing the proximal tibia as a three-column or a four-quadrant structure should also be evaluated in a future study [34, 35]; and 6) as per local policy, grossly deformed limbs are aligned before radiographs are taken in order to protect vascularization of the injured limb. This implies that the radiographs may not reflect the initial deformity. However, one could expect that realigning the limb by gentle manipulation may not be sufficient to highly alter initial fracture displacement.

Conclusions

Early recognition of injuries at risk of ACS is essential in the screening and treatment of tibial plateau fractures. Two parameters related to the occurrence of ACS in such fractures were highlighted in this study: the presence of a non-contiguous tibia fracture or knee dislocation (this parameter had not been reported yet), and higher AO/OTA classification. They may be especially useful when clinical findings are difficult to assess (doubtful clinical signs, obtunded, sedated or intubated patients), and should rise the suspicion level of the treating surgeon. In these cases, regular clinical examinations and/or ICP measurements should be performed before and after the surgery to monitor the soft tissue state even if the initial assessments were unremarkable regarding the eventual presence of ACS. However, they should not replace clinical examination that is paramount in the diagnosis of ACS in alert patients. Larger prospective studies are mandatory to confirm and refine both factors in predicting the occurrence of ACS.

Abbreviations

95% CI: 95% confidence intervals; ACS: Acute compartment syndrome; FDR: Femoral displacement ratio; ICC: Intraclass correlation coefficient; ICP: Intra-compartmental pressure; ISS: Injury Severity Score; OR: Odds ratios (OR); TWR: Tibial widening ratio

Acknowledgements

Not applicable.

Funding

There was no external source of funding or financial support for this study.

Authors' contributions

AG carried out the conception and design of the study, contributed to the acquisition and interpretation of data, participated to the interobserver and intraobserver reliability study, and drafted and critically revised the manuscript. AL participated in the conception and design of the study, performed the statistical analysis, and drafted and critically revised the manuscript. PB contributed to the acquisition and interpretation of data and critically revised the manuscript. PH participated in the conception and design of the study and critically revised the manuscript. TVP performed the statistical analysis and critically revised the manuscript. MZ contributed to the acquisition and interpretation of data, participated to the interobserver reliability study, and critically revised the manuscript. GC contributed to the acquisition and interpretation of data and critically revised the manuscript. All authors read and approved the final manuscript.

Consent for publication

Not applicable.

Competing interests

The authors declare that they have no competing interests.

Author details

[1]Department of Surgery, Division of Orthopaedic and Trauma Surgery, University Hospitals of Geneva, 4 Rue Gabrielle-Perret-Gentil, CH-1211 Geneva 14, Switzerland. [2]Division of Clinical Epidemiology, University Hospitals of Geneva, 4 Rue Gabrielle-Perret-Gentil, CH-1211 Geneva 14, Switzerland.

References

1. Court-Brown CM, Caesar B. Epidemiology of adult fractures: A review. Injury. 2006;37:691–7.
2. Marsh JL, Slongo TF, Agel J, Broderick JS, Creevey W, DeCoster TA, Prokuski L, Sirkin MS, Ziran B, Henley B, Audigé L. Fracture and dislocation classification compendium - 2007: Orthopaedic Trauma Association classification, database and outcomes committee. J Orthop Trauma. 2007; 21(Suppl):S1–133.
3. Schatzker J, McBroom R, Bruce D. The tibial plateau fracture. The Toronto experience 1968-1975. Clinical Orthop Relat Res. 1979;138:94–104.
4. Cole P, Levy B, Watson JT, Schatzker J. Tibial plateau fractures. In: Browner BD, Jupiter JB, Levine AM, Trafton PG, Krettek C, editors. Skeletal trauma: basic science, management, and reconstruction. 4th ed. Philadelphia: Saunders Elsevier; 2009. p. 2201–87.
5. Marsh JL. Tibial plateau fractures. In: Bucholz RW, Court-Brown CM, Heckman JD, Tornetta 3rd P, editors. Rockwood and Green's fractures in adult. 7th ed. Philadelphia: Lippincott Williams & Wilkins; 2010. p. 1780–831.
6. Watson JT, Wiss DA. Tibial plateau fractures: open reduction internal fixation. In: Wiss DA, editor. Master techniques in orthopaedic surgery: Fracture. 2nd ed. Philadelphia: Lippincott Williams & Wilkins; 2006. p. 407–37.
7. Borrelli J Jr. Management of soft tissue injuries associated with tibial plateau fractures. J Knee. 2014;27:5–9.
8. Allmon C, Greenwell P, Paryavi E, Dubina A, O'Toole RV. Radiographic predictors of compartment syndrome occurring after tibial fracture. J Orthop Trauma. 2016;30:387–91.
9. Menetrey J, Peter R. Acute compartment syndrome in the post-traumatic leg. Rev Chir Ortho Reparatrice Appar Mot. 1998;84:272–80.
10. Park S, Ahn J, Gee AO, Kuntz AF, Esterhai JL. Compartment syndrome in tibial fractures. J Orthop Trauma. 2009;23:514–8.
11. Ziran BH, Becher SJ. Radiographic predictors of compartment syndrome in tibial plateau fractures. J Orthop Trauma. 2013;27:61–5.
12. Barei DP, Nork SE, Mills WJ, Henley MB, Benirschke SK. Complications associated with internal fixation of high-energy bicondylar tibial plateau fractures utilizing a two-incision technique. J Orthop Trauma. 2004;18: 649–57.
13. Egol KA, Tejwani NC, Capla EL, Wolinsky PL, Koval KJ. Staged management of high-energy proximal tibia fractures (OTA types 41): the results of a prospective, standardized protocol. J Orthop Trauma. 2005;19:448–55.
14. Stark E, Stucken C, Trainer G, Tornetta P 3rd. Compartment syndrome in Schatzker type VI plateau fractures and medial condylar fracture-dislocations treated with temporary external fixation. J Orthop Trauma. 2009;23:502–6.
15. Wahlquist M, Iaguilli N, Ebraheim N, Levine J. Medial tibial plateau fractures: a new classification system. J Trauma. 2007;63:1418–21.
16. Gorczyca JT, Roberts CS, Pugh KJ, Ring D. Review of treatment and diagnosis of acute compartment syndrome of the calf: current evidence and best practices. Instr Course Lect. 2011;60:35–42.
17. Mauser N, Gissel H, Henderson C, Hao J, Hak D, Mauffrey C. Acute lower-leg compartment syndrome. Orthopedics. 2013;36:619–24.
18. Blick SS, Brumback RJ, Poka A, Burgess AR, Ebraheim NA. Compartment syndrome in open tibial fracture. J Bone Joint Surg Am. 1986;68-A:1348–53.
19. DeLee JC, Stiehl JB. Open tibia fracture with compartment syndrome. Clinical Orthop Relat Res. 1981;160:175–84.
20. Amendola A, Twaddle BC. Compartment syndromes. In: Browner BD, Jupiter JB, Levine AM, Trafton PG, Krettek C, editors. Skeletal trauma: basic science, management, and reconstruction. 3rd ed. Philadelphia: Saunders Elsevier; 2003. p. 268–92.
21. Südkamp NP. Soft-tissue injury: pathophysiology and its influence on fracture management - Evaluation/classification of closed and open injuries. In: Rüedi TP, Murphy WM, editors. AO principles of fracture management. 2nd ed. Stuttgart: Thieme; 2007. p. 86–113.
22. Gustilo RB, Anderson JT. Prevention of infection in the treatment of one thousand and twenty-five open fractures of long bones: retrospective and prospective analyses. J Bone Joint Surg Am. 1976;58-A:453–8.
23. Gustilo RB, Mendoza RM, Williams DN. Problems in the management of type III (severe) open fractures: a new classification of type III open fractures. J Trauma. 1984;24:742–6.
24. Doornberg JN, Rademakers MV, van den Bekerom MP, Kerkhoffs GM, Ahn J, Steller EP, Kloen P. Two-dimensional and three-dimensional computed tomography for the classification and characterisation of tibial plateau fractures. Injury. 2011;42:1416–25.
25. Moore TM. Fracture-dislocation of the knee. Clinical Orthop Relat Res. 1981; 156:128–40.
26. Fleiss JL, Cohen J. The equivalence of weighted kappa and the intraclass correlation coefficient as measures of reliability. Educ Psychol Meas. 1976;33: 613–9.
27. Landis JR, Koch GG. The measurement of observer agreement for categorical data. Biometrics. 1977;33:159–74.
28. Andrews JR, Tedder JL, Godbout BP. Bicondylar tibial plateau fracture complicated by compartment syndrome. Orthop Rev. 1992;21:317–9.
29. Röding F, Lindkvist M, Bergström U, Lysholm J. Epidemiologic patterns of injuries treated at the emergency department of a Swedish medical center. Injury Epidemiology. 2015;2:3.
30. Trauma Register DGU®. 20 Years of trauma documentation in Germany-Actual trends and developments. Injury. 2014;45(Suppl 3):S14–9.
31. Tejwani NC, Achan P. Staged management of high-energy proximal tibia fractures. Bull Hosp Jt Dis. 2004;62:62–6.
32. Unno F, Lefaivre KA, Osterhoff G, Guy P, Broekhuyse HM, Blachut PA, O'Brien P. Is early fixation of bicondylar tibial plateau fractures safe? An observational cohort study. J Orthop Trauma. 2017;31:151–7.
33. Haller JM, Holt D, Rothberg DL, Kubiak EN, Higgins TF. Does early versus delayed spanning external fixation impact complication rates for high-energy tibial plateau and plafond fractures? Clin Orthop Relat Res. 2016;474: 1436–44.
34. Chang SM, Hu SJ, Zhang YQ, Yao MW, Ma Z, Wang X, Dargel J, Eysel P. A surgical protocol for bicondylar four-quadrant tibial plateau fractures. Int Orthop. 2014;38:2559–64.
35. Luo CF, Sun H, Zhang B, Zeng BF. Three-column fixation for complex tibial plateau fractures. J Orthop Trauma. 2010;24:683–92.

22

Prediction of fracture load and stiffness of the proximal femur by CT-based specimen specific finite element analysis

Michiaki Miura*, Junichi Nakamura, Yusuke Matsuura, Yasushi Wako, Takane Suzuki, Shigeo Hagiwara, Sumihisa Orita, Kazuhide Inage, Yuya Kawarai, Masahiko Sugano, Kento Nawata and Seiji Ohtori

Abstract

Background: Finite element analysis (FEA) of the proximal femur has been previously validated with large mesh size, but these were insufficient to simulate the model with small implants in recent studies. This study aimed to validate the proximal femoral computed tomography (CT)-based specimen-specific FEA model with smaller mesh size using fresh frozen cadavers.

Methods: Twenty proximal femora from 10 cadavers (mean age, 87.1 years) were examined. CT was performed on all specimens with a calibration phantom. Nonlinear FEA prediction with stance configuration was performed using Mechanical Finder (mesh,1.5 mm tetrahedral elements; shell thickness, 0.2 mm; Poisson's coefficient, 0.3), in comparison with mechanical testing. Force was applied at a fixed vertical displacement rate, and the magnitude of the applied load and displacement were continuously recorded. The fracture load and stiffness were calculated from force–displacement curve, and the correlation between mechanical testing and FEA prediction was examined.

Results: A pilot study with one femur revealed that the equations proposed by Keller for vertebra were the most reproducible for calculating Young's modulus and the yield stress of elements of the proximal femur. There was a good linear correlation between fracture loads of mechanical testing and FEA prediction ($R^2 = 0.6187$) and between the stiffness of mechanical testing and FEA prediction ($R^2 = 0.5499$). There was a good linear correlation between fracture load and stiffness ($R^2 = 0.6345$) in mechanical testing and an excellent correlation between these ($R^2 = 0.9240$) in FEA prediction.

Conclusions: CT-based specimen-specific FEA model of the proximal femur with small element size was validated using fresh frozen cadavers. The equations proposed by Keller for vertebra were found to be the most reproducible for the proximal femur in elderly people.

Keywords: Finite element analysis, Proximal femoral fracture, Validation study, Fresh frozen cadaver, Osteoporosis

* Correspondence: michi.m.55@gmail.com
Department of Orthopedic Surgery, Graduate School of Medicine, Chiba University, 1-8-1 Inohana, Chuo-ku, Chiba city, Chiba 260-8677, Japan

Background

Proximal femoral neck fracture is a major cause of high morbidity and mortality in elderly people with osteoporosis [1, 2]. A decline in the bone mineral density (BMD) is associated with fracture; hence, to predict fracture risk, dual energy x-ray absorptiometry and quantitative computed tomography (CT) have been widely used to measure BMD [3–7]. However, BMD is correlated only with bone strength and cannot indicate other mechanical properties of the proximal femur [8]. Furthermore, its ability to predict bone strength varies [9–11]. CT-based finite element analysis (FEA) can account for various aspects of the bone, such as bone geometry, cortical and trabecular bone distribution, and loading direction, and can improve the predictive accuracy of bone strength. The first validation study was conducted by Keyak et al. [12], and several studies have reported the accuracy and usefulness of CT-based FEA of the proximal femur in the stance configuration [13–17].

Recently, a large number of studies using FEA of the proximal femur have been reported as a postoperative evaluation with small implants like screws, plates, and the femoral stem [18–23]. In future, these studies may be useful for preoperative planning to select the most suitable implant or fixation methods. However, FEA for the bone behavior with implants is controversial because mesh sizes of models that were used in previous validation studies were relatively larger than implant sizes. Thus, FEA models should be validated with a smaller mesh size to improve their reliability.

This study aimed to document a proximal femoral FEA model using fresh frozen cadavers with smaller mesh size and to verify the accuracy of FEA prediction using CT-based specimen-specific FEA compared with mechanical testing.

Methods

Specimen

Twenty femora (right, 10 and left, 10) from 10 fresh frozen cadavers (males, 5 and females, 5) were obtained from the Clinical Anatomy Laboratory in our university. The mean age was 87.1 years [range, 74–101 years; standard deviation (SD), 9.13]. Subjects underwent no previous hip surgeries. The cause of death included pneumonia ($n = 3$); senility ($n = 2$); heart failure ($n = 2$); and chronic renal failure, breast cancer, and pancreatic cancer ($n = 1$ each). Cadavers were stored at −22 °C, and after thawing at room temperature, whole femurs were retrieved from the body and all soft tissues were removed. CT was performed using Aquilion ONE (Toshiba Medical Systems, Tokyo, Japan) with imaging parameters including 320-row detector; 120 kV; 200 mA; slice thickness, 0.5 mm; and pixel width, 0.3 mm. A calibration phantom (QRM-BDC, QRM, Möhrendorf, DE) containing three hydroxyapatite rods (0, 100, and 200 mg/cm^3) was tested together with the specimen in water. The proximal femora were then sawed 12 cm distal from the tip of the greater trochanter, sloping 20° in the coronal plane to the shaft axis. Specimens were sprayed with a saline solution to maintain their moisture during the procedure and were not refrozen.

Mechanical testing

To verify fracture load assessment, quasi-static compression testing was conducted. Specimens were loaded using a universal testing machine (Autograph AG-20kN X Plus; Shimadzu, Kyoto, Japan). The distal 3-cm portion of each specimen parallel to the sawed surface was fixed using resin cement (resin box), and a resin cap was molded on the femoral head to apply a uniform compressive load (Fig. 1). The force was applied on the resin cap at a fixed vertical displacement rate of 5 mm/min until proximal femoral fracture occurred. The magnitude of the applied load and displacement were continuously recorded, and mechanical fracture was identified when the slope of the force–displacement curve (stiffness) rapidly decreased. Mechanical stiffness was calculated between 20% and 80% of the maximum fracture load using the force–displacement curve.

Nonlinear FEA prediction

Model development

Data from CT were transferred to an HP Z400 workstation (Hewlett-Packard, Palo Alto, CA, USA). The proximal femur model (12 cm distal from the tip of the greater trochanter) was made using FEA software (Mechanical Finder, Research Center for Computational Mechanics, Tokyo, Japan). All femoral trabecular bone and inner parts of the cortex were meshed using linear tetrahedral elements with 1.5-mm global edge length and overlaid with 1.5 × 1.5 × 0.2-mm triangular shell elements simulating the outer cortex.

Material properties

CT value of each element was set as the average of the voxels contained in one element. Mechanical properties of each element were calculated in Hounsfield units (HU) [24]. There are several equations for calculating the Young's modulus and yield stress for proximal femur. Therefore, we first performed a pilot study using CT DICOM data from an 85-year-old male to determine the most reproducible equations for proximal femur at this mesh size, and the most reproducible equations were adopted in subsequent tests. Modulus values of <0.01 MPa were designated as 0.01 MPa, and those >20 GPa as 20 GPa [25]. Young's modulus and yield stress of the shell element were calculated, assuming its CT value was 1000 HU. Drucker–Prager equivalent criterion was adopted for

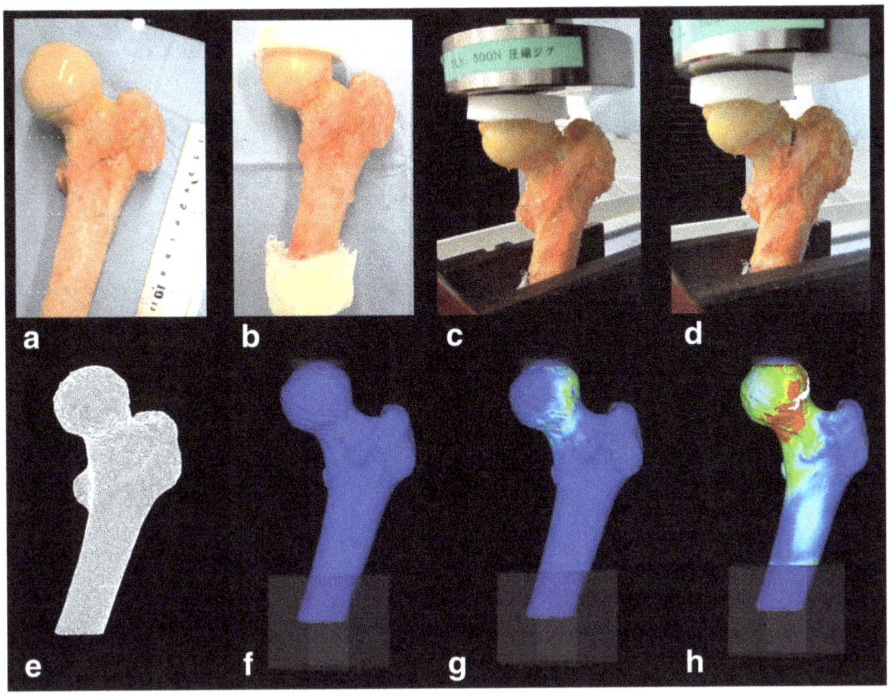

Fig. 1 Process of mechanical testing and finite element analysis. A proximal femur is sawed 12 cm distal from the tip of the greater trochanter, sloping 20° in the coronal plane to the shaft axis (**a**). The distal 3 cm of the specimen is fixed using resin cement and a 'resin cap' is placed on the femoral head (**b**). The force is applied at a fixed vertical displacement (**c**) until the proximal femoral fracture occurs (**d**). The model of the proximal femur is made (**e**), is angled and fixed at the distal end with a resin cap on the femoral head (**f**). A compressive load was applied (**g**) until predicted fracture (**h**)

the yield of the element [26]. The tensile yield stress was assumed to be 0.8 times the compressive yield stress, in agreement with previous studies [15, 27, 28]. Poisson's coefficient for each element was set at 0.3 [29].

To reproduce the real mechanical testing, the FEA model was sloped at 20° in the coronal plane to the shaft axis and fixed with a resin box 3 cm distally, and a resin cap was placed on the femoral head. A uniaxial compressive load with a uniform distribution was applied on the resin cap. The degree of displacement and the reaction force of each point were recorded, and the force–displacement curve was determined. FEA-predicted fracture load was defined as the load when stiffness had declined by >20% of the estimated values, and FEA-predicted stiffness was calculated in the same way as for the actual mechanical test.

Statistical analysis

Fracture load and stiffness were compared in mechanical testing and by FEA prediction using Student's *t* tests and Pearson χ2 tests (SPSS 16.0, SPSS, Inc., Chicago, Illinois, USA). Age, gender, and side differences were calculated using multiple regression analysis as predictive factors for the fracture load in the proximal femur. A *p*-value of <0.05 was considered significant.

Results

Pilot study

The force–displacement curves obtained from mechanical testing and FEA prediction using equations proposed by Keyak [11] (Fig. 2a), Carter [30] (Fig. 2b), Minamisawa [31] (Fig. 2c), and Keller for vertebra [32] (Fig. 2d) are shown. Considering the fracture load (the tip of the curve) and stiffness (the slope of the curve), we concluded that Keller's equation for vertebra was the most reproducible for the proximal femur. The following specific equations were used:

Young's modulus (E, MPa).

$$E = 0.001\ (\rho = 0)$$

$$E = 1890\,\rho^{1.92}\ (\rho < 0).$$

Yield stress (σ, MPa).

$$\sigma = 1.0 \times 10^{20}\ (\rho \leq 0.2).$$

$$\sigma = 284\,\rho^{2.27}\ (\rho > 0.2).$$

Accuracy of FEA prediction in fracture load

The mean fracture loads from mechanical testing and FEA prediction using Keller's equations for vertebra were 3435.8 N (SD, 1802.1) and 4520.3 N (SD, 1879.0),

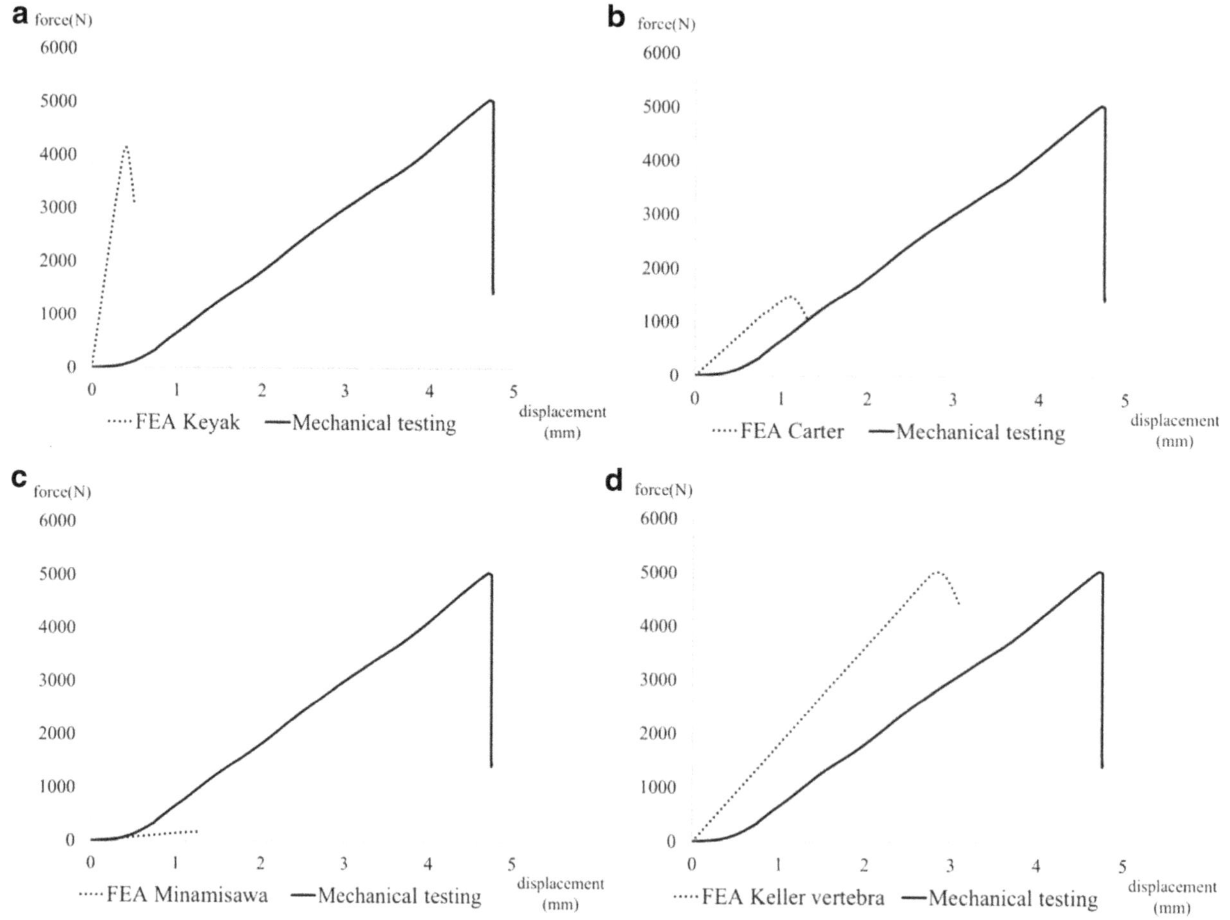

Fig. 2 Preliminary force-displacement curves from mechanical testing and FEA prediction. The equations proposed by Keyak (**a**), Carter (**b**), Minamisawa (**c**), and Keller for vertebra (**d**). Predicted fracture load and stiffness were 0.82 times and 9.74 times (**a**), 0.29 times and 1.28 times (**b**), 0.16 times and 0.13 times (**c**), and 0.97 times and 1.57 times (**d**) larger than those from mechanical testing, respectively

respectively. There was a good linear correlation between these values (Fig. 3).

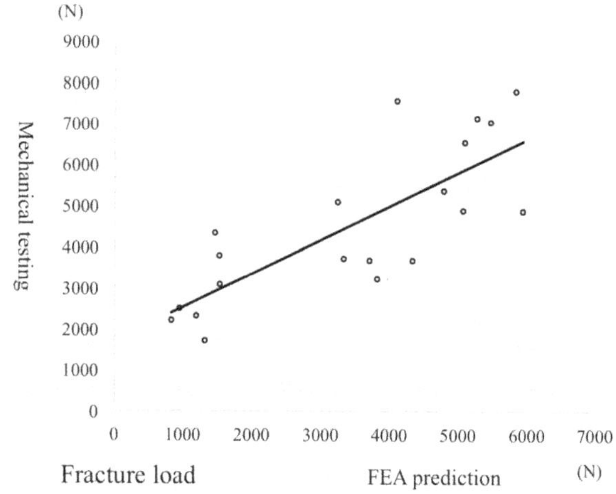

Fig. 3 Relationship of fracture load between mechanical testing and the FEA prediction. (Mechanical fracture load) = 0.8201× (FEA predicted fracture load) + 1702.6, $R^2 = 0.6187$, $p = 0.001$

Accuracy of FEA prediction in stiffness

The mean stiffness from mechanical testing and FEA prediction were 1280 N/mm (SD, 847) and 1566 N/mm (SD, 664), respectively. There was also a good linear correlation between these values (Fig. 4).

Correlation between fracture load and stiffness

There was a significant linear correlation between fracture load and stiffness in mechanical testing (Fig. 5a) and an excellent correlation between these in FEA prediction (Fig. 5b).

Laterality in mechanical testing and FEA prediction

Fracture load and stiffness were not significantly different between the right and left femora for both mechanical testing and FEA prediction (Table 1).

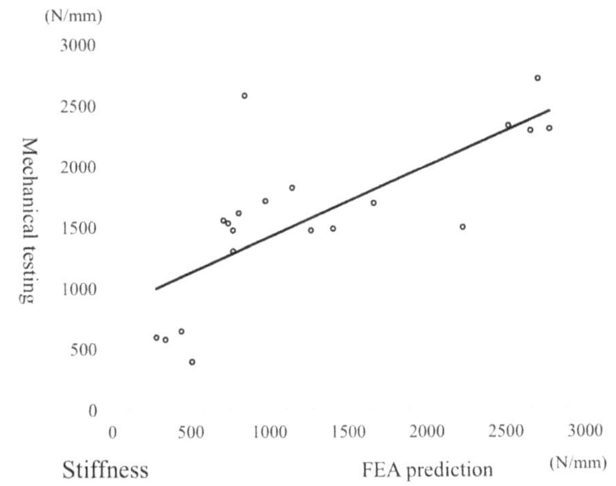

Fig. 4 Relationship of stiffness between mechanical testing and the FEA prediction. (Mechanical stiffness) = 0.5810 × (FEA predicted stiffness) + 0.8223, $R^2 = 0.5499$, $p = 0.001$

Effect of age on mechanical testing and FEA prediction

There was a significant linear correlation between fracture load and age from mechanical testing; the load declined 142.6 N per year (Fig. 6a). FEA prediction also produced a significant linear correlation between fracture load and age, with load declining by 153.8 N per year (Fig. 6b).

Discussion

FEA prediction was validated with a CT-based subject-specific proximal femoral FEA model with a smaller element size using fresh frozen cadavers. This study adopted a finer size tetrahedral element (1.5 mm) for the entire model than that reported in previous studies [13–17]. FEA models in previous studies used a 3.0-mm cube-shaped element [13], a 1.5-mm cube-shaped element only below the lesser trochanter [14], a 3.0-mm tetrahedral element [15], or a 1.5–4.0-mm tetrahedral element [16, 17]. These element sizes are no longer sufficient to match the progress of modern implant technology and are insufficient to analyze the proximal femur with small screws or a stem-inserted model of the femur. Cube-shaped elements can make a mechanically precise model, but the model cannot be automatically made and is time-consuming to construct. An adequate model can be made using tetrahedral elements. At least 1.5-mm tetrahedral elements of the entire model are essential to simulate the proximal femur with small implants.

Preliminary testing revealed that Keller's equations for vertebra were the most reproducible for calculating Young's modulus and yield stress for the proximal femur. Although Keller's equations for vertebra predicted approximately 1.6 times greater stiffness than mechanical testing, Keyak's equations, which were adopted in several previous studies, predicted approximately 10 times greater stiffness than mechanical testing. We consider the error of Keller's equations for vertebra to be acceptable and better than that reported in other studies. The correspondence between the proximal femur and vertebra derives from the high proportion of sponge-like cancellous bone with a thin cortical bone shell in both. Moreover, both proximal femur and vertebra present comparable risks for fracture in people with osteoporosis.

Correlations between mechanical testing and FEA prediction were significant for both fracture load and stiffness in this study. However, previous studies have shown extremely high correlations (fracture load, $R^2 = 0.73–0.96$ and stiffness, $R^2 = 0.62–0.82$) [13–17]. These discrepancies in the results may probably be due to differences in the equations adopted for FEA models. Smaller element size might be

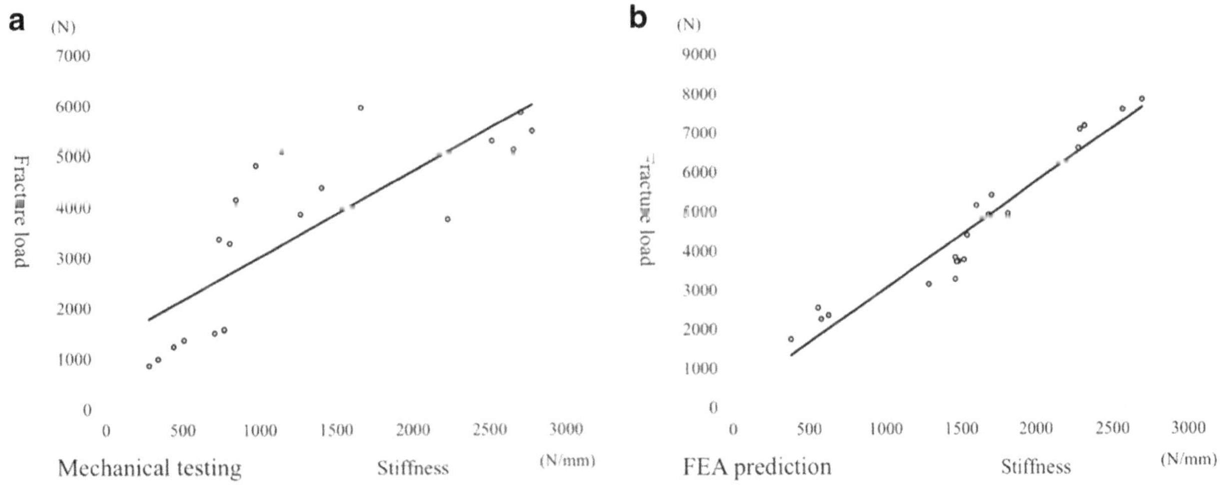

Fig. 5 Relationship between fracture load and stiffness. Mechanical testing (**a**): (fracture load) = 1.6943 × (stiffness) + 1266.9, $R^2 = 0.6345$, $p = 0.001$. FEA prediction (**b**): (fracture load) = 2.7207 × (stiffness) + 259.65, $R^2 = 0.9240$, $p = 0.001$

Table 1 Laterality in mechanical testing and FEM prediction

	Right	Left	*p*
Mechanical testing			
Fracture load	3537.6 ± 1779.3	3333.9 ± 1914.9	0.762
Rigidity	1368.0 ± 880.5	1192.0 ± 850.2	0.706
FEM prediction			
Fracture load	4515.1 ± 2055.6	4525.5 ± 1796.5	0.940
Rigidity	1572.0 ± 712.1	1560.0 ± 650.5	0.821

Mean ± standard deviation
Mann-Whitney U test

another reason for the discrepancy. It has been shown that differences in element size influence the results of FEA predictions [15, 33]. We adopted a compressive displacement condition to reproduce the results from mechanical testing, not to simulate the actual fracture situation, which may also have influenced the results. Furthermore, bone strength is determined not only by BMD but also by bone quality. Bone quality includes bone turnover, microarchitecture, collagen quality, mineralization, microdamage, and bone matrix and mineral composition [34–36]. Approximately 70% of bone strength is dependent on BMD and 30% on bone quality [37]. CT-based FEA can calculate the influence of BMD, but it does not consider all aspects of bone quality, which suggests that there is some systematic error inherent to FEA prediction. Nevertheless, we believe that our results are an acceptable estimate of mechanical behavior.

Good correlations between fracture load and stiffness have been reported previously [16]. This suggests that the fracture load of each specimen depends on its stiffness rather than on the degree of displacement at the point of fracture. The correlation between load and stiffness was far higher with FEA prediction than with mechanical testing. Bone quality, which was not considered in CT-based FEA, might have influenced these results.

Our study had certain limitations. First, most subjects were aged >80 years; hence, these results cannot be applied to younger people. However, FEA prediction of proximal femoral mechanical properties is most useful for elderly people at the risk of proximal femoral fractures. Second, we did not examine the fall configuration that was the most suitable to simulate actual hip fracture with a high correlation between mechanical and FEA-predicted values [12, 16, 38–40]. We only adopted the one-legged stance configuration to examine the behavior of the proximal femur because our focus was to validate the model and make it possible to analyze the model with small implants. Recent studies using FEA prediction of the proximal femur with small implants have provided much important knowledge [18–23]; however, the validation was insufficient. Third, we did not compare mechanical fracture sites with FEA-predicted fracture sites because most mechanical fracture sites were not obvious macroscopically or with CT imaging. The fracture sites could be evaluated with micro CT, but it was not practical or necessary for this study.

Conclusion

FEA model of the proximal femur with small element size was validated using fresh frozen cadavers. The equations proposed by Keller for vertebra were found to be the most reproducible for the proximal femur in elderly people.

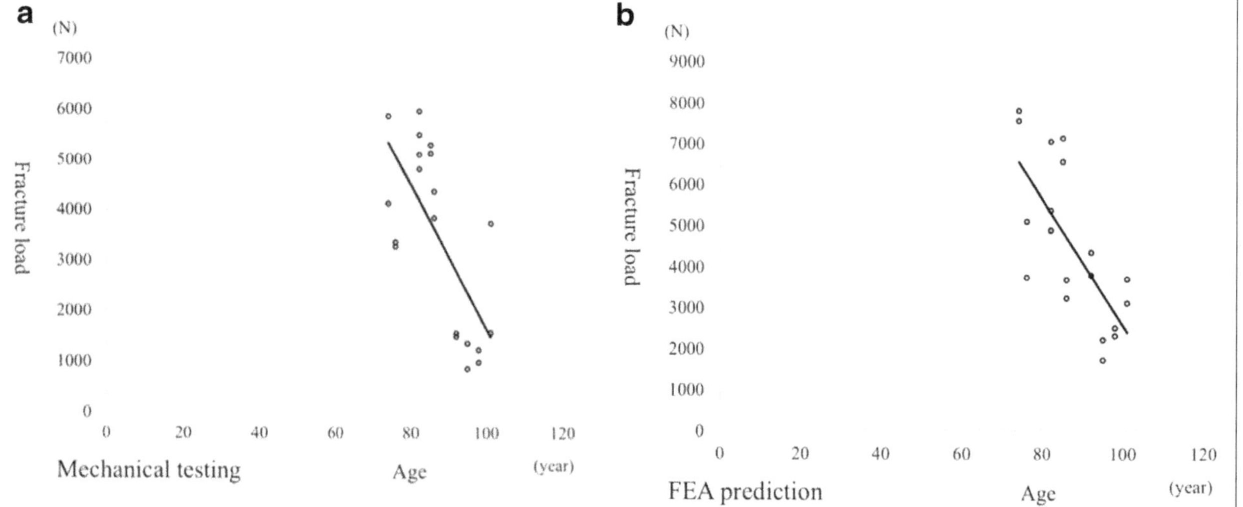

Fig. 6 Relationship between fracture load and age. Mechanical testing (**a**): (fracture load) = −142.6 × (age) + 15,856, $R^2 = 0.4949$, $p = 0.001$. FEA prediction (**b**): (fracture load) = −153.8 × (age) + 17,915, $R^2 = 0.5295$, $p = 0.001$

Abbreviations
BMD: Bone mineral density; CT: Computed tomography; FEA: Finite element analysis; HU: Hounsfield units

Acknowledgements
Not applicable.

Funding
Junichi Nakamura received JSPS KAKENHI Grant Number 25870125. Study sponsors had no involvement in study design, data collection or interpretation, writing of the manuscript. The other authors have nothing to disclose.

Authors' contributions
MM performed all testing and analysis, interpreted the date and wrote manuscript as corresponding author. JN and YM conceived of this study, participated in its design and coordination, and helped to draft the manuscript. YW and TS participated in obtaining the specimens from the cadavers and performing mechanical testing. SH, SO1 (Sumihisa Orita), KI, YK, MS and KN participated in the design and performed the statistical analysis. SO2 (Seiji Ohtori) contributed to the design and interpreting the date, and finally revised and gave the approval of this manuscript. All authors have read and approved this final submitted manuscript.

Consent for publication
Not applicable.

Competing interests
The authors declare that they have no competing interests.

References
1. Johnell O, Kanis JA. An estimate of the worldwide prevalence and disability associated with osteoporotic fractures. Osteoporos Int. 2006 Dec;17(12): 1726–33.
2. Cummings SR, Melton LJ. Epidemiology and outcomes of osteoporotic fractures. Lancet. 2002 May 18;359(9319):1761–7.
3. Hayes WC. Biomechanics of cortical and trabecular bone: implications for assessment of fracture risk. In: Hayes WC, editor. Basic orthopaedics biomechanics. Raven press; 1991. p. 93–142.
4. Assessment of fracture risk and its application to screening for postmenopausal osteoporosis. Report of a WHO Study Group. World Health Organ Tech Rep Ser. 1994;843:1–129. Review.
5. Adams JE. Quantitative computed tomography. Eur J Radiol. 2009 Sep;71(3): 415–24.
6. Black DM, Bouxsein ML, Marshall LM, Cummings SR, Lang TF, Cauley JA, Ensrud KE, Nielson CM, Orwoll ES. Osteoporotic fractures in men (MrOS) research group. Proximal femoral structure and the prediction of hip fracture in men: a large prospective study using QCT. J Bone Miner Res. 2008 Aug;23(8):1326–33.
7. Bousson VD, Adams J, Engelke K, Aout M, Cohen-Solal M, Bergot C, Haguenauer D, Goldberg D, Champion K, Aksouh R, Vicaut E, Laredo JD. Vivo discrimination of hip fracture with quantitative computed tomography: results from the prospective European femur fracture study (EFFECT). J Bone Miner Res. 2011 Apr;26(4):881–93.
8. Ammann P, Rizzoli R. Bone strength and its determinants. Osteoporos Int. 2003;14(Suppl 3):S13–8.
9. Bouxsein ML, Coan BS, Lee SC. Prediction of the strength of the elderly proximal femur by bone mineral density and quantitative ultrasound measurements of the heel and tibia. Bone. 1999 Jul;25(1):49–54.
10. Lochmüller EM, Müller R, Kuhn V, Lill CA, Eckstein F. Can novel clinical densitometric techniques replace or improve DXA in predicting bone strength in osteoporosis at the hip and other skeletal sites? J Bone Miner Res. 2003 May;18(5):906–12.
11. Faulkner KG, Cummings SR, Black D, Palermo L, Glüer CC, Genant HK. Simple measurement of femoral geometry predicts hip fracture: the study of osteoporotic fractures. J Bone Miner Res. 1993 Oct;8(10):1211–7.
12. Keyak JH, Rossi SA, Jones KA, Skinner HB. Prediction of femoral fracture load using automated finite element modeling. J Biomech. 1998 Feb;31(2):125–33.
13. Keyak JH. Improved prediction of proximal femoral fracture load using nonlinear finite element models. Med Eng Phys. 2001 Apr;23(3):165–73.
14. Cody DD, Gross GJ, Hou FJ, Spencer HJ, Goldstein SA, Fyhrie DP. Femoral strength is better predicted by finite element models than QCT and DXA. J Biomech. 1999 Oct;32(10):1013–20.
15. Bessho M, Ohnishi I, Matsuyama J, Matsumoto T, Imai K, Nakamura K. Prediction of strength and strain of the proximal femur by a CT-based finite element method. J Biomech. 2007;40(8):1745–53.
16. Dall'Ara E, Luisier B, Schmidt R, Kainberger F, Zysset P, Pahr D. A nonlinear QCT-based finite element model validation study for the human femur tested in two configurations in vitro. Bone. 2013 Jan;52(1):27–38.
17. Dragomir-Daescu D, Salas C, Uthamaraj S, Rossman T. Quantitative computed tomography-based finite element analysis predictions of femoral strength and stiffness depend on computed tomography settings. J Biomech. 2015 Jan 2; 48(1):153–61.
18. Noda M, Saegusa Y, Takahashi M, Tezuka D, Adachi K, Naoi K. Biomechanical study using the finite element method of internal fixation in Pauwels type III vertical femoral neck fractures. Arch Trauma Res. 2015 Aug 26;4(3):e23167.
19. Hrubina M, Horak Z, Skotak M, Letocha J, Baca V, Dzupa V. Assessment of complications depending on the sliding screw position - finite element method analysis. Bratisl Lek Listy. 2015;116(5):302–10.
20. Chang CW, Chen YN, Li CT, Peng YT, Chang CH. Role of the compression screw in the dynamic hip-screw system: a finite-element study. Med Eng Phys. 2015 Dec;37(12):1174–9.
21. Leonidou A, Moazen M, Lepetsos P, Graham SM, Macheras GA, Tsiridis E. The biomechanical effect of bone quality and fracture topography on locking plate fixation in periprosthetic femoral fractures. Injury. 2015 Feb;46(2):213–7.
22. Peng MJ, Chen HY, Hu Y, Ju X, Bai B. Finite element analysis of porously punched prosthetic short stem virtually designed for simulative uncemented hip arthroplasty. BMC Musculoskelet Disord. 2017 Jul 11;18(1):295.
23. Burchard R, Braas S, Soost C, Graw JA, Schmitt J. Bone preserving level of osteotomy in short-stem total hip arthroplasty does not influence stress shielding dimensions - a comparing finite elements analysis. BMC Musculoskelet Disord. 2017 Aug 7;18(1):343.
24. Les CM, Keyak JH, Stover SM, Taylor KT, Kaneps AJ. Estimation of material properties in the equine metacarpus with use of quantitative computed tomography. J Orthop Res. 1994;12:822–33.
25. Keyak JH, Rossi SA, Jones KA, Les CM, Skinner HB. Prediction of fracture location in the proximal femur using finite element models. Med Eng Phys. 2001;23:657–64.
26. Drucker DC, Prager W. Soil mechanics and plastic analysis of limit design. Q Appl Math. 1952;10:157–65.
27. Kaneko TS, Pejcic MR, Tehranzadeh J, Keyak JH. Relationships between material properties and CT scan data of cortical bone with and without metastatic lesions. Med Eng Phys. 2003 Jul;25(6):445–54.
28. Keaveny TM, Wachtel EF, Ford CM, Hayes WC. Differences between the tensile and compressive strengths of bovine tibial trabecular bone depend on modulus. J Biomech. 1994;27:1137–46.
29. Matsuura Y, Kuniyoshi K, Suzuki T, Ogawa Y, Sukegawa K, Rokkaku T, Thoreson AR, An KN, Takahashi K. Accuracy of specimen-specific nonlinear finite element analysis for evaluation of radial diaphysis strength in cadaver material. Comput Methods Biomech Biomed Engin. 2015;18(16):1811–7.
30. Carter DR, Hayes WC. The compressive behavior of bone as a two-phase porous structure. J Bone Joint Surg Am. 1977 Oct;59(7):954–62.
31. Minamisawa T. Japanese only. 1981.
32. Keller TS. Predicting the compressive mechanical behavior of bone. J Biomech. 1994 Sep;27(9):1159–68.

33. Keyak JH, Skinner HB. Three-dimensional finite element modelling of bone: effects of element size. J Biomed Eng. 1992;14:483–9.
34. Fonseca H, Moreira-Gonçalves D, Coriolano HJ, Duarte JA. Bone quality: the determinants of bone strength and fragility. Sports Med. 2014 Jan;44(1):37–53.
35. Gourion-Arsiquaud S, Faibish D, Myers E, Spevak L, Compston J, Hodsman A, Shane E, Recker RR, Boskey ER, Boskey AL. Use of FTIR spectroscopic imaging to identify parameters associated with fragility fracture. J Bone Miner Res. 2009 Sep;24(9):1565–71.
36. Riggs BL, Hodgson SF, O'Fallon WM, Chao EY, Wahner HW, Muhs JM, Cedel SL, Melton LJ 3rd. Effect of fluoride treatment on the fracture rate in postmenopausal women with osteoporosis. N Engl J Med 1990 Mar 22; 322(12):802–809.
37. NIH Consensus Development Panel on Osteoporosis Prevention, Diagnosis, and Therapy. Osteoporosis prevention, diagnosis, and therapy. JAMA 2001 Feb 14;285(6):785–795. Review.
38. Varga P, Schwiedrzik J, Zysset PK, Fliri-Hofmann L, Widmer D, Gueorguiev B, Blauth M, Windolf M. Nonlinear quasi-static finite element simulations predict in vitro strength of human proximal femora assessed in a dynamic sideways fall setup. J Mech Behav Biomed Mater. 2016 Apr;57:116–27.
39. Dragomir-Daescu D, Op Den Buijs J, McEligot S, Dai Y, Entwistle RC, Salas C, Melton LJ 3rd, Bennet KE, Khosla S, Amin S. Robust QCT/FEA models of proximal femur stiffness and fracture load during a sideways fall on the hip. Ann Biomed Eng 2011 Feb;39(2):742–755.
40. Nishiyama KK, Gilchrist S, Guy P, Cripton P, Boyd SK. Proximal femur bone strength estimated by a computationally fast finite element analysis in a sideways fall configuration. J Biomech. 2013 Apr 26;46(7):1231–6.

Comparison of the direct and indirect reduction techniques during the surgical management of posterior malleolar fractures

Hong-fei Shi[1], Jin Xiong[1*], Yi-xin Chen[1*], Jun-fei Wang[1], Xu-Sheng Qiu[1], Jie Huang[2], Xue-yang Gui[2], Si-yuan Wen[3] and Yin-he Wang[1]

Abstract

Background: The optimal method for the reduction and fixation of posterior malleolar fracture (PMF) remains inconclusive. Currently, both of the indirect and direct reduction techniques are widely used. We aimed to compare the reduction quality and clinical outcome of posterior malleolar fracture managed with the direct reduction technique through posterolateral approach or the indirect reduction technique using ligamentotaxis.

Methods: Patients with a PMF involving over 25% of the articular surface were recruited and assigned to the direct reduction (DR) group or the indirect reduction (IR) group. Following reduction and fixation of the fracture, the quality of fracture reduction was evaluated in post-operative CT images. Clinical and radiological follow-ups were performed at 6 weeks, 3 months, 6 months, 12 months, and then at 6 month-intervals postoperatively. Functional outcome (AOFAS score), ankle range of motion, and Visual Analog Scale (VAS) were evaluated at the last follow-up. Statistical differences were compared between the DR and IR groups considering the patient demographics, quality of fracture reduction, AOFAS score, and VAS.

Results: Totally 116 patients were included, wherein 64 cases were assigned to the DR group and 52 cases were assigned to the IR group. The quality of fracture reduction was significant higher in the DR group ($P = 0.038$). In the patients who completed a minimum of 12 months' follow-up, a median AOFAS score of 87 was recorded in the DR group, which was significantly higher than that recorded in the IR group (a median score of 80). The ankle range of motion was slightly better in the DR group, with the mean dorsiflexion restriction recorded to be 5.2° and 6.1° in the DR and IR group respectively ($P = 0.331$). Similar VAS score was observed in the two groups ($P = 0.419$).

Conclusions: The direct reduction technique through a posterolateral approach provide better quality of fracture reduction and functional outcome in the management of PMF over 25% of articular surface, as compared with the indirect reduction technique using ligamentotaxis.

Trial registration: NCT02801474 (retrospectively registered, June 2016, ClinicalTrails.gov).

Keywords: Posterior malleolar fracture, Posterolateral approach, Buttress plate, Ligamentotaxis

* Correspondence: dr.xiongjin@gmail.com; dr.chenyixin@gmail.com
[1]Department of Orthopaedics, Nanjing Drum Tower Hospital, The Affiliated Hospital of Nanjing University Medical School, No. 321 Zhongshan Road, Nanjing, China
Full list of author information is available at the end of the article

Background

The incidence of the posterior malleolar fracture (PMF) was reported to be 7 to 44% of all ankle fractures [1]. Despite of the evidence provided by anatomical and biomechanical studies that the posterior malleolus serves as an important contributor to the stability of ankle mortise and syndesmosis, the indication of surgical reduction and fixation of PMF remains controversial [2–4]. Fragment size is frequently used as a reference for surgical intervention, and the posterior malleolar fracture involves more than 25% of articular surface is generally recommended to be reduced and fixed to prevent instability and reduce the risk of post-traumatic degenerative changes [1].

The optimal method for the reduction and fixation of PMF remains inconclusive. Often, the posterior fragment, also known as Volkmann's fragment, reduces simultaneously via ligamentotaxis of the posteroinferior tibiofibular ligament (PITL) following an anatomical reduction of the lateral malleolus [5]. Following this indirect reduction procedure, percutaneous screw fixation can be achieved through a stab incision. Alternatively, the posterior malleolus fragment can be direct visualized and reduced through a posterolateral approach with the patient in a prone position [6]. Buttress plate or lag screws can then be placed to stabilize the fragment.

Currently, both of the indirect and direct reduction techniques are widely used among orthopaedic surgeons during the operative treatment of PMF, while conflicting data has been published regarding the subsequent clinical outcomes [7–10]. Few studies could be found comparing the quality of fracture reduction, as well as the functional and clinical outcomes between the indirect and direct reduction techniques. In this study, we aimed to compare the reduction quality and clinical outcome of PMF managed with the direct reduction technique through a posterolateral approach or the indirect reduction technique using ligamentotaxis.

Methods

This study was approved by the ethics committee of the authors' institution (Ref. No. 115690). Between January 2012 and December 2014, patients with a posterior malleolus fracture were recruited as candidates for this prospective study. Following screening by two of the senior surgeons (HFS and XSQ), the patients were finally included meeting the inclusion criteria of (1) age between18 to 70 years, (2) unstable and displaced (more than 2 mm) posterior malleolar fractures requiring surgical management, (3) posterior malleolar fragment involving over 25% of the articular surface measured in preoperative lateral view radiographs and sagittal reconstruction of CT images. Patients with open fractures, pathological fractures, delayed fractures, or additional ipsilateral lower extremity fractures were excluded. Informed-consent documents were obtained from all the eligible patients that stated the aim and protocol of this study. Preoperative anteroposterior (AP), lateral, and mortise view radiographs as well as computed tomography (CT) scans were routinely obtained to evaluate the characteristic of the fracture according to the Lauge-Hansen classification and AO/OTA classification. The injury mechanism was recorded as low-energy injury (a small-level fall or a sprain) or high-energy injury (a motor-vehicle accident or a fall from a height > 1 meter). Patients were then assigned to the direct reduction (DR) group or the indirect reduction (IR) group by monthly turns.

All the patients were operated on by two of the senior surgeons (JX and YXC). During operation, patients received general or spinal anesthesia, with a thigh tourniquet applied to prevent bleeding. In the DR group, the posterior and lateral malleoli were accessed via a posterolateral approach with the patients in prone position [11]. Care was taken to protect the sural nerve and lesser saphenous vein during superficial dissection [12]. With the peroneal tendons retracted medially, the fibular fracture was exposed and reduced anatomically in the first place. Posteriorly placed one-third tubular plate, reconstruction plate, or laterally placed posterolateral distal fibula plate (Synthes, Switzerland) was used to stabilize the fibular fracture. The posterior malleolus was then exposed between the fiexor halluces longus and peroneus longus interval. The PITL was carefully preserved. Articular impaction was inspected and reduced if any. The posterior malleolar fragment was then reduced with reference to the typical metaphyseal-diaphyseal spike of the posterior malleolus. If comminution occurred, the fracture reduction was performed in a lateral-to-medial manner. One-third tubular plate, reconstruction plate, or distal radius plate (Synthes, Switzerland) were applied spanning the fracture in a buttress mode (Fig. 1). One or multiple 4.0 mm cannulated screws could also be used if applicable. A separate medial approach was then performed to address the medial osseous and/or ligamentous injuries. Anatomical reduction and fixation of the medial malleolus was achieved under direct visualization and verified using intraoperative C-arm.

In the IR group, the lateral and/or medial malleolar fractures received open reduction and internal fixation (ORIF) using standard AO (Arbeitsgemeinschaft für Osteosynthesefragen) osteosynthesis technique with the patients in supine position. Anatomical reduction of the lateral and/or medial malleolus was confirmed under fluoroscopy. The posterior malleolus was then reduced through ligamentotaxis with the ankle in dorsiflexion. If necessary, percutaneously applied pointed reduction forceps, bone hook, K-wire, or periosteal elevator was used

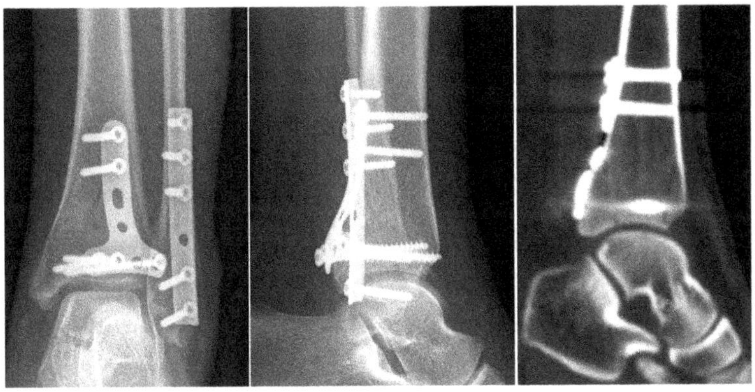

Fig. 1 For the patient presented in Fig. 4, a distal radius plate was applied spanning the fracture in a buttress mode to fix the PMF. The postoperative sagittal reconstruction of CT images confirmed an excellent (anatomical) reduction of the posterior fragment

to reduce the posterior malleolar fragment anatomically [13, 14]. Intraoperative lateral view radiographs were taken using C-arm to verify the reduction. One or two 4.0 mm cannulated screws were then used to fix the posterior malleolar in anterior-to-posterior direction.

In both groups, intraoperative external rotation stress test and Cotton test were performed to evaluate the stability of syndesmosis following reduction and fixation of the fractures. Syndesmotic screws were placed when positive results were observed in the external rotation stress test (increased medial clear space at the ankle mortise) or in the Cotton test (>2 mm of lateral migration of the lateral malleolus) [15, 16].

Postoperatively, all the fractures were stabilized with a short leg splint for 2 weeks, followed by 4 weeks of non-weight-bearing rehabilitation focusing on the range of motion. Regular clinical and radiological assessments were performed at 6 weeks, 3 months, 6 months, 12 months, and then at 6 month-intervals according to our routine follow-up regime. Progressive weight bearing and strengthening was initiated since 6 weeks postoperatively, with reference to the healing status checked in follow-up radiographs. The syndesmotic screws were removed, if any, at 3 months postoperatively.

Postoperative radiographs and CT scan were obtained routinely to evaluate the quality of fracture reduction. The maximum residual displacement of the posterior malleolus, the gap in the joint surface, and/or the articular step-off were measured in sagittal cuts of the CT scan. The quality of fracture reduction was graded as excellent (less than 1 mm), good (1 to 2 mm), or poor (more than 2 mm) as described in literature [17].

Functional outcome was evaluated according to the American Orthopaedic Foot and Ankle Society ankle-hindfoot score (AOFAS) at the last follow-up [18]. The ankle range of motion (ROM) was measured, and the difference of the dorsiflexion between the injured and uninjured side was calculated and presented as dorsiflexion restriction [19, 20]. Visual Analog Scale (VAS) was used to evaluate local pain.

All the evaluations were performed by two of the senior surgeons (JFW and YHW) independently. The interobserver quantitative data were averaged for further statistical analysis. IBM SPSS version 19.0 software (SPSS Inc., Chicago, IL) was used with the statistical significance set at a P value of less than 0.05. The assumption of normal distribution of the parametric data was testified using Q-Q plots. Demographics of the two groups were compared using independent t test or Chi-Square test. The quality of fracture reduction were compared using Chi-Square test. The AOFAS score and VAS were analyzed using Mann-Whitney U test to compare the difference between groups.

Results

The demographics of the two groups were presented in Table 1. Totally 116 patients (116 fractures) were included in this investigation, among which 64 cases were assigned to the DR group and 52 cases were assigned to the IR group. No significant difference was detected between the groups considering the age ($P = 0.751$), gender ($P = 0.097$), Lauge-Hansen classification ($P = 0.647$), AO/OTA classification ($P = 0.344$), injury mechanism ($P = 0.642$), and the time from trauma to surgery ($P = 0.733$).

As measured in the postoperative radiographs and CT scan, 34 (53.1%) and 16 (30.8%) patients achieved excellent fracture reduction in the DR and IR group respectively (Table 1). The percentage of excellent fracture reduction was 22.3% higher in the DR group than in the IR group. A good fracture reduction was observed in 25 (39.1%) patients in the DR group and in 27 (51.9%) patients in the IR group. The percentage of excellent or good reduction was 9.5% higher in the DR group than in the IR group. More than 2 mm residual fracture displacement and/or articular step-off were found in 5 (7.8%) patients in the DR group and in 9 (17.3%)

Table 1 Patient demographics and results

	Direct reduction group	Indirect reduction group	*P* value
No. of patients	64	52	
Gender			
Male	28	31	0.097
Female	36	21	
Lauge-Hansen classification			
Pronation-external rotation	12	12	0.647
Supination-external rotation	52	40	
AO/OTA classification			
44B3	47	35	0.344
44C1	4	3	
44C2	11	13	
44C3	2	1	
Injury mechanism			
Low-energy	50	43	0.642
High-energy	14	9	
Age (*Yr.*)	49.0 ± 12.4	48.1 ± 15.2	0.751
Time before surgery (days)	4.3 ± 2.0	4.5 ± 2.8	0.733
Quality of reduction			
Excellent	34 (53.1%)	16 (30.8%)	0.038*
Good	25 (39.1%)	27 (51.9%)	
Poor	5 (7.8%)	9 (17.3%)	
Follow-up duration (months)	19.9 ± 5.2	20.0 ± 5.8	0.882
AOFAS	87 (58 to 95)	80 (59 to 95)	0.034*
Dorsiflexion restriction (°)	5.2 ± 4.5	6.1 ± 4.3	0.331
VAS	2 (0 to 7)	2 (0 to 7)	0.419

*$P < 0.05$

patients in the IR group. The quality of fracture reduction was significant higher in the DR group compared with that in the IR group ($P = 0.038$).

Totally 89 patients (48 in the DR group and 41 in the IR group) completed a minimum of 12 months' follow-up with the clinical outcome evaluated in the outpatient clinic (Figs. 2 and 3). The mean follow-up duration was 19.9 (12 to 32) months and 20.0 (12 to 36) months in the DR and IR group respectively ($P = 0.882$). The other 27 patients were lost to follow-up due to different kind of reasons. At the last follow-up, a median AOFAS score of 87 was recorded in the DR group, which was significantly higher than that recorded in the IR group (a median score of 80). The ROM of the ankle was slightly better in the DR group, with the mean dorsiflexion restriction recorded to be 5.2° and 6.1° in the DR and IR group respectively

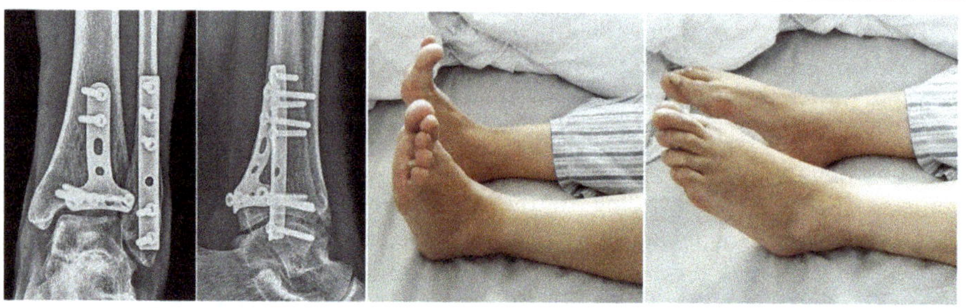

Fig. 2 For the patient presented in Fig. 4, the AOFAS score was 94 at the last follow-up (24 months postoperatively). Satisfied ankle range of motion were achieved

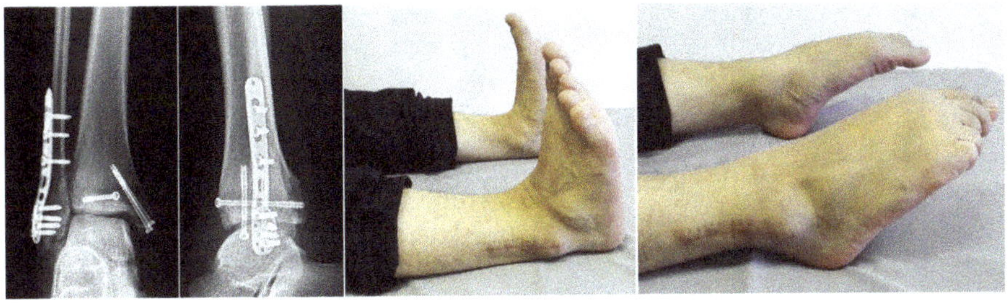

Fig. 3 For the patient presented in Fig. 5, the AOFAS score was 88 at the last follow-up (12 months postoperatively). Satisfied ankle range of motion were achieved

($P = 0.331$). Besides, similar VAS score was observed in the two groups ($P = 0.419$).

No major intraoperative complications was observed. Two patient in the DR group developed superficial infection postoperatively. Both of them were managed successfully with local dressing changes and oral antibiotics. Calf muscle vein thrombosis was diagnosed in one patient in the DR group and two patients in the IR group during follow-up. Therapeutic dosages of low-molecular-weight heparins (LMWH) was prescribed till thrombolysis confirmed using color duplex Doppler ultrasound. Fracture nonunion, implant loosening or failure was not observed in each of the groups.

Discussion

Surgical management of ankle fractures aims to achieve articular congruity, ankle alignment and stability with maximal functional recovery. Unlike the studies on the management of lateral and medial malleolar fractures, the surgical indication and optimal technique for the management of PMF remains inconclusive. In the study, we compared the radiological and functional outcome of PMF managed with the direct or indirect reduction technique. Higher quality of fracture reduction and better functional outcome were achieved when the PMF was treated with direct reduction technique through a posterolateral approach, while similar ankle range of motion and VAS score were observed when compared with the patients managed with the indirect reduction technique using ligamentotaxis.

Currently, the recommended indication for posterior malleolar fixation is when the fracture affecting over 25% of the articular surface, displacement over 2 mm, ankle instability, and persistent subluxation of the talus [4]. In our study, we included the patients with a posterior malleolar fragment involving over 25% of the articular surface measured in preoperative lateral view radiographs or sagittal reconstruction of CT images (Figs. 4 and 5). The debate continues whether the fragment less than 25% should be anatomically reduced and fixed. Some authors reported negative relationships between the fixation of small posterior malleolar fragment and the functional outcome, while others believed that the fixation of small posterior malleolar fragment would contribute to the stability of syndesmosis [2, 4, 21, 22]. Recent anatomical and clinical studies provide evidence that the morphology of the fracture fragment might be more important than the fragment size [1, 23]. A thorough study of the morphology of the fracture fragment in reconstructed CT images might provide information about the injury mechanisms, and hence guided different way of reduction and fixation [9, 24].

One important finding of our study was that the direct reduction technique through a posterolateral approach led to significant higher quality of fracture reduction, as evaluated in postoperative CT images, than the indirect reduction technique using ligamentotaxis. Since plain

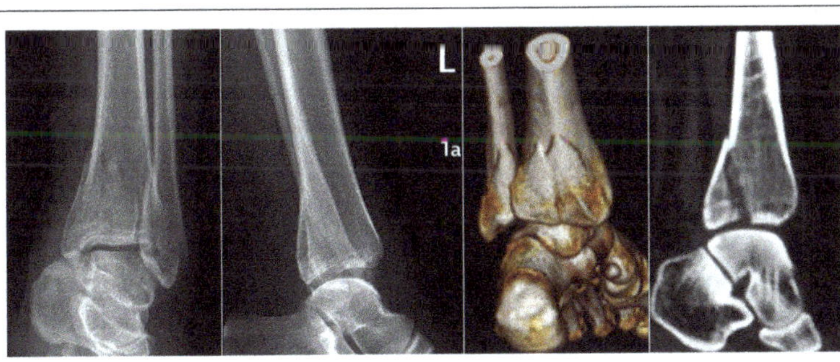

Fig. 4 The 56-year-old female patient treated using direct reduction technique. Preoperative AP and lateral radiograph showed a pilon-type PMF. Preoperative 3D and sagittal reconstruction of CT images provided more precise determination of the morphology and size of the posterior fragments

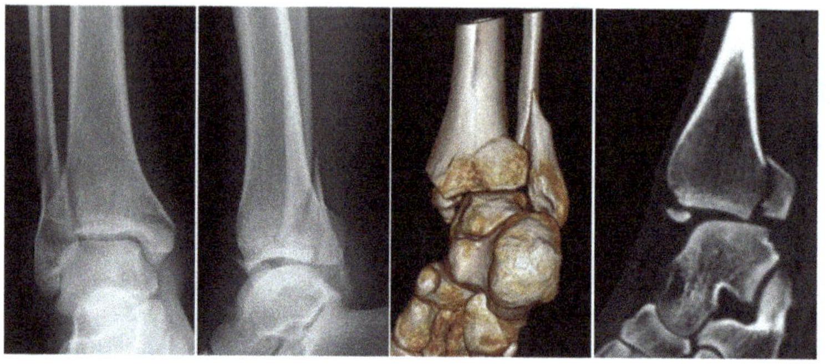

Fig. 5 The 55-year-old male patient treated using indirect reduction technique. Preoperative radiographs and CT images showed a displaced PMF

radiography was considered inaccurate with poor reliability in the assessment of PMF, postoperative CT scan was routinely performed in our institution to evaluate the quality of fracture reduction [25, 26]. The rate of excellent (or anatomical) reduction were observed to be 53.1% (34/64) and 30.8% (16/52) in the DR and IR group respectively. In Huber's study, the rate of anatomical reduction of PMF was reported to be 27% via indirect reduction, while 83% of the patients achieved anatomical reduction using direct posterior approach [6]. A possible reason for the remarkable lower rate of anatomical reduction observed in our study compared with that in Huber's study was that CT scan might provide more precise determination of residual fracture gap and articular step-off of posterior malleolus [9] (Fig. 6).

Several factors might contribute to the better quality of fracture reduction achieved via the direct reduction technique. First, it's more convenient to use the typical metaphyseal-diaphyseal spike of the posterior malleolus as reference to reduce the posterior fragment when exposed through the posterolateral approach. Second, fixation of small posterior malleolar fragment to larger distal tibia might be biomechanically stronger than anterior-to-posterior screw fixation, which would help to achieve better interfragmentary compression and reduce gaps between the posterior fragment and distal tibia [6]. Gravity would also help to reduce the talus and PMF in prone position. In case of the occurrence of articular impaction, the posterior lateral approach might provide adequate visualization of the posterior fragment compared with the indirect reduction technique. The impacted articular fragment could then be meticulously accessed and reduced through fracture line or via cortical window.

Despite of the advantages described above, the direct reduction technique did not prevail over the indirect reduction technique in clinical practice [7]. It was reported that 83% of posterior malleolar fractures were fixed using anterior-to-posterior screws with indirect reduction technique. [8] Some authors believed that indirect reduction and percutaneous screw fixation were less traumatic, while posterolateral approach might increase the risk of posterior scarring, tendon impingement, and sural nerve injury [27, 28]. Provided that PITL was intact, the posterolateral fragment could be easily reduced

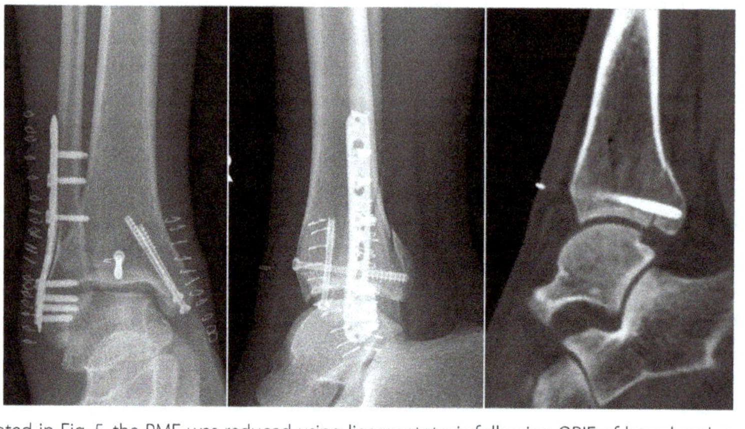

Fig. 6 For the patient presented in Fig. 5, the PMF was reduced using ligamentotaxis following ORIF of lateral and medial malleoli. Percutaneous screw fixation of PMF was achieved through a stab incision. The postoperative sagittal reconstruction of CT images provided more precise determination of residual articular step-off of the posterior malleolus which could be easily ignored in radiographs

using ligamentotaxis following anatomical reduction of the fibula [1]. However, when the PMF was severely comminuted, impacted, or accompanied by medial extension (described as Haraguchi type-II fracture), direct reduction technique was preferred [29] (Fig. 1).

Functional outcome of ankle fractures was believed to be associated with fracture morphology, articular involvement, fracture fragment size, severity of comminution, and residual step-off or gaps. In our study, provided a better quality of fracture reduction, the DR group presented significantly higher AOFAS score than the IR group. The ankle range of motion, on the other hand, was only slightly better in the DR group, as reflected by the recorded dorsiflexion restriction. In literature, very different results were reported considering the functional outcome of PMF following surgical reduction and fixation. Choi reported a mean AOFAS score of 90.6 following ORIF of PMF through a modified posterolateral approach [28]. Erdem achieved a mean AOFAS score of 94.1 of PMF following posterior-to-anterior lag screw fixation or buttress plate fixation through posterolateral approach [30]. Compared with our study, the patients with a PMF smaller than 25% of articular surface were included in these studies, which might contribute to the higher AOFAS scores reported in these studies. Besides, the pilon-type PMFs, characterized by posteromedial fracture extension to the medial malleolus with varying articular impaction, were exclude from Erdem's study [29]. The pilon-type PMFs were generally believed to lead to inferior functional outcomes than regular ankle fractures [31–33]. Evers and Drijfhout van Hooff reported mean AOFAS scores of 70.9 and 81 in their studies respectively, wherein the PMFs greater than 25% of the joint surface were fixed [9, 20]. These results were similar with our study, while detailed techniques of fracture reduction and fixation, unfortunately, were not described in these two studies.

In this study, as one of the limitations, the radiographic osteoarthritis status was not graded or compared between groups due to limited time of follow-up [10]. Theoretically, an anatomically reduced and fixed posterior malleolus would provide important buttress to contain the talus, stabilize syndesmosis, and reduce the risk of post-traumatic osteoarthritis [20]. Future study with long-term follow-up results would provide further information considering the influence of different rate of anatomical reduction on the grade of post-traumatic arthrosis between the DR and the IR groups.

Conclusions

In conclusion, the direct reduction technique through a posterolateral approach provide better quality of fracture reduction and functional outcome in the management of PMF over 25% of articular surface, as compared with the indirect reduction technique using ligamentotaxis.

Abbreviations

AOFAS: American Orthopaedic Foot and Ankle Society; AP: Anteroposterior; CT: Computed tomography; DR: Direct reduction; IR: Indirect reduction; LMWH: Low-molecular-weight heparins; ORIF: Open reduction and internal fixation; PITL: Posteroinferior tibiofibular ligament; PMF: Posterior malleolar fracture; ROM: Range of motion; VAS: Visual Analog Scale

Acknowledgements

We would like to thank Li-ping Chen, Xiao-xia Zhong, and Bei Cheng for their assistance during patient recruitment and data collection.

Funding

This study was supported by the National Natural Science Foundation of China (81401793, 81572132, and 81271997) and the Six Talent Peeks Project in Jiangsu Province (2016-WSW-060).

Authors' contributions

All authors read and agreed with the contents of the manuscript. HFS and JX participated in the study design. The patients included in this study were screened by HFS and XSQ, and then were operated on by JX and YXC. JFW and YHW performed the radiographic evaluations and functional assessments. HFS was in charge of interpreting the data analysis and drafting the manuscript. JH, XYG and SYW assisted in revising the manuscript.

Competing interests

There's no competing interest. No benefits in any form have been received or will be received from a commercial party related directly or indirectly to the subject of this article.

Consent to publication

Written informed consent was obtained from each patient for publication, along with any accompanying images.

Author details

[1]Department of Orthopaedics, Nanjing Drum Tower Hospital, The Affiliated Hospital of Nanjing University Medical School, No. 321 Zhongshan Road, Nanjing, China. [2]Nanjing Medical University, Nanjing, China. [3]Nanjing University Medical School, Nanjing, China.

References

1. Irwin TA, Lien J, Kadakia AR. Posterior malleolus fracture. J Am Acad Orthop Surg. 2013;21(1):32–40.
2. Gardner MJ, Brodsky A, Briggs SM, Nielson JH, Lorich DG. Fixation of posterior malleolar fractures provides greater syndesmotic stability. Clin Orthop Relat Res. 2006;447:165–71.
3. Bartonicek J, Rammelt S, Kostlivy K, Vanecek V, Klika D, Tresl I. Anatomy and classification of the posterior tibial fragment in ankle fractures. Arch Orthop Trauma Surg. 2015;135(4):505–16.
4. Odak S, Ahluwalia R, Unnikrishnan P, Hennessy M, Platt S. Management of Posterior Malleolar Fractures: A Systematic Review. J Foot Ankle Surg. 2016; 55(1):140–5.
5. Mak KH, Chan KM, Leung PC. Ankle fracture treated with the AO principle-an experience with 116 cases. Injury. 1985;16(4):265–72.
6. Huber M, Stutz PM, Gerber C. Open reduction and internal fixation of the posterior malleolus with a posterior antiglide plate using a postero-lateral approach-a preliminary report. Foot Ankle Surg. 1996;2(2):95–103.
7. Gardner MJ, Streubel PN, McCormick JJ, Klein SE, Johnson JE, Ricci WM. Surgeon practices regarding operative treatment of posterior malleolus fractures. Foot Ankle Int. 2011;32(4):385–93.
8. Mingo-Robinet J, Lopez-Duran L, Galeote JE, Martinez-Cervell C. Ankle fractures with posterior malleolar fragment: management and results. J Foot Ankle Surg. 2011;50(2):141–5.
9. Evers J, Barz L, Wahnert D, Gruneweller N, Raschke MJ, Ochman S. Size matters: The influence of the posterior fragment on patient outcomes in trimalleolar ankle fractures. Injury. 2015;46 Suppl 4:S109–13.

10. O'Connor TJ, Mueller B, Ly TV, Jacobson AR, Nelson ER, Cole PA. "A to p" screw versus posterolateral plate for posterior malleolus fixation in trimalleolar ankle fractures. J Orthop Trauma. 2015;29(4):e151–6.
11. Talbot M, Steenblock TR, Cole PA. Posterolateral approach for open reduction and internal fixation of trimalleolar ankle fractures. Can J Surg. 2005;48(6):487–90.
12. Jowett AJ, Sheikh FT, Carare RO, Goodwin MI. Location of the sural nerve during posterolateral approach to the ankle. Foot Ankle Int. 2010;31(10): 880–3.
13. Lee HJ, Kang KS, Kang SY, Lee JS. Percutaneous reduction technique using a Kirschner wire for displaced posterior malleolar fractures. Foot Ankle Int. 2009;30(2):157–9.
14. Strenge KB, Idusuyi OB. Technique tip: percutaneus screw fixation of posterior malleolar fractures. Foot Ankle Int. 2006;27(8):650–2.
15. Van Heest TJ, Lafferty PM. Injuries to the ankle syndesmosis. J Bone Joint Surg Am. 2014;96(7):603–13.
16. Gardner MJ, Graves ML, Higgins TF, Nork SE. Technical Considerations in the Treatment of Syndesmotic Injuries Associated With Ankle Fractures. J Am Acad Orthop Surg. 2015;23(8):510–8.
17. Ketz J, Sanders R. Staged posterior tibial plating for the treatment of Orthopaedic Trauma Association 43C2 and 43C3 tibial pilon fractures. J Orthop Trauma. 2012;26(6):341–7.
18. Kitaoka HB, Alexander IJ, Adelaar RS, Nunley JA, Myerson MS, Sanders M. Clinical rating systems for the ankle-hindfoot, midfoot, hallux, and lesser toes. Foot Ankle Int. 1994;15(7):349–53.
19. Verhage SM, Schipper IB, Hoogendoorn JM. Long-term functional and radiographic outcomes in 243 operated ankle fractures. J Foot Ankle Res. 2015;8:45.
20. van Hooff Drijfhout CC, Verhage SM, Hoogendoorn JM. Influence of fragment size and postoperative joint congruency on long-term outcome of posterior malleolar fractures. Foot Ankle Int. 2015;36(6):673–8.
21. De Vries JS, Wijgman AJ, Sierevelt IN, Schaap GR. Long-term results of ankle fractures with a posterior malleolar fragment. J Foot Ankle Surg. 2005;44(3): 211–7.
22. Donken CC, Goorden AJ, Verhofstad MH, Edwards MJ, van Laarhoven CJ. The outcome at 20 years of conservatively treated 'isolated' posterior malleolar fractures of the ankle: a case series. J Bone Joint Surg. 2011;93(12): 1621–5.
23. Mangnus L, Meijer DT, Stufkens SA, Mellema JJ, Steller EP, Kerkhoffs GM, Doornberg JN. Posterior Malleolar Fracture Patterns. J Orthop Trauma. 2015; 29(9):428–35.
24. Yao L, Zhang W, Yang G, Zhu Y, Zhai Q, Luo C. Morphologic characteristics of the posterior malleolus fragment: a 3-D computer tomography based study. Arch Orthop Trauma Surg. 2014;134(3):389–94.
25. Buchler L, Tannast M, Bonel HM, Weber M. Reliability of radiologic assessment of the fracture anatomy at the posterior tibial plafond in malleolar fractures. J Orthop Trauma. 2009;23(3):208–12.
26. Meijer DT, Doornberg JN, Sierevelt IN, Mallee WH, van Dijk CN, Kerkhoffs GM, Stufkens SA, Ankle Platform Study Collaborative - Science of Variation G. Guesstimation of posterior malleolar fractures on lateral plain radiographs. Injury. 2015;46(10):2024–9.
27. Gonzalez TA, Watkins C, Drummond R, Wolf JC, Toomey EP, DiGiovanni CW. Transfibular Approach to Posterior Malleolus Fracture Fixation: Technique Tip. Foot Ankle Int. 2015;37(4):440–5.
28. Choi JY, Kim JH, Ko HT, Suh JS. Single Oblique Posterolateral Approach for Open Reduction and Internal Fixation of Posterior Malleolar Fractures With an Associated Lateral Malleolar Fracture. J Foot Ankle Surg. 2015;54(4):559–64.
29. Haraguchi N, Haruyama H, Toga H, Kato F. Pathoanatomy of posterior malleolar fractures of the ankle. J Bone Joint Surg (Am Vol). 2006;88(5): 1085–92.
30. Erdem MN, Erken HY, Burc H, Saka G, Korkmaz MF, Aydogan M. Comparison of lag screw versus buttress plate fixation of posterior malleolar fractures. Foot Ankle Int. 2014;35(10):1022–30.
31. Weber M. Trimalleolar fractures with impaction of the posteromedial tibial plafond: implications for talar stability. Foot Ankle Int. 2004;25(10):716–27.
32. Klammer G, Kadakia AR, Joos DA, Seybold JD, Espinosa N. Posterior pilon fractures: a retrospective case series and proposed classification system. Foot Ankle Int. 2013;34(2):189–99.
33. Ruokun H, Ming X, Zhihong X, Zhenhua F, Jingjing Z, Kai X, Jing L. Postoperative radiographic and clinical assessment of the treatment of posterior tibial plafond fractures using a posterior lateral incisional approach. J Foot Ankle Surg. 2014;53(6):678–82.

24

Morphological characteristics of the posterior malleolar fragment according to ankle fracture patterns: a computed tomography-based study

Young Yi[1†], Dong-Il Chun[2†], Sung Hun Won[2], Suyeon Park[3], Sanghyeon Lee[4] and Jaeho Cho[4*]

Abstract

Background: The posterior malleolar fragment (PMF) of an ankle fracture can have various shapes depending on the injury mechanism. The purpose of this study was to evaluate the morphological characteristics of the PMF according to the ankle fracture pattern described in the Lauge-Hansen classification by using computed tomography (CT) images.

Methods: We retrospectively analyzed CT data of 107 patients (107 ankles) who underwent surgery for trimalleolar fracture from January 2012 to December 2014. The patients were divided into two groups: 76 ankles in the supination-external rotation (SER) stage IV group and 31 ankles in the pronation-external rotation (PER) stage IV group. The PMF type of the two groups was assessed using the Haraguchi and Jan Bartonicek classification. The cross angle (α), fragment length ratio (FLR), fragment area ratio (FAR), sagittal angle (θ), and fragment height (FH) were measured to assess the morphological characteristics of the PMF.

Results: The PMF in the SER group mainly had a posterolateral shape, whereas that in the PER group mainly had a posteromedial two-part shape or a large posterolateral triangular shape ($P = 0.02$). The average cross angle was not significantly different between the two groups (SER group = 19.4°, PER group = 17.6°). The mean FLR and FH were significantly larger in the PER group than in the SER group ($P = 0.024$, $P = 0.006$). The mean fragment sagittal angle in the PER group was significantly smaller than that in the SER group ($P = 0.017$).

Conclusions: With regard to the articular involvement, volume, and vertical nature, the SER-type fracture tends to have a smaller fragment due to the rotational force, whereas the PER-type fracture tends to have a larger fragment due to the combination of rotational and axial forces.

Keywords: Ankle fracture, Computed tomography, Posterior malleolar fragment, Morphology

Background

Ankle fractures commonly occur with an overall age- and sex-adjusted incidence rate of 187 per 100,000 person-years [1]. Trimalleolar fracture with the posterior malleolar fragment (PMF) accounted for 7% of ankle fractures [2]. Clinical studies have shown that the presence of a posterior malleolar fragment (PMF) is important as a prognostic factor or functional outcome in the treatment of ankle fractures [3–6]. Although fixation is recommended for fragments involving 25–30% of articular surface based on the articular involvement of the overall trimalleolar fracture, technical treatment strategies, such as indication or method for fixation of the PMF, remain controversial [7–10].

To understand the pathoanatomy or morphology of the PMF, some studies have been undertaken using plain radiographs [11–13], computed tomography (CT) cross-section [14–16], and 3-D reconstruction CT [17, 18]. However, most studies had proven that using plain

* Correspondence: hohotoy@nate.com
†Equal contributors
4Department of Orthopaedic Surgery, Chuncheon Sacred Heart Hospital, Hallym University, 77, Sakju-ro, Chuncheoni-si, Gangwon-do 200-704, Republic of Korea

radiographs are inadequate to properly understand the pathoanatomy of this PMF. In a few studies that examined PMFs using CT, the authors concluded that PMFs resulted from ankle and pilon fractures. To date, two classification systems [14, 17] of assessing PMF morphology of ankle fractures have been addressed through CT-based studies. Despite the fact that these two classification systems [14, 17] were able to describe the pathoanatomy or morphology of the PMF in ankle fracture, neither classification described the morphological characteristics of the PMF according to the ankle fracture pattern or injury mechanism. Therefore, a better understanding of morphological characteristics of the PMF depending on the mechanism of the injury could be useful to surgeon on planning the fixation of the PMF and may provide a basis for prognosis.

The most commonly used classification systems of ankle fractures are the Lauge-Hansen and Dannis-Weber/AO classification systems. The Dannis-Weber/AO classification system is simple to understand due to the coordinating role of the fibula and syndesmosis of the ankle joint. On the other hand, the Lauge-Hansen classification system is complex and cumbersome due to the need to understand the different stages of pathological damage in addition to the fracture pattern depending on the injury mechanism. For these reasons, the Dannis-Weber/AO classification system has more reliability and reproducibility compared to the Lauge-Hansen classification system [19]. Despite these shortcomings, the Lauge-Hansen system provided the most clinically relevant information, because the ankle fractures are categorized as basis for injury mechanism using a combination of foot position and direction force [1].

The aim of the present study was to evaluate the morphological characteristics of the posterior malleolar fragment (PMF) according to the ankle fracture pattern described in the Lauge-Hansen classification on the basis of a comprehensive CT.

Methods

We retrospectively reviewed consecutive patients who underwent surgery for ankle fracture from January 2012 to December 2014. The following are the exclusion criteria in this study: patients who did not undergo a CT exam before surgery; had fractures without a PMF; were below 18 years old; had previous deformity; and had a significant vertical shift or comminuted PMF, which was unavailable for measurement. We retrospectively analyzed CT data of 107 patients (107 ankles) who underwent surgery for trimalleolar fracture including PMF. Two orthopedic surgeons (JC; orthopedic surgeons, foot and ankle expert, 9 years of experience and SL; orthopedic resident, trauma semi-expert, 3 years of experience) divided the patients into the following groups (according to the Lauge-Hansen classification): 76 ankles in the supination-external rotation (SER) stage IV group and 31 ankles in the pronation-external rotation (PER) stage IV group.

To assess the PMF morphological characteristics of the ankle fractures of each group according to the abovementioned classification systems, all cases from both groups were respectively categorized by the same two orthopedic surgeons using the Haraguchi [14] and Jan Bartonicek [17] classification. Based on the Haraguchi classification, the cases were categorized into three types: type I, the posterolateral-oblique type; type II, the medial-extension type; and type III, the small-shell type. Based on the Jan Bartonicek classification, the cases were categorized into five types: type 1, the extraincisural fragment with an intact fibularnotch; type 2, the posterolateral fragment extending into the fibular notch; type 3, the posteromedial two-part fragment involving the medial malleolus; type 4, the large posterolateral triangular fragment (involving more than one-third of the notch); and type 5, the nonclassified, irregular, osteoporotic fragments.

To assess the morphological characteristics of the PMF using CT images, five measurements, which have been used in previous studies [14, 18], were utilized: cross angle (α), fragment length ratio (FLR), fragment area ratio (FAR), sagittal angle (θ), and fragment height (FH). The CT examinations of the ankles were all performed using a conventional 64-channel CT (Toshiba Aquilion TSX-101A 64 channel, Toshiba Medical System, Tokyo, Japan). Axial, sagittal, and coronal (reconstruction thickness of 2 mm) bone window reformation images were used for the measurements. Using the Picture Archiving and Communication System (PACS) system, all measurements were reviewed independently by the two orthopedic surgeons. The cross angle (α, Fig. 1a), FLR (Fig. 1b), and FAR (Fig. 1c) were measured using the axial images. The bimalleolar axis was defined as the center of the fibula and the distal part of the tibia. The cross angle (α) was the angle between the bimalleolar axis and the major fracture line of the PMF on the image at the level of the tibial plafond. The FLR was defined as the ratio between the length of the fragment and the capital diameter of the tibial plafond on the image at the level of the tibial plafond. The length of the fragment and the capital diameter of the tibial plafond were measured by moving the bimalleolar axis parallel from the posterior tibial lip to the anterior tibial lip. The distance between the apex of the fragment and the posterior tibial lip was defined as the length of the fragment (l). The capital diameter of the tibial plafond (L) was measured in the same manner between the anterior and posterior tibial lips. The FAR was measured using a tool in the

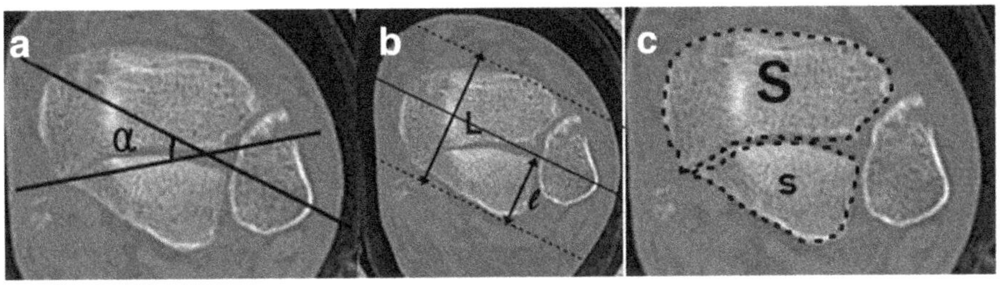

Fig. 1 The radiographicmeasurements on the cross section. **a** The cross angle (α) wasdetermined by measuring theangle between the bimalleolaraxis and the major fracture line. **b** The fragment lengthratio (FLR) was determined by calculatingthe percent of length (l)/length (L). **c** The fragment arearatio (FAR) was determined bycalculating the percent of area(s)/area (s + S)

PACS system, which was used to measure the posterior fragment area (s) and the remaining cross-sectional area of the tibia (S) at the level of the tibial plafond. We calculated the ratio of the fragment area to the total cross-sectional area of the tibial plafond.

Using the CT sagittal reconstruction images, we identified a neutral axis (NA) based on the bisection of the midshaft of the tibia. The sagittal angle (θ) (Fig. 2a) was measured relative to the neutral axis and the major fracture line of the posterior fragment on the sagittal reconstruction images. A line parallel to the neutral axis (NA') was drawn through the apex of the posterior fragment on the sagittal reconstruction views. The FH (Fig. 2b) was defined as the largest distance from the apex of the fragment to the point that was across the joint and the NA' on the consecutive sagittal reconstruction views. The FH was measured on the sagittal reconstruction views.

Statistical analysis

Inter- and intraobserver reliabilities were obtained for all radiographic parameters using the intraclass correlation coefficient (ICC). According to the definitions of Landis and Koch [20], ICCs of 0.81–1.00, 0.61–0.80, 0.41–0.60, 0.21–0.40, and 0.00–0.20 were interpreted as excellent, good, moderate, fair, and poor, respectively. A p value of < 0.05 was considered statistically significant. The Pearson's chi-square and Student's t tests were used to compare sex, age, and radiologic measurements between the SER and PER groups. The Fisher's exact test was used to compare the morphological difference in PMF morphology of the ankle fractures between the two groups according to the two classification systems. The p values on the comparison of the radiologic measurements between the SER and PER groups were calculated using the analysis of covariance adjusted for age and Jan Bartonicek classification.

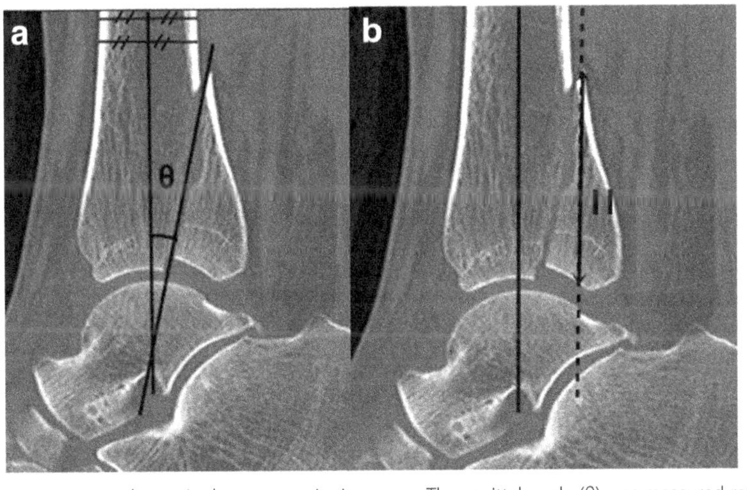

Fig. 2 The radiographic measurements on the sagittal reconstructionimages. **a** The sagittal angle (θ) was measured relative to the neutralaxis and the major fracture line of the posterior fragment on thesagittal reconstruction images. **b** The largest distance from the apexof the fragment to the point which is crossed by the dotted line andthe articular surface on consecutive sagittal reconstruction views isdefined as the fragment height (FH)

This study was completed with appropriate institutional review board approval.

Results

Intraclass correlation coefficients were generated for all radiographic measurements. All measurements were higher than 0.75 (indicating acceptable reliability) and were employed in the study. There was no significant difference in terms of sex between the SER and PER groups, but age was significantly different between these groups. When the two groups were only categorized using the Jan Bartonicek classification, there was a significant difference between the SER and PER groups. The PMF in the SER group mainly had a posterolateral shape, whereas that in the PER group mainly had a posteromedial two-part shape or a large posterolateral triangular shape ($p = 0.02$). These results are shown in Table 1.

The mean (95% CI) and p value of the difference between the two groups with regard to radiographic measurements are shown in Table 2. The mean cross angle (α) was not significantly different between the two groups (SER group = 19.4°, PER group = 17.6°). The mean FLR and the mean FH were significantly larger in the PER group than in the SER group ($p = 0.024$, $p = 0.006$). The mean fragment sagittal angle (θ) in the PER group was significantly smaller than that in the SER group ($p = 0.017$).

Table 1 Demographic Data and CategorizingResults using Haraguchi and Jan BartonicekClassification

	SER (n = 76)		PER (n = 31)		P-value†
Sex					0.2692
Male	28	(36.8%)	15	(48.4%)	
Female	48	(63.2%)	16	(51.6%)	
Age	49.8	±15.8	38.7	±15.0	0.0011
Haraguchi classification					0.0851
1	58	(76.3%)	18	(58.1%)	
2	17	(22.4%)	13	(41.9%)	
3	1	(1.3%)	0	(0.0%)	
Jan Bartonicek classification					0.0203
1	1	(1.3%)	0	(0.0%)	
2	42	(55.3%)	8	(25.8%)	
3	17	(22.4%)	13	(41.9%)	
4	16	(21.1%)	10	(32.3%)	

Values are number of patients (%) or mean ± SD unless otherwise indicated
SER supination-external rotation, *PER* pronation-external rotation
† *P*-values are calculated by Pearson chi-square test, Fisher's exact test or Student's t-test as appropriate

Table 2 Comparison Results ofRadiographic Measurements between SER and PER Groups

	SER (n = 76)			PER (n = 31)			P-value†
Alphaangle	13.1	(8.9	17.4)	13.6	(8.6	18.7)	0.7869
FLR	24.7	(21.0	28.4)	28.3	(24.0	32.7)	0.0249
FAR	12.2	(8.8	15.7)	15.0	(10.9	19.1)	0.0762
Fagittal angle	21.2	(17.7	24.7)	17.5	(13.4	21.7)	0.0173
Fragment height	17.6	(14.4	20.9)	21.6	(17.7	25.5)	0.0062

Values are mean (95% CI) adjusted by age and Jan Bartonicek classification
SER supination-external rotation, *PER* pronation-external rotation, *FLR* fragment length ratio, *FAR* fragment area ratio
† *P*-values are calculated by analysis of covariance adjusted for age and Jan Bartonicek classification

Discussion

The PMF is a lesion involving the posterior tibial plafond, including extra-articular osseous avulsions, posterolateral triangular fragment, and impaction of the entire posterior lip [11]. These fragments can commonly occur in various injury patterns, such as ankle fractures, tibia pilon fractures, and tibial spiral shaft fractures [18]. It has been reported that ankle fractures with PMF have a less satisfactory clinical outcome compared to uni- and bimalleolar ankle fractures [3]. Nevertheless, the optimal treatment algorithm of posterior malleolar fractures remains controversial. In recent years, there has been increasing interest on the morphological classification of these injuries and consensus for surgical fixation. Although two classification systems [14, 17] associated with PMF in ankle fractures were reported, both classifications could not distinguish the morphological differences of the PMF according to the injury mechanism of the ankle fracture. Our study aimed at providing the morphological characteristics of the PMF according to the ankle fracture pattern described in the Lauge-Hansen classification, which is useful in determining the type of fixation method to be used.

Traditionally, the lateral view of a plain radiograph has been used to identify the PMF in ankle fractures. However, it has been reported that plain radiographic assessment of the PMF is poorly reliable and accurate although the PMF's size involving tibial articular surface can be estimated [11, 13]. Accordingly, CT should be required to accurately assess the size and shape of the PMF. In accordance with other studies [14, 17, 18, 21], the authors in the present study used preoperative CT to evaluate the morphology of the PMF, including the fragment size, degree of articular involvement, and FH.

In ankle fractures, Haraguchi et al. [14] were the first to classify 57 cases of PMFs into three types: type I, the posterolateral-oblique type (67%); type II, the medial-extension type (19%); and type III, the small-shell type (14%). However, this classification was based on the fragment size using only a transverse CT scan. Through the investigation performed using CT-based PMF mapping in a series of 45 patients, Mangnus et al. [21] suggested that the morphology of the PMF might be more important than the fragment size alone in making clinical decisions, and they identified Haraguchi type II as a separate fracture pattern. Bartonicek et al. [17] proposed an alternative classification with five categories; the authors argued that a part of type II (the medial-extension type by Haraguchi et al. [14] would be considered a tibial pilon fracture. Moreover, some authors [15, 22] addressed the term posterior pilon variant; this fracture is characterized by a posterior malleolar fracture with posteromedial fragment, such as the medial-extension type II described by Haraguchi et al. [14]. The results of our present study showed that the medial-extension type was more common in the PER group than in the SER group, although the difference was not statistically significant. Bartonicek et al. [17] suggested that the type 3 cases (the posteromedial two-part fragment involving the medial malleolus) could have been caused by the combination of compression force and avulsion, and the type 4 cases (the large posterolateral triangular fragment involving more than one-third of the notch) were probably caused by compression force or as part of a tibia pilon fracture variant. In the present study, when two groups were categorized according to the Jan Bartonicek classification, types 3 and 4 were more statistically and significantly frequent in the PER group than in the SER group. Therefore, this can indicate that the PMF morphological classification presented previously may differ according to the classification of ankle fracture based on the injury mechanism.

Our study showed that the mean FLR and FH were significantly larger in the PER group than in the SER group. Also, the mean fragment sagittal angle (θ) in the PER group was significantly smaller than that in the SER group (p = 0.017). In a previous study [18], the area of articular involvement for tibia plafond was significantly associated with FLR. In addition, the fragment sagittal angle (θ) was considered as the vertical nature of the PMF, which can be affected by the shearing force transmitted by the loading. When interpreting our results with reference to the previous study, it can be assumed that the volume of the PMF was larger in the PER group than in the SER group and that the PMF of the PER group has a more vertical nature than that of the SER group.

Knowing the precise mechanism of ankle fractures is important for surgeons to be able to accurately assess the fracture pattern. The Lauge-Hansen classification describes, firstly, the position of the foot at the time of injury and, secondly, the deforming force on the ankle [23]. The ankle may be in one of following positions at the time of trauma: pronation (eversion) and supination (inversion). Three deforming forces may occur: abduction, adduction, and external rotation, which determine the following mechanisms of injury: pronation-abduction (PA), PER, supination-adduction (SA), and SER. The posterior malleolar fracture may occur in both PER and SER injury mechanisms. In stage IV of the PER injury mechanism, posterior malleolar and fibular fracture may occur with or without medial malleolar fracture. However, posterior malleolar and fibular fracture may occur without medial malleolar fracture in stage III of the SER injury mechanism or trimalleolar fracture may occur in stage IV of the SER injury mechanism. In the present study, we compared the PMF morphology of the trimalleolar fracture in stage IV of both the SER and PER injury mechanisms to minimize the bias, which was achieved by adjusting the degree of the deforming force causing the fracture and the type of fracture as equally as possible.

The differences in the PMF morphological characteristics according to the ankle fracture pattern are presumed to be caused by the different foot positions at the time of trauma. In the sequence of supination injuries, fracture of the posterior malleolus may have occurred mainly due to the pulling force of the intact posterior inferior tibiofibular ligament (PITFL) in addition to the rupture of the intact anterior inferior tibiofibular ligament (AITFL) and a fibular spiral fracture. The occurrence of posterior malleolar fractures in the SER injury is mainly caused by the transverse plane rotation. On the other hand, the posterior malleolar fracture in the sequence of pronation injuries may have occurred due to the pushing force of the foot combined with the pulling force in addition to the medial malleolar fracture, involvement of the AITFL with extension into the interosseous membrane, and a spiral or oblique high fibular fracture (Fig. 3). This form of pronation injury is affected not only by the pronation force, but also by the posterior displacement stress combined with lateral malleolar displacement [21, 24] and axial compression force by the talus [25]. In this case, the unstable or large displaced posterior malleolar fracture could be presented. Therefore, the differences of morphological characteristics of the PMF by direction force may be clinically relevant to the different methods for fixation of the PMF. The treatment strategy proposed by the authors is that the smaller fragment due to the rotational force is enough to position the screw, while the larger fragment due to a combination of rotational and axial forces require direct open reduction and internal fixation.

This study has some limitations. The number of patients in the SER group was more than double of that in the PER group. Supination external rotation type has

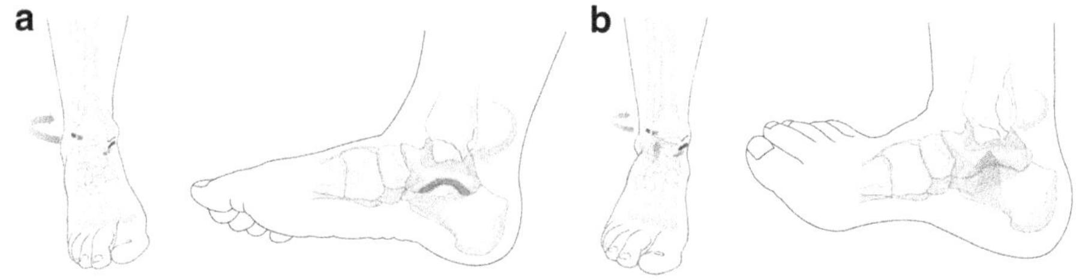

Fig. 3 a The occurrence of posteriormalleolar fractures in the supination-external rotation stage IV injury is mainly caused by the rotational force. **b** The posterior malleolar fracture in the pronation-external rotationstage IV injury may have occurreddue to a combination of rotational and axial forces

been reported as the most common mechanism of fracture, accounting for 40–70% of all ankle fractures [26]. For this reason, it is presumed that the difference in the number of patients was shown by the two groups. On the other hand, statistically, a compromise power analysis could be performed to determine the appropriate sample size for this study. The control group showed a power (1-β err prob) of 0.845 for detecting a noncentrality parameter δ of 2.03 at a critical t level of 1.019. Thus, this study has a statistically meaningless difference in the number of samples between the two groups, but this difference could lead to reader confusion. The radiographic measurement of the small fragment may have poor precision. Moreover, the definition that distinguishes ankle fractures involving the tibial plafond and tibial pilon fractures is not yet clear. These factors may increase the systematic bias in the present research. Furthermore, the assessment based on CT may be somewhat insufficient to quantify the morphological characteristics of the PMF. In the future, quantification of three-dimensional CT is required to support the results presented in this study.

Conclusions

The morphological characteristics of the PMF in trimalleolar fracture may differ according to the ankle fracture pattern based on the injury mechanism. With regard to the articular involvement, volume, and vertical nature, the SER-type fracture tends to have a smaller fragment due to the rotational force, whereas the PER-type fracture tends to have a larger fragment due to a combination of rotational and axial forces.

Abbreviations

AITFL: Anterior inferior tibiofibular ligament; CT: Computed tomography; FAR: Fragment area ratio; FH: Fragment height; FLR: Fragment length ratio; ICC: Intraclass correlation coefficient; PA: Pronation-abduction; PACS: picture archiving and communication system; PER: Pronation-external rotation; PITFL: Posterior inferior tibiofibular ligament; PMF: Posterior malleolar fragment; SA: Supination-adduction; SER: Supination-external rotation

Acknowledgements

Not applicable.

Funding

This research was supported by Hallym University Research Fund 2016 (HURF-2016-22). Moreover, this work was supported by Soonchunhyang University Hospital.

Authors' contributions

YY and DIC conceived the study, participated in its design and coordination, and helped draft the manuscript. SHW participated in the study design and helped to draft the manuscript. SP, as a consultant for statistical analysis, performed the statistical analysis. SL and JC analyzed and interpreted the data. JC was a major contributor in writing the manuscript and gave assessment guidance during this study. All authors have read and approved the final manuscript.

Consent for publication

Not applicable.

Competing interests

The authors declare that they have no competing interests.

Author details

[1]Seoul Foot and Ankle Center, Inje University Seoul Paik Hospital, Seoul, Republic of Korea. [2]Department of Orthopedic Surgery, Seoul Hospital, Soonchunhyang University College of Medicine, Seoul, Republic of Korea. [3]Department of Biostatistics, Seoul Hospital, Soonchunhyang University College of Medicine, Seoul, Republic of Korea. [4]Department of Orthopaedic Surgery, Chuncheon Sacred Heart Hospital, Hallym University, 77, Sakju-ro, Chuncheoni-si, Gangwon-do 200-704, Republic of Korea.

References

1. Daly PJ, Fitzgerald RH Jr, Melton LJ, Ilstrup DM. Epidemiology of ankle fractures in Rochester, Minnesota. Acta Orthop Scand. 1987;58(5):539–44.
2. Court-Brown CM, McBirnie J, Wilson G. Adult ankle fractures–an increasing problem? Acta Orthop Scand. 1998;69(1):43–7.
3. Jaskulka RA, Ittner G, Schedl R. Fractures of the posterior tibial margin: their role in the prognosis of malleolar fractures. J Trauma. 1989;29(11):1565–70.
4. Langenhuijsen JF, Heetveld MJ, Ultee JM, Steller EP, Butzelaar RM. Results of ankle fractures with involvement of the posterior tibial margin. J Trauma. 2002;53(1):55–60.
5. Tejwani NC, Pahk B, Egol KA. Effect of posterior malleolus fracture on outcome after unstable ankle fracture. J Trauma. 2010;69(3):666–9.
6. Weber M, Ganz R. Malunion following trimalleolar fracture with posterolateral subluxation of the talus–reconstruction including the posterior malleolus. Foot Ankle Int. 2003;24(4):338–44.
7. Gardner MJ, Streubel PN, McCormick JJ, Klein SE, Johnson JE, Ricci WM. Surgeon practices regarding operative treatment of posterior malleolus fractures. Foot Ankle Int. 2011;32(4):385–93.
8. Miller AN, Carroll EA, Parker RJ, Helfet DL, Lorich DG. Posterior malleolar stabilization of syndesmotic injuries is equivalent to screw fixation. Clin Orthop Relat Res. 2010;468(4):1129–35.

9. Rammelt S, Heim D, Hofbauer LC, Grass R, Zwipp H. Problems and controversies in the treatment of ankle fractures. Unfallchirurg. 2011; 114(10):847–60.
10. van den Bekerom MP, Haverkamp D, Kloen P. Biomechanical and clinical evaluation of posterior malleolar fractures. A systematic review of the literature. J Trauma. 2009;66(1):279–84.
11. Buchler L, Tannast M, Bonel HM, Weber M. Reliability of radiologic assessment of the fracture anatomy at the posterior tibial plafond in malleolar fractures. J Orthop Trauma. 2009;23(3):208–12.
12. Ebraheim NA, Mekhail AO, Haman SP. External rotation-lateral view of the ankle in the assessment of the posterior malleolus. Foot Ankle Int. 1999; 20(6):379–83.
13. Ferries JS, DeCoster TA, Firoozbakhsh KK, Garcia JF, Miller RA. Plain radiographic interpretation in trimalleolar ankle fractures poorly assesses posterior fragment size. J Orthop Trauma. 1994;8(4):328–31.
14. Haraguchi N, Haruyama H, Toga H, Kato F. Pathoanatomy of posterior malleolar fractures of the ankle. J Bone joint Surg Am Vol. 2006;88(5): 1085–92.
15. Klammer G, Kadakia AR, Joos DA, Seybold JD, Espinosa N. Posterior pilon fractures: a retrospective case series and proposed classification system. Foot Ankle Int. 2013;34(2):189–99.
16. Magid D, Michelson JD, Ney DR, Fishman EK. Adult ankle fractures: comparison of plain films and interactive two- and three-dimensional CT scans. AJR Am J Roentgenol. 1990;154(5):1017–23.
17. Bartonicek J, Rammelt S, Kostlivy K, Vanecek V, Klika D, Tresl I. Anatomy and classification of the posterior tibial fragment in ankle fractures. Arch Orthop Trauma Surg. 2015;135(4):505–16.
18. Yao L, Zhang W, Yang G, Zhu Y, Zhai Q, Luo C. Morphologic characteristics of the posterior malleolus fragment: a 3-D computer tomography based study. Arch Orthop Trauma Surg. 2014;134(3):389–94.
19. Yin MC, Yuan XF, Ma JM, Xia Y, Wang T, Xu XL, Yan YJ, Xu JH, Ye J, Tong ZY, et al. Evaluating the reliability and reproducibility of the AO and Lauge-Hansen classification Systems for Ankle Injuries. Orthopedics. 2015;38(7): e626–30.
20. Landis JR, Koch GG. The measurement of observer agreement for categorical data. Biometrics. 1977;33(1):159–74.
21. Mangnus L, Meijer DT, Stufkens SA, Mellema JJ, Steller EP, Kerkhoffs GM, Doornberg JN. Posterior malleolar fracture patterns. J Orthop Trauma. 2015; 29(9):428–35.
22. Weber M. Trimalleolar fractures with impaction of the posteromedial tibial plafond: implications for talar stability. Foot Ankle Int. 2004;25(10):716–27.
23. Lauge-Hansen N. Fractures of the ankle. III. Genetic roentgenologic diagnosis of fractures of the ankle. Am J Roentgenol Radium Therapy, Nucl Med. 1954;71(3):456–71.
24. Warner SJ, Schottel PC, Hinds RM, Helfet DL, Lorich DG. Fracture-dislocations demonstrate poorer postoperative functional outcomes among pronation external rotation IV ankle fractures. Foot Ankle Int. 2015;36(6):641–7.
25. Switaj PJ, Weatherford B, Fuchs D, Rosenthal B, Pang E, Kadakia AR. Evaluation of posterior malleolar fractures and the posterior pilon variant in operatively treated ankle fractures. Foot Ankle Int. 2014;35(9):886–95.
26. Michelson J, Solocoff D, Waldman B, Kendell K, Ahn U. Ankle fractures. The Lauge-Hansen classification revisited. Clin Orthop Relat Res. 1997; 345:198–205.

25

Is additional balloon Kyphoplasty safe and effective for acute thoracolumbar burst fracture?

Ping-Jui Tsai[1,2], Ming-Kai Hsieh[1,2,3*], Kuo-Feng Fan[1,2], Lih-Huei Chen[1,2], Chia-Wei Yu[1,2], Po-Liang Lai[1,2], Chi-Chien Niu[1,2], Tsung-Ting Tsai[1,2] and Wen-Jer Chen[1,2]

Abstract

Background: Burst fracture is a common thoracolumbar injury that is treated using posterior pedicle instrumentation and fusion combined with transpedicular intracorporeal grafting after reduction. In this study, we compared the outcome of these two techniques by using radiologic imaging and functional outcome.

Methods: Sixty-one patients with acute thoracolumbar burst fracture were operated with kyphoplasty (n = 31) or vertebroplasty (n = 30) and retrospectively reviewed in our institution between 2011 and 2014. All 61 patients underwent surgery within 5 days after admission to the hospital and then followed-up for 12 to 24 months after surgery.

Results: Significant improvement was found in the anterior vertebral height (92 ± 8.9% in the kyphoplasty group, 85.6 ± 7.2% in the vertebroplasty group, $p < 0.01$) at 1 month post-operatively and (89 ± 7.9% in the kyphoplasty group, 78 ± 6.9% in the vertebroplasty group, $p < 0.01$) at the 24-month follow-up. Significant improvement was also observed in the kyphotic angle (1.2 ± 0.5° in the kyphoplasty group, 10.5 ± 1.2° in the vertebroplasty group, $p < 0.01$) at 1 month post-operatively and (5.4 ± 1.2° in the kyphoplasty group, 11.5 ± 8.5° in the vertebroplasty group, p < 0.01) at the 24-month follow-up. Both operations led to significant improvement of the patients' pain and the Oswestry disability index (p < 0.01). Cement leakage was noted in 29% of patients after kyphoplasty and 77% of patients after vertebroplasty (p < 0.01). Only one implant failure (3.3%), which required further surgical intervention, was reported in the vertebroplasty group.

Conclusions: Reduction with additional balloon at the fractured site is better than indirect reduction only by posterior instrumentation. The better reduction of kyphotic angle and the lower cement leakage rate in the kyphoplasty group indicate that additional balloon kyphoplasty is safe and effective for acute thoracolumbar burst fracture.

Keywords: Burst fracture, Vertebroplasty, Kyphoplasty, Calcium sulfate/phosphate cement, Acute thoracolumbar burst fracture

Background

Burst fracture is a common thoracolumbar injury that occurs because of failure of the anterior and middle columns due to axial loading [1]. When anterior vertebral body height loss exceeds 50%, when the spinal canal is compromised by more than 50%, or when angulation is greater than 20° [1], surgical intervention should be considered. Recently, Thoracolumbar Injury Classification and Severity Score (TLICSS), which included fracture morphology, neurological injury and the integrity status of posterior ligamentous complex to determine stability and to decide operative or nonoperative treatment [2]. According to this classification, operative treatment is recommended for a score ≥ 5 points, and conservative nonoperative treatment for a score ≤ 3 points [2, 3].

Posterior pedicle instrumentation and fusion combined with transpedicular intracorporeal grafting after reduction

* Correspondence: mk660628@gmail.com
[1]Department of Orthopedic Surgery, Chang Gung Memorial Hospital and Chang Gung University, Taoyuan, Taiwan
[2]Bone and Joint Research Center, Chang Gung Memorial Hospital, Linkou, Taiwan

is a well-known surgical technique [4, 5]. Several different types of grafts exist, including autogenous bone grafts, allogenous bone grafts, and artificial bone grafts; these bone grafts are composed of polymethylmethacrylate (PMMA) or calcium sulfate, and calcium phosphate, among others [6–8]. Because of the complications at the donor site with autogenous bone grafts [9] and the risk of infection with allogenous bone grafts, artificial bone grafts are now more widely used. In addition, studies have shown that artificial bone grafts are as efficient as autogenous bone grafts [10].

Balloon kyphoplasty is a relatively effective technique to reduce the fracture site [11–14]. Reduction by balloon is speculated to effectively correct vertebral body height and angle. Another advantage of balloon kyphoplasty is decreased cement leakage, which is often a problem with vertebroplasty. Few researches [15] have compared the effects of balloon kyphoplasty with traditional vertebroplasty in acute thoracolumbar burst fracture. Our study aimed to compare the radiologic and functional outcomes of these two techniques.

Methods

Sixty-one patients with acute thoracolumbar burst fracture with or without neurologic deficit were treated with balloon kyphoplasty (n = 31) or vertebroplasty (n = 30) between 2011 and 2014 (Table 1). The Chang Gung Medical Foundation Institutional Review Board approved this study (103-3387B) and waived the requirement for informed consent because of the retrospective nature of the study. All the patients were treated with transpedicular intracorporeal grafting with calcium sulfate/phosphate cement and stabilization with pedicle-screw instrumentation. The results were compared in a retrospective, nonrandomized cohort study.

Table 1 Patient demographics data

Characteristic	Kyphoplasty	Vertebroplasty	*p* value
Number of patients	31	30	0.91
Age	35.5 ± 6.5	41.2 ± 6.8	0.814
Gender: female (%)	14 (54%)	12 (48%)	0.258
Location of fractured vertebrae			
Thoracic (T8–T10)	4	2	
T–L (T11–L1)	21	19	0.390
Lumbar (L2–L3)	6	9	
Neurological status (ASIA⁺)			
A	1	6	
B	0	2	
C	2	2	0.456
D	2	1	
E	26	19	
Hospital stay	12.5 ± 2.55	13 ± 3	0.551

ASIA⁺: American Spine Injury Association impairment scale [17]

Operation was indicated when the patient had a thoracolumbar injury classification and severity score [16] greater than 5. Additional balloon kyphoplasty was favored in the presence of kyphotic vertebrae and disruption of the posterior vertebral cortex, where higher-viscosity cement can be injected. All 61 patients underwent surgery within 5 days after admission to the hospital and were followed up for at least 24 months after surgery. Each patient underwent neurologic assessment by using a rating scale based on the American Spine Injury Association (ASIA) impairment scale [17]. The treatment outcomes were assessed with special reference to the anterior vertebral height (AVH), kyphotic angle, degree of back pain (visual analog scale or VAS), the Oswestry disability index (ODI) at pre-operative and post-operative follow-up after 1, 3, 6, 12, and 24 months. Complications including cement leakage and implant failure were also assessed. Beginning on the day after surgery and continuing for 3 months, patients were encouraged to ambulation while wearing a Taylor's brace. Unrestricted activity was permitted after considering the individual patient's neurologic situation.

Operative technique

All operative procedures were performed with the patients under general anesthesia with endotracheal intubation. All patients were placed in a prone position on a radiolucent frame. Long or short constructs were planned and instrumented according to the level of the burst fracture. Long instrumentation (2 vertebrae above and 2 vertebrae below the fracture) was used for fractures between T11 and L2 (26 patients). Short instrumentation (One vertebra above and one vertebra below the fracture) was used if the fractured vertebra was located above T10 or below L3 (35 patients) (Table 2).

Pedicle screws (SmartLoc® Spinal Fixation System, A-Spine Asia Co, Ltd., Taiwan) of the proper diameter were placed down into the pedicles of selected nonfractured vertebrae above and below the fractured vertebra using a standard posterior midline approach. Ligamentotaxis was achieved by proper longitudinal rod contouring [18] with distraction used along the entire area of instrumentation. Kyphoplasty was performed as follows: a cannula and an expander were inserted into the pedicle, and then a drill was inserted through the cannula. A balloon (Versys; SI Medical Co, Ltd., Korea) was inserted unilaterally into the fractured vertebral body and inflated slowly with initial bulk pressure [19]. Subsequently, the inflated balloon was deflated and withdrawn, then the intravertebral cavity was filled with calcium sulfate/phosphate cement (PRO-DENSE® Bone Graft Substitute, Wright Medical Technology, Arlington, TN,

Table 2 Operative data

Operative Characteristic	Kyphoplasty	Vertebroplasty	*p* value
Short (1 above and 1 below fractured vertebra)	19	16	0.312
Long (2 above and 2 below fractured vertebra)	12	14	
Blood loss (ml)	265 ± 25	215 ± 85	0.058
Operative time (minutes)	125 ± 26	115 ± 14	0.25
Follow-up	29.5 ± 5.5	28.5 ± 4.5	0.462
Volume injected (ml)	12 ± 2.5	6.5 ± 1.5	<0.01

USA) [20]. This calcium phosphate cement product in a radiopaque liquid that was injected anteriorly into the void produced by the balloon inflation (Figs. 1, 2). Vertebroplasty was performed with a cannula inserted into the fractured vertebra. Under the fluoroscopic monitoring, the calcium sulfate/phosphate cement was injected when the cannula reached the defect of the fractured vertebra (Figs. 3, 4). Decompressive laminectomy was performed in patients with neurological deficit. Posterior or posterolateral fusions were not performed in either group. Union was defined as continuous trabeculae of bridging anterior osteophytes on plain films with absence of halo signs of screws. Probable fusion was defined as unclear trabecular bone with no radiolucent screws. Radiolucent screws or osteolysis of augmented artificial bone was labeled as nonunion [21]. Complications included cement leakages, wound infection, cardiopulmonary embolism and nonunion were recorded and analyzed. Cement leakages were classified into three types: type S, via the segmental vein; type B, via the basivertebral vein; and type C, through a cortical defect [22].

Statistical analysis

Data from both groups were analyzed with SPSS statistical software package (SPSS Inc., Chicago, IL, USA). Tests of hypotheses between both groups were conducted using a Student t-test for numerical data (including age, follow-up period, operation time, estimated blood loss, AVH, kyphotic angle, presence of back pain [VAS], and the ODI). *P*-values <0.05 were defined as statistically significant.

Results

No significant difference was observed in age, gender, location of fractured vertebrae, neurological status,

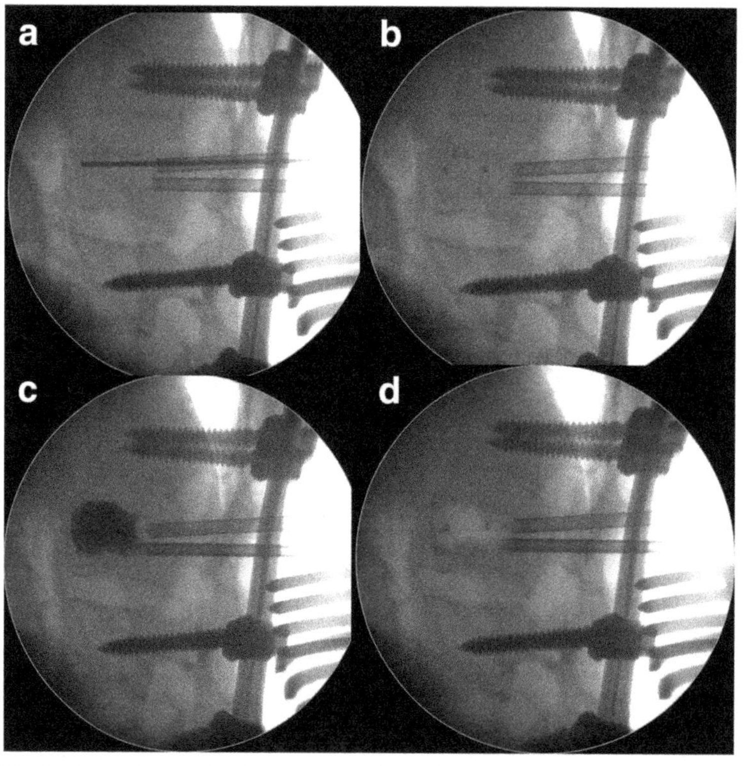

Fig. 1 Radiographic image of kyphoplasty technique. Kyphoplasty was performed using a cannula and an expander, which were inserted into the pedicle, as well as a drill, which was inserted through the cannula. A needle pipe and pin was placed parallel to the superior endplate in the lateral view (**a**). The balloon was slowly inflated with initial bulk pressure (**b** and **c**). The volume of the balloon was carefully controlled to restore the fractured vertebra until adequate kyphotic angle reduction was obtained or the inflation pressure reached 220 psi [19]. The operator should record the amount of injected fluid to predict the cement volume. The balloon was deflated and withdrawn (**d**), and the created cavity was filled with cement [19]

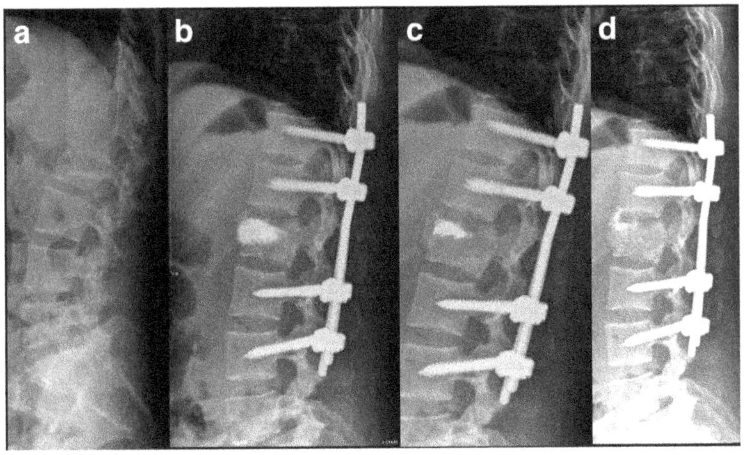

Fig. 2 Radiographic image of one patient who received kypoplasty and long instrumentation. **a**. Lateral roentgenogram of a 25-year-old female patient showing a burst fracture of L2; the kyphotic angle is 30°. **b**. Postoperative lateral X-ray 3 days after surgery showing excellent restoration after kyphoplasty and long instrumentation; the kyphotic angle is −6°. **c**. Intact implant and kyphotic angle is −3° three months after surgery. **d**. Solid anterior fusion (continuous trabeculae of bridging anterior osteophytes without halo signs of screws) was achived and kyphotic angle was 0° 12 months after surgery

and hospital stay in both groups (Table 1). According to the ASIA neurologic grading scale, 7 patients had grade A, 2 patients had grade B, 4 patients had grade C, 3 patients had grade D, and 45 patients had grade E. All 9 patients with incomplete neurologic deficit had at least 1 ASIA grade neurologic improvement at the 24-month follow-up.

The mean operative time in the kyphoplasty group was 125 min (range, 99–151 min) and 115 min in the vertebroplasty group (range, 101–129 min) which was

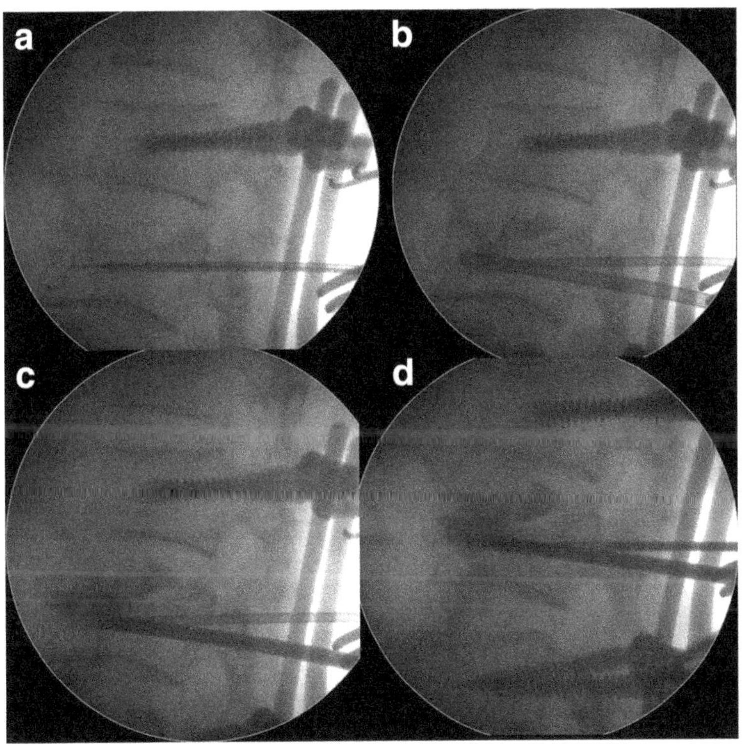

Fig. 3 Vertebroplasty technique and cement leakage. Vertebroplasty was performed by inserting a cannula into the fractured vertebra (**a**). Calcium sulfate/phosphate cement was injected when the cannula tip reached the defect of the fractured vertebra under fluoroscopic monitoring (**b**, **c**). Intradiscal leakage and poor body reduction were noted during vertebroplasty (**d**)

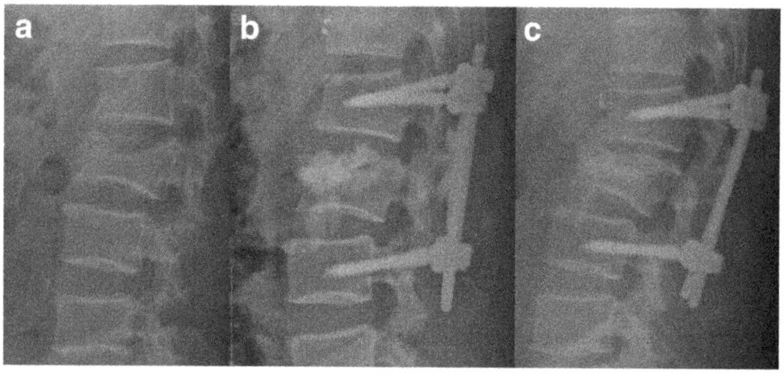

Fig. 4 Radiographic image of one patient who received vetebralplasty and short instrumentation. **a**. Lateral roentgenogram of a 35-year-old male patient showing a L3 burst fracture; the kyphotic angle is 20°. **b**. Postoperative lateral roentgenogram showing good reduction (the kyphotic angle is 0 degree) through vertebroplasty and short instrumentation with intradiscal and paraspinal leakages 3 days after surgery. **c**. The kyphotic angle is −3° 12months after surgery and solid anterior fusion (continuous trabeculae of bridging anterior osteophytes without halo signs of screws) was achived. But the kyphotic angle is 12 degree and the rod was bended 12 months after surgery

not statistically significant difference(p = 0.25). The total volume of blood loss was 265 ml in the kyphoplasty group (range, 240–290 ml) and 215 ml in the vertebroplasty group (range, 130–300); the difference was also not statistically significant (p = 0.058). All patients were observed in an average follow-up of 29 months (range, 24–36 months). The volume of cement injected in the kyphoplasty group was 12 ml (range, 9.5–14.5 ml) and 6.5 ml in the vertebroplasty group (range, 5–8 ml); the difference was statistically significant ($p < 0.01$) (Table 2).

Significant improvement in the AVH (92 ± 8.9% in the kyphoplasty group, 85.6 ± 7.2% in the vertebroplasty group, p < 0.01) was found at 1 month post-operatively and (89 ± 7.9% in the kyphoplasty group, 78 ± 6.9% in the vertebroplasty group, p < 0.01) at the 24-month follow-up. The kyphotic angle between the two groups was also significant with 1.2 ± 0.5° in the kyphoplasty group and 10.5 ± 1.2° in the vertebroplasty group ($p < 0.01$) at 1 month post-operatively, and 5.4 ± 1.2° in the kyphoplasty group and 11.5 ± 8.5° in the vertebroplasty group ($p < 0.01$) at the 24-month follow-up (Fig. 5a, b). Both surgical procedures resulted in improvement of the patients' pain and the ODI without statistical significance between the two groups (Fig. 5).

Complications.

The three patterns in C-type leakage are paraspinal, intradiscal, and posterior. Cement leakage was observed in 29% of patients in the kyphoplasty group (including 6% leakages via the segmental vessels, 10% through a paraspinal cortical defect, and 13% through a intradiscal cortical defect) and in 77% of patients after vertebroplasty (including 3% leakages via the basivertebral vein, 10% via segmental vein, 20% leakages through a paraspinal cortical defect, 30% through a intradiscal cortical defect, and 14% through the posterior cortical wall) ($p < 0.01$) (Fig. 6). There is no intraoperative cardiogenic hypotension, pulmonary embolism, or deteriorated neurological deficit in the 32 patients (9 and 23 in the kyphoplasty and vertebroplasty groups, respectively) with cement leakage. Superficial wound infection or deep wound infection was not found in our series. At the final follow-up, 60 of the 61 patients exhibited union or probable union. Nonunion was only in one implant (3.3%) in the vertebroplasty group, which required further surgical intervention. There is no adjacent vertebral fractures in the 2-year follow-up.

Discussion

In this study, long instrumentation were performed in T11-L1 fractured vertebrae. 9 patients with T11-L1 fractured vertebrae in kyphoplasty group and 5 patients in vertebroplasty group were performed short instrumentation because of strong bone screw purchase. However, the results of many studies [10, 23–25] showed that lack of anterior support may lead to a high percentage of early implant failure. A large cavity in fractured vertebrae is created during posterior instrumented construct after application of a distraction force, and thus may lead to reduction site collapse and worsened clinical outcomes. The materials used for anterior reconstruction includes autogenous and artificial bone grafts. The results of several studies have shown that artificial bone grafts produce similar success rates to autogenous bone grafts. In addition, the use of artificial bone grafts may lead to shorter operation time and less blood loss [10].

Many techniques have been used to establish anterior vertebral support. Vertebroplasty, which was first used in 1987 [26], became an efficient method for treating compression fractures [27]. Balloon-assisted kyphoplasty is a developed technique [19, 28, 29] to restore the vertebral body height and to treat local kyphosis which also contributes to anterior column stability. In the

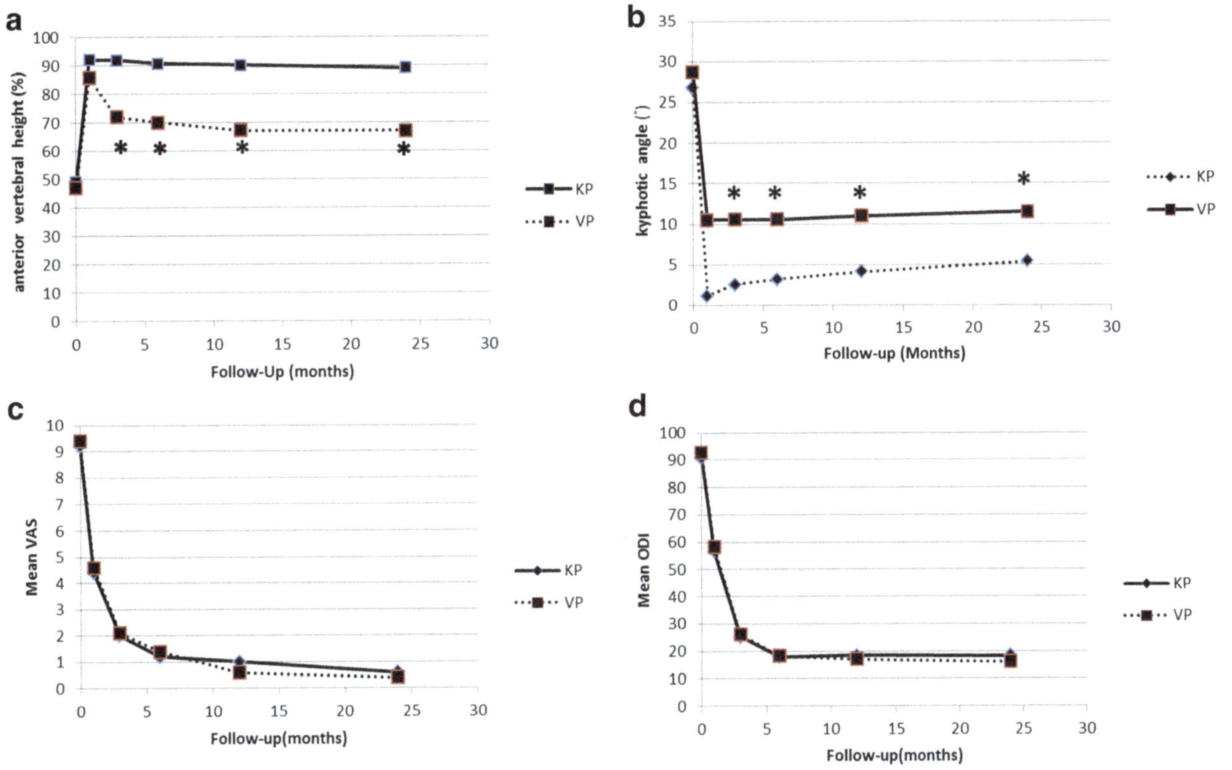

Fig. 5 Comparisons of the kyphoplasty and vertebroplasty in anterior vertebral height (**a**), kyphotic angle (**b**), mean VAS (**c**) and ODI (**d**) at baseline and follow-up. Group calculated means and 95% confidence intervals are shown in panels A, B, C and D. In panels A and B, the treatment p value refers to the average treatment effect difference (*, $p < 0.05$) at 3, 6, 12, and 24 months follow-up. In panels C and D, no clinical treatment effect difference was found at pre-operative and post-operative follow-up

present study, posterior screw fixation combined with kyphoplasty for anterior support produced significantly better kyphosis angle correction and better vertebral body height, as shown during the 24-month follow-up. Using posterior distraction, reduction of fractured vertebrae is improved indirectly by ligamentotaxis but distraction force also increases kyphotic angle. The distraction force applied in the kyphoplasty patients may be lower in the vertebroplasty patients, and thus post-operative lordotic angle may be better in the kyphoplasty

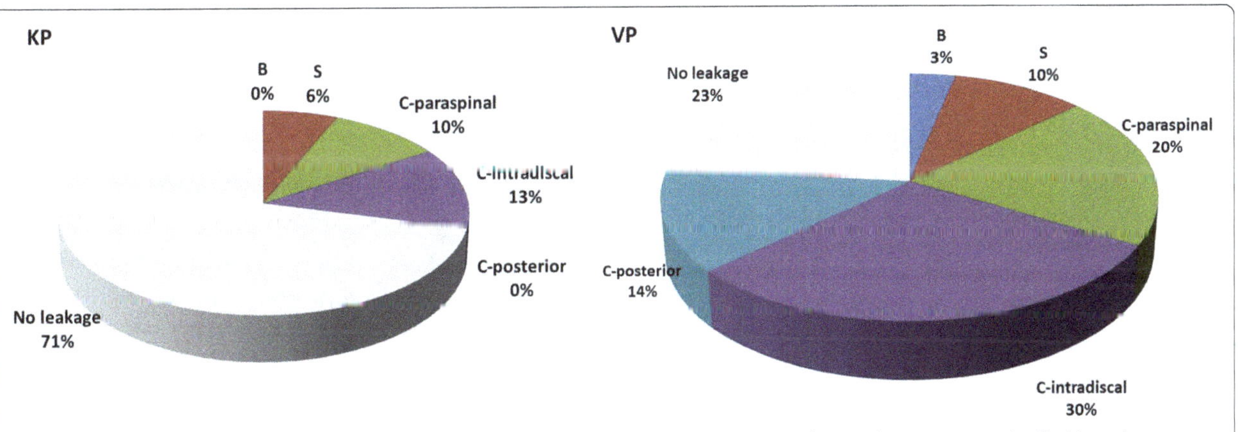

Fig. 6 Comparisons of cement leakage between the kyphoplasty and vertebroplasty groups. Leakages of cement were classified into three different types [22]: type B, through the basivertebral vein; type S, through the segmental vein; and type C, through a cortical defect including three patterns in C-type leakage (i.e., paraspinal, intradiscal, and posterior). Kyphoplasty resulted in considerably less cement extravasation (29%) than vertebroplasty (77%). In our series, leakage into the spinal canal (C-posterior type leakage) is significant in the vertebroplasty group (14% in the vertebroplasty group to 0% in the kyphoplasty group)

group. The reported kyphotic angle correction with transpedicular bone grafting and short pedicle fixation techniques ranges from 64% to 105% [18, 30–33]. The average corrections of 92% in the kyphoplasty group and 85.6% in vertebroplasty group are within the previous reported range. The average loss of correction after posterior short segment instrumentation plus transpedicular augmentation with biodegradable bone cement is not significantly different from that following traditional anterior and posterior spinal operations [18, 30, 34], with the loss of correction ranging from 1° to 4.2°.

Posterior instrumentation is speculated to fail due to the large bone defect created inside the fractured vertebra after indirect height restoration through distraction and ligamentotaxis force applied during surgery [35]. Because the majority of patients with burst fractures in our series were aged between 29 and 48 years, the use of a more biocompatible bone cements (e.g.,calcium phosphate and hydroxyapatite) is preferred [30, 36, 37]. Self-hardening calcium sulfate/phosphate bone cements have been developed as alternatives to avoid long-term side effects of PMMA [38–40] because of the biocompatibility, no local heat or toxic effect on surrounding bone tissues [41, 42] and can stimulate bone formation at the bone–cement interface [43]. Korovessis P. [44] reported an improvement of kyphotic angle from preoperative 16° to postoperative 1° at final follow-up and the AVH ratio from 0.6 to 0.9 in 29 thoracolumbar burst fracture patients using kyphoplasty with calcium phosphate cement and pedicle screws instrumentation and reported a similar result in 18 thoracolumbar burst fracture patients [45] using balloon kyphoplasty with calcium phosphate cement combined with posterior short segmental fixation. In both of their study, they didn't use vertebroplasty as a control group which is difficult to make a conclusion that the reduction using balloon at the site of the fractured vertebra is better than the indirect reduction by means of distraction provided only by instrumentation. We also doubt this similar data [44, 45] because of the distraction force applied in open surgery should be larger than minimal invasive method so that radiological result in open surgery should be better.

The reason why significant improvements were noted in kyphotic angle and AVH at post-operative one month, but decreased in the 24-month follow-up in our study, because of the calcium sulfate/phosphate cement was partial resorption.

In this study, the volume injected in the kyphoplasty group was significantly higher than that in the vertebroplasty group (12 ± 2.5 cm^3 vs. 6.5 ± 1.5 cm^3, $p < 0.01$) because the void space in fractured vertebrae was created by balloon kyphoplasty, and thus, the vertebral height and kyphotic angle will be better and maintained in the 24-month follow-up in the kyphoplasty group.

According to the previous studies, balloon assisted kyphoplasty results in considerably less cement extravasation, compared to vertebroplasty [46–48]. In a systematic review of clinical studies, the rate of cement leakage was 9% in kyphoplasty groups and 41% in vertebroplasty groups [49]. In a meta-analysis study, cement extravasation were observed in 7% of patients after kyphoplasty, but in 20% of patients after vertebroplasty [50]. In the present study, 29% of the kyphoplasty group had cement leakage, compared to 77% in the vertebroplasty group (Fig. 6). The higher leakage rate may be due to acute burst fracture in young patients instead of osteoporotic compression in older patients. The lower rate of cement leakage in the kyphoplasty group proved the fact that injection of high-viscosity cement at low pressure into a created cavity is a significant improvement over the injection of low-viscosity cement at high pressure into an unreduced fractured vertebra (Fig. 7) [19, 29, 49]. In our series, leakage into the spinal canal was significant in the vertebroplasty group (16% in the vertebroplasty group to 0% in the kyphoplasty group), indicating that kyphoplasty is a considerably safe procedure in the treatment of thoracolumbar burst fractures. Only one implant failure (3.3%), which required further surgical intervention, was found in the vertebroplasty group.

In our series, a larger amount of cement was injected into the vertebrae of the kyphoplasty group; this group exhibited better eventual stability than the vertebroplasty group. The authors believe that the reduction with additional balloon at the fractured site is better than the indirect reduction through distraction force provided by posterior instrumentation. Additional balloon kyphoplasty is safe and effective for acute thoracolumbar burst fracture.

There are several limitations in this study. 1) This is a retrospective study and mean follow-up was 29 months. The long-term effectiveness of this technique still needs

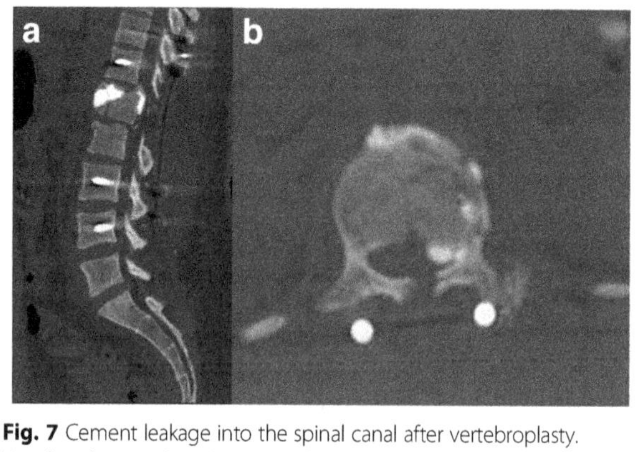

Fig. 7 Cement leakage into the spinal canal after vertebroplasty. Vertebroplasty without balloon inflation causes cement leakage through the cortical disruption as detected on postoperative computed tomography scanning (**a**, **b**)

to be evaluated. 2) The surgical indication is different in kyphoplasty group and vertebroplasty group. 3) The numbers of the patients in both groups were limited.

Conclusions

Balloon kyphoplasty and vertebroplasty with injection of calcium sulfate/phosphate cement combined with posterior fixation for acute thoracolumbar burst fractures both provided immediate stability and reduction of post-traumatic segmental kyphosis. In addition, the use of additional balloon kyphoplasty led to better reduction of fractured vertebrae, less cement leakage, and better stability than in patients who only received vertebroplasty.

Acknowledgements
We thank the Department of Orthopaedic Surgery for their contribution to the study.

Funding
This work was supported by Chang Gung Memorial Hospital (grant No. CMRPG3F2051).

Authors' contributions
P-JT, K-FF and M-KH participated in the study design, in collecting the data, the statistically analyses and drafting of the manuscript. L-HC, C-CN, P-LL, W-JC, T-TT and C-WY participated in the study design. M-KH advised and assisted drafting of the manuscript. All authors read and approved the final manuscript.

Consent for publication
Not applicable.

Competing interests
TT-T is a member of the Editorial Board of BMC Musculoskeletal Disorders. The remaining authors have no competing interests.

Author details
[1]Department of Orthopedic Surgery, Chang Gung Memorial Hospital and Chang Gung University, Taoyuan, Taiwan. [2]Bone and Joint Research Center, Chang Gung Memorial Hospital, Linkou, Taiwan. [3]5, Fu-Hsin Street, Kweishan Shiang, Taoyuan ,333, Linkou, Taiwan.

Reference

1. Benson DR, Burkus JK, Montesano PX, Sutherland TB, McLain RF. Unstable thoracolumbar and lumbar burst fractures treated with the AO fixateur interne. J Spinal Disord. 1992;5:335–43.
2. Patel AA, Dailey A, Brodke DS, Daubs M, Harrop J, Whang PG, Vaccaro AR. Spine trauma study G: Thoracolumbar spine trauma classification: the Thoracolumbar injury classification and severity score system and case examples. J Neurosurg Spine. 2009;10:201–6.
3. Hitchon PW, Abode-Iyamah K, Dahdaleh NS, Shaffrey C, Noeller J, He W, Moritani T. Nonoperative Management in Neurologically Intact Thoracolumbar Burst Fractures: clinical and radiographic outcomes. Spine (Phila Pa 1976). 2016;41:483–9.
4. Mermelstein LE, McLain RF, Yerby SA. Reinforcement of thoracolumbar burst fractures with calcium phosphate cement. A biomechanical study. Spine (Phila Pa 1976). 1998;23:664–70.
5. Kramer DL, Rodgers WB, Mansfield FL. Transpedicular instrumentation and short-segment fusion of thoracolumbar fractures: a prospective study using a single instrumentation system. J Orthop Trauma. 1995;9:499–506.
6. Wu XT, Jiang XJ, Zhang SD, Yang HL. Biomechanical evaluation of vertebroplasty using calcium sulfate cement for thoracolumbar burst fractures. Chin J Traumatol. 2007;10:327–33.
7. Yang H, Zou J. Filling materials used in kyphoplasty and vertebroplasty for vertebral compression fracture: a literature review. Artif Cells Blood Substit Immobil Biotechnol. 2011;39:87–91.
8. Zaryanov AV, Park DK, Khalil JG, Baker KC, Fischgrund JS. Cement augmentation in vertebral burst fractures. Neurosurg Focus. 2014;37:E5.
9. Arrington ED, Smith WJ, Chambers HG, Bucknell AL, Davino NA. Complications of iliac crest bone graft harvesting. Clin Orthop Relat Res. 1996;329:300–9.
10. Liao JC, Fan KF, Keorochana G, Chen WJ, Chen LH. Transpedicular grafting after short-segment pedicle instrumentation for thoracolumbar burst fracture: calcium sulfate cement versus autogenous iliac bone graft. Spine (Phila Pa 1976). 2010;35:1482–8.
11. Deramond H, Wright NT, Belkoff SM. Temperature elevation caused by bone cement polymerization during vertebroplasty. Bone. 1999;25:17–21.
12. Togawa D, Kovacic JJ, Bauer TW, Reinhardt MK, Brodke DS, Lieberman IH. Radiographic and histologic findings of vertebral augmentation using polymethylmethacrylate in the primate spine: percutaneous vertebroplasty versus kyphoplasty. Spine (Phila Pa 1976). 2006;31:E4–10.
13. Kasperk C, Hillmeier J, Noldge G, Grafe IA, Dafonseca K, Raupp D, Bardenheuer H, Libicher M, Liegibel UM, Sommer U, et al. Treatment of painful vertebral fractures by kyphoplasty in patients with primary osteoporosis: a prospective nonrandomized controlled study. J Bone Miner Res. 2005;20:604–12.
14. Molloy S, Sewell MD, Platinum J, Patel A, Selvadurai S, Hargunani R, Kyriakou C. Is balloon kyphoplasty safe and effective for cancer-related vertebral compression fractures with posterior vertebral body wall defects? J Surg Oncol. 2016;113:835–42.
15. Boonen S, Van Meirhaeghe J, Bastian L, Cummings SR, Ranstam J, Tillman JB, Eastell R, Talmadge K, Wardlaw D. Balloon kyphoplasty for the treatment of acute vertebral compression fractures: 2-year results from a randomized trial. J Bone Miner Res. 2011;26:1627–37.
16. Wood KB, Li W, Lebl DR, Ploumis A. Management of thoracolumbar spine fractures. Spine J. 2014;14:145–64.
17. American Spinal Injury Association/International Medical Society of Paraplegia. International standards for neurological and functional classification of spinal cord injury-revised 2000. Chicago: ASIA; 2002.
18. Korovessis P, Baikousis A, Zacharatos S, Petsinis G, Koureas G, Iliopoulos P. Combined anterior plus posterior stabilization versus posterior short-segment instrumentation and fusion for mid-lumbar (L2-L4) burst fractures. Spine (Phila Pa 1976). 2006;31:859–68.
19. Yu CW, Hsieh MK, Chen LH, Niu CC, Fu TS, Lai PL, Chen WJ, Chen WC, Lu ML. Percutaneous balloon kyphoplasty for the treatment of vertebral compression fractures. BMC Surg. 2014;14:3.
20. Kotnis NA, Parasu N, Finlay K, Jurriaans E, Ghert M. Chronology of the radiographic appearances of the calcium sulphate-calcium phosphate synthetic bone graft composite following resection of bone tumours–a preliminary study of the normal post-operative appearances. Skelet Radiol. 2011;40:563–70.
21. Christensen FB, Laursen M, Gelineck J, Eiskjaer SP, Thomsen K, Bunger CE. Interobserver and intraobserver agreement of radiograph interpretation with and without pedicle screw implants: the need for a detailed classification system in posterolateral spinal fusion. Spine (Phila Pa 1976). 2001;26:538–43.
22. Yeom JS, Kim WJ, Choy WS, Lee CK, Chang BS, Kang JW. Leakage of cement in percutaneous transpedicular vertebroplasty for painful osteoporotic compression fractures. J Bone Joint Surg Br. 2003;85:83–9.
23. McLain RF, Sparling E, Benson DR. Early failure of short-segment pedicle instrumentation for thoracolumbar fractures. A preliminary report. J Bone Joint Surg Am. 1993;75:162–7.

24. Olerud S, Karlstrom G, Sjostrom L. Transpedicular fixation of thoracolumbar vertebral fractures. Clin Orthop Relat Res. 1988;227:44–51.
25. Ebelke DK, Asher MA, Neff JR, Kraker DP. Survivorship analysis of VSP spine instrumentation in the treatment of thoracolumbar and lumbar burst fractures. Spine (Phila Pa 1976). 1991;16(Suppl 8):428–32.
26. Galibert P, Deramond H, Rosat P, Le Gars D. Preliminary note on the treatment of vertebral angioma by percutaneous acrylic vertebroplasty. Neurochirurgie. 1987;33:166–8.
27. Kroon F, Staples M, Ebeling PR, Wark JD, Osborne RH, Mitchell PJ, Wriedt CH, Buchbinder R. Two-year results of a randomized placebo-controlled trial of vertebroplasty for acute osteoporotic vertebral fractures. J Bone Miner Res. 2014;29:1346–55.
28. Coumans JV, Reinhardt MK, Lieberman IH. Kyphoplasty for vertebral compression fractures: 1-year clinical outcomes from a prospective study. J Neurosurg. 2003;99:44–50.
29. Heini PF, Orler R. Kyphoplasty for treatment of osteoporotic vertebral fractures. Eur Spine J. 2004;13:184–92.
30. Toyone T, Tanaka T, Kato D, Kaneyama R, Otsuka M. The treatment of acute thoracolumbar burst fractures with transpedicular intracorporeal hydroxyapatite grafting following indirect reduction and pedicle screw fixation: a prospective study. Spine (Phila Pa 1976). 2006;31:E208–14.
31. Shen WJ, Liu TJ, Shen YS. Nonoperative treatment versus posterior fixation for thoracolumbar junction burst fractures without neurologic deficit. Spine (Phila Pa 1976). 2001;26:1038–45.
32. Li KC, Li AF, Hsieh CH, Chen HH. Transpedicle body augmenter in painful osteoporotic compression fractures. Eur Spine J. 2007;16:589–98.
33. Li KC, Hsieh CH, Lee CY, Chen TH. Transpedicle body augmenter: a further step in treating burst fractures. Clin Orthop Relat Res. 2005;436:119–25.
34. McDonough PW, Davis R, Tribus C, Zdeblick TA. The management of acute thoracolumbar burst fractures with anterior corpectomy and Z-plate fixation. Spine (Phila Pa 1976). 2004;29:1901–9.
35. Daniaux H. Transpedicular repositioning and spongioplasty in fractures of the vertebral bodies of the lower thoracic and lumbar spine. Unfallchirurg. 1986;89:197–213.
36. Gelb H, Schumacher HR, Cuckler J, Ducheyne P, Baker DG. In vivo inflammatory response to polymethylmethacrylate particulate debris: effect of size, morphology, and surface area. J Orthop Res. 1994;12:83–92.
37. San Millan Ruiz D, Burkhardt K, Jean B, Muster M, Martin JB, Bouvier J, Fasel JH, Rufenacht DA, Kurt AM. Pathology findings with acrylic implants. Bone. 1999;25(Suppl 2):85–90.
38. Lim TH, Brebach GT, Renner SM, Kim WJ, Kim JG, Lee RE, Andersson GB, An HS. Biomechanical evaluation of an injectable calcium phosphate cement for vertebroplasty. Spine (Phila Pa 1976). 2002;27:1297–302.
39. Tomita S, Molloy S, Jasper LE, Abe M, Belkoff SM. Biomechanical comparison of kyphoplasty with different bone cements. Spine (Phila Pa 1976). 2004;29:1203–7.
40. Cho DY, Lee WY, Sheu PC. Treatment of thoracolumbar burst fractures with polymethyl methacrylate vertebroplasty and short-segment pedicle screw fixation. Neurosurgery. 2003;53:1354–60.
41. Bai B, Jazrawi LM, Kummer FJ, Spivak JM. The use of an injectable, biodegradable calcium phosphate bone substitute for the prophylactic augmentation of osteoporotic vertebrae and the management of vertebral compression fractures. Spine (Phila Pa 1976). 1999;24:1521–6.
42. Chow LC, Takagi S, Constantino PD, et al. Self-setting calcium phosphate cements. Mat Res Soc Symp Proc. 1991;179:1–24.
43. LeGeros RZ. Properties of osteoconductive biomaterials: calcium phosphates. Clin Orthop Relat Res. 2002;395:81–98.
44. Korovessis P, Repantis T, Petsinis G, Iliopoulos P, Hadjipavlou A. Direct reduction of thoracolumbar burst fractures by means of balloon kyphoplasty with calcium phosphate and stabilization with pedicle-screw instrumentation and fusion. Spine (Phila Pa 1976). 2008;33:E100–8.
45. Korovessis P, Hadjipavlou A, Repantis T. Minimal invasive short posterior instrumentation plus balloon kyphoplasty with calcium phosphate for burst and severe compression lumbar fractures. Spine (Phila Pa 1976). 2008;33:658–67.
46. Garfin SR, Yuan HA, Reiley MA. New technologies in spine: kyphoplasty and vertebroplasty for the treatment of painful osteoporotic compression fractures. Spine (Phila Pa 1976). 2001;26:1511–5.
47. Ledlie JT, Renfro MB. Kyphoplasty treatment of vertebral fractures: 2-year outcomes show sustained benefits. Spine (Phila Pa 1976). 2006;31:57–64.
48. Lieberman IH, Dudeney S, Reinhardt MK, Bell G. Initial outcome and efficacy of "kyphoplasty" in the treatment of painful osteoporotic vertebral compression fractures. Spine (Phila Pa 1976). 2001;26:1631–8.
49. Hulme PA, Krebs J, Ferguson SJ, Berlemann U. Vertebroplasty and kyphoplasty: a systematic review of 69 clinical studies. Spine (Phila Pa 1976). 2006;31:1983–2001.
50. Eck JC, Nachtigall D, Humphreys SC, Hodges SD. Comparison of vertebroplasty and balloon kyphoplasty for treatment of vertebral compression fractures: a meta-analysis of the literature. Spine J. 2008;8:488–97.

26

A new anatomic locking plate for the treatment of posterolateral tibial plateau fractures

Zhen Jian[1†], Rongguang Ao[1†], Jianhua Zhou[1], Xinhua Jiang[1], Dianying Zhang[2*] and Baoqing Yu[1*]

Abstract

Background: Posterolateral tibial plateau fractures have become more common, and their treatment is of great importance to knee function. Additionally, there is no available literature detailing specialized anatomic locking plate for tibial plateau fractures. Therefore, the aim of the study was to evaluate the safety and clinical efficacy of an innovative anatomic locking plate for treatment of posterolateral tibial plateau fractures.

Methods: Between March 2014 and January 2016, 12 patients with posterolateral tibial plateau fracture underwent surgery with the anatomic locking plate for the posterolateral tibial plateau via the posterolateral approach. Relevant operational data for clinical evaluation were collected.

Results: The mean follow-up time was 26 months, and the mean age was 35 years for 12 patients. The mean interval between the time of injury and the surgery was 6.1 days. Radiological fracture union was evident in all patients at 12 weeks. During surgery, the blood loss ranged from 100 to 300 mL, and the duration ranged from 55 to 90 min. The Tegner–Lysholm functional score ranged from 85 to 97 at the final follow-up. Moreover, the final Rasmussen functional score ranged from 25 to 29, and Rasmussen anatomical score ranged from 13 to 18.

Conclusions: The newly designed anatomic locking plate for the posterolateral tibial plateau provided adequate fixation along the posterolateral tibial plateau. It proved to be safe and effective in a small-sample-size population (12 patients) during a 12- to 34-month follow-up.

Keywords: Posterolateral tibial plateau fractures, Anatomic locking plate, Posterolateral approach

Background

Tibial plateau fractures are commonly encountered in clinical practice, whereas posterolateral tibial plateau fractures have rarely been reported in the past. However, posterolateral tibial plateau fractures have been reported in up to 7% of all tibial plateau fractures with increased high-energy trauma and use of computed tomography (CT) [1–3].

Good reduction and firm fixation are vital for treatment of posterolateral tibial plateau fractures. Many authors recommend surgical treatment to restore joint congruity and mechanical stability and further guarantee the best prognosis [4, 5]. However, the operative treatment of posterolateral tibial plateau fractures remains a challenge due to the fibular head and ligamentous structures that impede adequate exposure of the posterolateral joint surface. Although many approaches have been reported [4, 6–9] to achieve appropriate exposure, there is no general consensus.

Recent studies [7–9] on the treatment of posterolateral tibial plateau fractures have focused on surgical approaches. There is no literature to our knowledge about a specialized anatomic locking plate for posterolateral tibial plateau fractures. Surgeons usually have to choose buttress plate systems such as L-shaped plates and T-plates used in the fixation of distal radius. However, due to the irregular bony structure of the region, the plates often require contouring during surgery to fit the posterolateral tibial plateau, which may potentially lead to longer operative duration, higher

* Correspondence: zdy8016@163.com; doctorybq@163.com
†Zhen Jian and Rongguang Ao contributed equally to this work.
[2]Department of Orthopedics, Peking University People's Hospital, Beijing 100044, China
[1]Department of Orthopaedics, Shanghai Pudong Hospital, Shanghai Fudan Univercity Pudong Medical Center, Shanghai 201399, China

blood loss, and decreased mechanical strength of the plate. Additionally, the proximal locking screws in these plates may not achieve the "raft" effect to support the articular surface of the posterolateral tibial plateau fracture. Therefore, details of an innovative anatomic locking plate for the posterolateral tibial plateau (Fig. 1) and the clinical outcomes were reported to evaluate the safety and clinical efficacy of this innovative plate.

Methods

General data

This retrospective study was conducted after obtaining the approval of the institutional review board. Between March 2014 and January 2016, 12 patients with a posterolateral tibial plateau fracture (ages 18–45 years) underwent surgery with the anatomic locking plate for the posterolateral tibial plateau. Patients with osteofascial compartment syndrome, open fracture, multiple trauma, pathologic fractures, autoimmune diseases, blood disorder, and surgical contraindications were excluded. All patients received anteroposterior and lateral radiographs and three-dimensional computed tomography reconstruction images of the tibial plateau before surgery. Additionally, all patients were followed up either by clinic review or by telephone as required.

According to the CT reconstruction images, the main fragments were located in the posterior half of the lateral condyle and/or a fracture line impacted the posterior aspect of the lateral plateau. According to three-column classification [10], all cases were fractures of the posterolateral column. Preoperative management included distal bony traction and splint. After the soft tissue condition was stable, all the fractures were exposed and reduced via the posterolateral approach by the same surgeon (Yu).

Plate details

The anatomic locking plate for the posterolateral tibial plateau (Fig. 2) was designed according to the structure of the posterolateral tibial plateau in a Chinese population. It was oblique "T" shaped to fit the posterolateral structure of the tibial plateau with a low profile and beveled edges. The angle between the plate head and the waist was 136°. It had five 30° universal locking holes to ensure precise screw insertion in the head, which fixed the plate with the posterolateral side of the tibial plateau. Especially three proximal row screws paralleled with the plateau could buttress powerfully as a "raft effect." Tiny holes in the top of the plate head were used in cases of a temporary fixation or comminuted fragment fixation by K-wire insertion and capsule sutures. When plate data was transefer into 3D computer-aided design (CAD) model, several patients' knee CT data were also integrated with the CAD model, implant placement was simulated in silico to check for accuracy. When we obtained the plate patent, the plate was made by a qualified custom-made plate manufacture (WASTON Medical Appliance Co, Ltd., China). All structure was made of titanium. Finally, the plates obtained were completely consistent with our design in terms of their shape and distribution and the orientation of screws.

Surgical technique and rehabilitation

All operations were performed using spinal anesthesia or general anesthesia with the patients in the prone position, and the lower limb tourniquet was inflated.

A posterolateral incision was placed over the biceps femoris muscle. Attention must be paid to identify and dissect the peroneal nerve posterior of the biceps femoris muscle. Then gently retracted laterally for the nerve

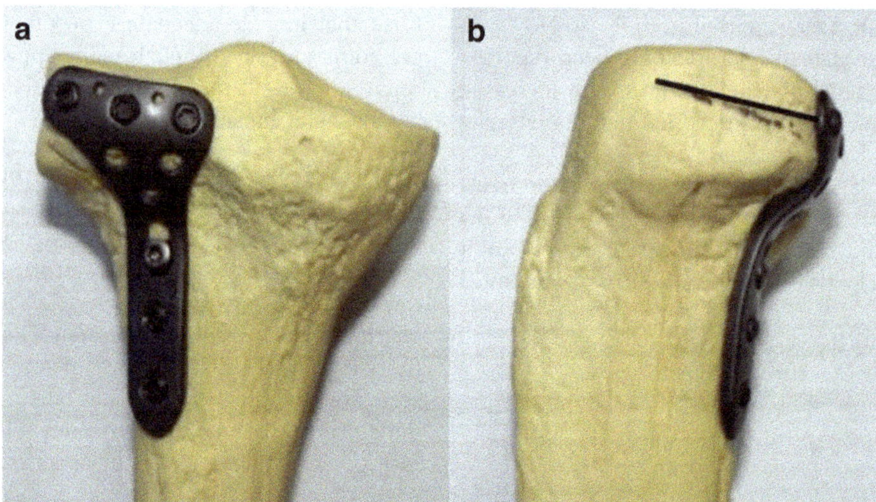

Fig. 1 The newly designed posterolateral anatomic locking plate which is specially used in posterolateral tibial plateau fracture. **a**, posterior view of the tibial plateau. **b**, lateral view of tibial plateau

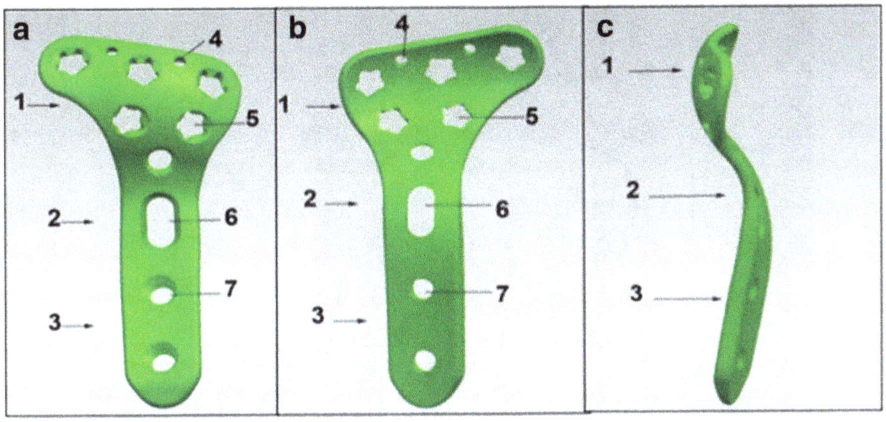

Fig. 2 Schematic figureof The newly designed posterolateral anatomic locking plate. **a**, posterior view; **b**, anterior view; **c**, lateral view(1.head, 2.waist, 3.body, 4.K-wires hole, 5.locking screw hole, 6.sliding compression hole, 7.locking screw hole)

protection during the operation. Medially retracted the lateral head of the gastrocnemius with the origin of the soleus elevated from the proximal section of tibia. The popliteus tendon could be retracted proximally to allow for fracture site visualization. The soleus was then detached from dorsal fibula with carefulness. Thereafter, the exposed capsule was incised to allow for the visualization of the entire lateral aspects of tibial plateau, including the posterolateral corner.

Temporary fix the fracture fragments with multiple K-wires. After elevation, the defect was filled with artificial bone graft. Then, screw formation of the posterolateral anatomic locking plate was attempted. Three "raft" proximal row locking screws were inserted parallel with the plateau joint surface. The reduction quality and location of internal fixation were further identified by fluoroscopic guidance. The physical examination of the knee stability was routinely conducted to exclude ligament injury.

Mobilization of the knee joint was encouraged immediately after surgery, and discharge was agreed when 90° was achieved, usually 5–10 days postoperatively. The knee motion range, as well as muscle strengthening was increased after surgical incision healing. Patients were initially allowed no weight bearing for 12 weeks to avoid early loss of reduction. Depending on radiographic signs of healing, partial weight bearing was advised and advanced to full weight bearing as soon as the patients can tolerate.

Clinical evaluation was performed using the Tegner–Lysholm functional score, Rasmussen functional score [4], and Rasmussen anatomical score [4]. The Rasmussen functional score was used to evaluate knee function primarily with special attention paid to the single plane stability and rotation stability. The Rasmussen functional score is a specific outcome index for postoperative evaluation of tibial plateau fractures. It consists of five categories, including pain (6 points), walking capacity (6 points), extension (6 points), total range of motion (6 points), and stability (6 points). The total score is the sum of these five items, and the higher scores indicate the greater function. A score of 30 points is defined as normal, 27–30 as excellent, 20–26 as good, 10–19 as fair, and 6–10 as poor. The Rasmussen anatomical score consists of three categories, including depression (6 points), condylar widening (6 points), and angulation (6 points). A score of 18 points is defined as excellent, 12–17 as good, 6–11 as fair, and 0–5 as poor. Medical image data of one patient is shown in Fig. 3.

Results

The average follow-up was 26 months (12–34 months). The average age of patients was 35 year-old (18–45 years). The general conditions of patients are listed in Table 1. The mean time from injury to surgery was 6.1 days (0–12 days). At 12 weeks, evidence of radiological fracture union was obtained in all patients (10–14 weeks).

During surgery, time and blood loss were recorded. No case of ligament reparation was found in the study because all patients with knee instability were excluded. Nine patients obtained anatomic articular surface reduction as well as three obtained good reduction.

Tegner-Lysholm function score, Rasmussen functional score, and Rasmussen anatomic score of final follow-up were recorded (Table 2). Radiograph showed intra-articular reduction loss of 2 mm step-off in one case, which might be caused by weight-bearing too early. No knee instability or pain was found in all cases. The average knee motion arc was 137° (122°–153°).

Incidence of CPN (Common Peroneal Nerve) injury was noted in none case. Lateral knee instability was seen in none case. No flexion contractures or extensor lag was seen. No deep vein thrombosis or graft site morbidity was seen at the follow-up. In addition, no case of incurred nonunion or internal fixation failure was reported. However,

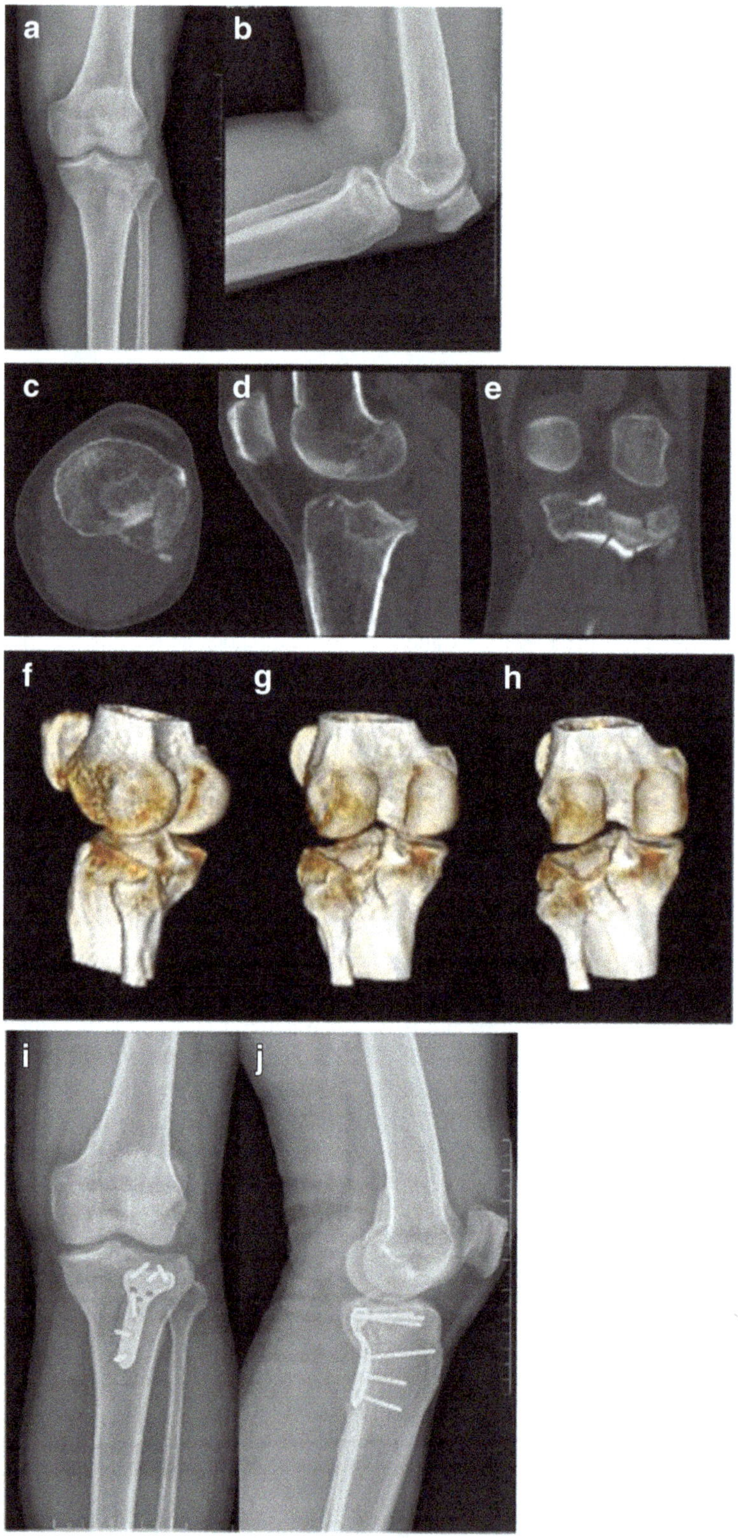

Fig. 3 One male patient with posterolateral tibial plateau fracture, 43y, caused by car-accident. **a**, **b** were preoperational anteroposterior and lateral radiographs of one posteroleteral tibial plateau fracture. **c**-**h** showed more fracture details by 3-D reconstruction of CT scan. **i**, **j** were anteroposterior and lateral radiographs of the patient acquired after open reduction and internal fixation with the plate

Table 1 General conditions

Case Number	Age(y)	Sex	Cause	Follow-up(mo)
1	18	Male	Veh.Acc.	12
2	43	Male	Veh.Acc.	18
3	42	Female	Fall	32
4	38	Male	Fall	22
5	45	Male	Fall	20
6	41	Female	Veh.Acc	24
7	39	Male	Fall	34
8	35	Male	Fall	31
9	33	Male	Veh.Acc	28
10	36	Female	Fall	33
11	33	Male	Fall	27
12	31	Female	Struck	31

one patient had superficial wound infection that recovered after treatment with antibiotics and local dressing changes.

Discussion

Patients with untreated posterolateral tibial plateau fracture may suffer from chronic pain, knee instability, and loss of function, especially when climbing the stairs, which even leads to malunion that needs surgery or re-surgery. Thus, many surgeons have agreed that open reduction and internal fixation should be preferred over non-operative treatment [1, 2, 4, 5]. Multiple approaches have been described given the complexity of the posterolateral tibial plateau anatomy [2].

Lobenhoffer et al. [9] introduced a posterolateral approach with fibular osteotomy with better visualization. An anterolateral approach with partial or full fibula head removed was developed by Yu [4], which do great benefit for reduction and fixation in the treatment of posterolateral tibial plateau fractures. However, fibular osteotomies may injury the common peroneal nerve and decrease the stability of the lateral knee joint [11]. Frosch et al. [8] described a posterolateral approach with a lateral arthrotomy for visualizing the joint surface. Posterolateral approach was modified by Tao [7] with an L-shaped incision. Fibular osteotomy was not required in this approach and it protected the soft tissue well, showing encouraging clinical outcomes. The posterolateral approach without fibular osteotomy was chosen in the present study.

Although surgical approaches have been well discussed in previous studies [4, 7–9], operative fixation in treatment of posterolateral tibial plateau fractures has rarely been reported. No specialized plate is used for the treatment due to the irregular shape of the posterolateral tibial plateau. The most widely used system is the distal radius locking plate [1]. The plate usually has to be contoured during surgery to achieve satisfying fitness, which may damage the locking hole and affect the angle stability. Moreover, the plate cannot achieve the "raft" effect due the fact that the proximal locking screws are parallel to the joint surface. This may lead to a higher risk of reduction failure, further comprising outcomes.

Cho et al. [3] reported a novel technique of 2.7-mm rim plating in tibial plateau fractures to address these problems. Rim plates function as positional plates (named "Hugging plates") rather than buttress plates. The rim plate maintains the posterolateral tibial fracture reduction with the collinear clamp used for a rigid maneuver reduction throughout the fixation procedure. This rim plating technique can be easily applied to isolated posterolateral fracture fragments. However, it is difficult to use in patients with posterolateral tibial comminution and posterolateral corner depression. Moreover,both anterior and posterior stripping to obtain an adequate operative field, together with less antiskid ability, limits its use.

The newly designed anatomic locking plate for the posterolateral tibial plateau, which is oblique "T" shaped, fits the posterolateral structure of the tibial plateau well

Table 2 Clinical findings

Case Number	Blood loss (ml)	Operation duration (min)	Tegner–Lysholmscore	Rasmussen functional score	Rasmussen anatomical score
1	250	70	97	29	18
2	100	55	93	28	16
3	160	55	87	27	14
4	200	60	89	28	15
5	230	70	85	25	13
6	200	65	95	26	16
7	210	80	90	26	15
8	240	80	91	28	16
9	150	75	93	27	16
10	300	90	88	28	15
11	180	75	88	27	16
12	220	70	89	26	15

enough that it reduces plate contouring during surgery, shortens operative duration, decreases blood loss, and potentially decreases plate failure. In our study, our new anatomic locking plate fit anatomically, requiring no additional manipulation. The beveled edges and low profile of the plate can reduce the risk of prominence, which always leads to secondary implant remove surgery. Further, the proximal row locking screws can achieve the "raft" effect, which provides firm strength holding the articular surface. The main limitation distally is the posterior tibial neurovascular bundle. It is difficult to safely achieve exposure beyond approximately 8–10 cm distal to the lateral joint line owing to vessel trifurcation that transverse the interosseous membrane and muscle mass medial to the fibula. However, the length of plate is appropriate to reach the distal border, ...without damaging the neuromuscular bundle. Thus, distal tibial exposure is not necessarily required. According to the Rasmussen functional/anatomical score, all patients achieved "good" results. The plate was proven to be safe and effective in a small-sample-size population (12 patients) during a 12- to 34-month follow-up.

The limitations of the study were the relatively small sample size; hence, large-sample studies need to be conducted to prove the efficacy of the technique. In addition, further biomechanical studies are required to evaluate buttress performance, compression forces, and comparative features against traditional buttress line plates via the posterolateral approach.

Conclusions

In conclusion, the newly designed anatomic locking plate for the posterolateral tibial plateau was proven to be safe and effective in a small-sample-size population (12 patients) during a 12- to 34-month follow-up. The plate fit the irregular posterolateral tibial plateau well, without requiring additional contouring. Therefore, this new plate may be used as a favorable internal fixation choice for treatment of posterolateral plateau fractures.

Abbreviations

CPN: Common Peroneal Nerve; CT: Computed tomography

Acknowledgments

We thank LetPub (www.letpub.com) for providing linguistic assistance during the preparation of this manuscript.

Funding

Research Grant for the Key Disciplines Group Construction Project of Pudong Health Bureau of Shanghai (Grant No. PWZxq2017-11), the Program for Medical Key Department of Shanghai (Grant No. ZK 2015B17), Program for Outstanding Leader of Shanghai (Grant No. 046), Health Science and Technology of Pudong Municipal Commission of Health and Family Planning of Shanghai (Grant No. PW2015A-15).

Authors' contributions

BY and DZ designed the plate and provided the data of patients. ZJ, RA, JZ and XJ analyzed the data. ZJ and RA wrote the paper. All authors read and approved the final manuscript.

Consent for publication

Written consent to publish the content of this report along with the accompanying images was obtained from all patients.

Competing interests

The authors declare that they have no competing interests.

References

1. Bhattacharyya T, McCarty LP 3rd, Harris MB, Morrison SM, Wixted JJ, Vrahas MS, et al. The posterior shearing tibial plateau fracture: treatment and results via a posterior approach. J Orthop Trauma. 2005;19:305–10.
2. Wang Y, Luo C, Hu C, Sun H, Zhan Y. An innovative intra-articular osteotomy in the treatment of posterolateral Tibial plateau fracture Malunion. The journal of knee surgery. 2016;
3. Cho JW, Samal P, Jeon YS, Oh CW, Oh JK. Rim plating of posterolateral fracture fragments (PLFs) through a modified anterolateral approach in Tibial plateau fractures. J Orthop Trauma. 2016;30:e362–e68.
4. Yu B, Han K, Zhan C, Zhang C, Ma H, Su J. Fibular head osteotomy: a new approach for the treatment of lateral or posterolateral tibial plateau fractures. Knee. 2010;17:313–8.
5. Waldrop JI, Macey TI, Trettin JC, Bourgeois WR, Hughston JC. Fractures of the posterolateral tibial plateau. Am J Sports Med. 1988;16:492–8.
6. Hu SJ, Chang SM, Zhang YQ, Ma Z, Du SC, Zhang K. The anterolateral supra-fibular-head approach for plating posterolateral tibial plateau fractures: a novel surgical technique. Injury. 2016;47:502–7.
7. Tao J, Hang DH, Wang QG, Gao W, Zhu LB, Wu XF, et al. The posterolateral shearing tibial plateau fracture: treatment and results via a modified posterolateral approach. Knee. 2008;15:473–9.
8. Frosch KH, Balcarek P, Walde T, Sturmer KM. A new posterolateral approach without fibula osteotomy for the treatment of tibial plateau fractures. J Orthop Trauma. 2010;24:515–20.
9. Lobenhoffer P, Gerich T, Bertram T, Lattermann C, Pohlemann T, Tscheme H. Particular posteromedial and posterolateral approaches for the treatment of tibial head fractures. Unfallchirurg. 1997;100:957–67.
10. Luo CF, Sun H, Zhang B, Zeng BF. Three-column fixation for complex tibial plateau fractures. J Orthop Trauma. 2010;24:683–92.
11. Pires RE, Giordano V, Wajnsztejn A, Oliveira Santana EJ, Pesantez R, Lee MA, et al. Complications and outcomes of the transfibular approach for posterolateral fractures of the tibial plateau. Injury. 2016;47:2320–5.

27

Evaluation of three patient reported outcome measures following operative fixation of closed ankle fractures

Andrew M. Garratt[1*], Markus G. Naumann[2], Ulf Sigurdsen[3], Stein Erik Utvåg[3,4] and Knut Stavem[4,5,6]

Abstract

Background: Several patient reported outcome measures (PROMs) are available for assessing the outcomes of ankle fracture but few have been compared for recommended measurement properties. This study compares the measurement properties of the Lower Extremity Function Scale (LEFS), Olerud Molander Ankle Score (OMAS) and Self-Reported Foot and Ankle Score (SEFAS) following ankle surgery.

Methods: The retrospective cohort study included 959 patients aged 18 years and over who underwent surgical treatment (ORIF) for unstable and closed ankle fractures in SE Norway. The PROMs were included in a postal questionnaire sent to patients' homes in 2015, three years after surgery. Missing data, structural validity, internal consistency, test-retest reliability and validity were assessed.

Results: Confirmatory factor analysis results showed model fit for the SEFAS and a bi-dimensional LEFS with scales of easy and difficult items. The OMAS performed less satisfactorily. Cronbach's alpha and test-retest correlations ranged from 0.82 to 0.96 and 0.91 to 0.93 respectively. The smallest detectable differences for group and individual comparisons were 14.1 to 20.6 and 0.93 to 1.55; SEFAS performed best. As hypothesised, instrument scores were highly correlated and with those for the EQ-5D and SF-36 physical functioning. Mean imputation where half or more items are completed increased usable scores by 1.4–15.7% without affecting measurement properties.

Conclusions: The three instruments largely performed satisfactorily in relation to important measurement properties but the LEFS had evidence for two dimensions relating to easier and more difficult aspects of function. Mean imputation where half or more items are completed increased the number of usable responses for all three instruments. The three instruments represent different approaches to measuring outcomes and their content should be considered carefully when choosing between them. The SEFAS is designed for a range of foot disorders including ankle fractures and has the best measurement properties in this population.

Keywords: Ankle, Patient reported outcome measures, PROMs, PROs, Validity, Reliability

Background

Ankle fracture constitutes approximately 9% of all fractures, have an incidence of 122 per 100,000 people [1] and incidence requiring hospitalisation of 83 per 100,000 people [2]. Following a systematic review it was concluded that there was insufficient evidence as to whether conservative management or surgery gives the best long-term outcomes in adult patients [1]. Moreover, the evidence derived from a systematic review of competing surgical technologies led to the conclusion that further evaluation, including greater consideration of long-term outcomes, was necessary [3].

Ankle fractures reduce quality of life and particularly in older people, may cause loss of independence. It is important that studies evaluating outcomes in these patients include valid and reliable patient reported outcome measures (PROMs) that reflect important concerns of patients [4]. There are a large number of ankle-specific PROMs [5] but few have been developed with the input of fracture patients or sufficiently evaluated

* Correspondence: andrew.garratt@fhi.no
[1]Division for Health Services, Norwegian Institute of Public Health, Oslo, Norway

for measurement properties [4]. Clinicians and researchers wishing to select an ankle specific PROM are faced with a confusing array of instruments with little information on measurement properties in ankle fracture patients. When a choice of instrument exists, the concurrent evaluation of their measurement properties in the patients and health care setting of interest is highly informative [6]. Systematic reviews of measurement properties are also informative, however, the two published reviews focus on ankle problems more generally [5] or ligament injuries [7].

The Lower Extremity Functional Scale (LEFS) [8], Olerud and Molander Ankle Score (OMAS) [9] and Self-Reported Foot and Ankle Score (SEFAS) [10] have been widely applied but have undergone limited testing for measurement properties in patients with ankle fractures. These three instruments represent different approaches to measuring outcomes in patients with ankle fractures; the LEFS focuses on lower limb, the OMAS is ankle fracture specific, and the SEFAS is foot and ankle specific. None of them have been tested for structural validity, which gives evidence supporting their scoring as unidimensional scales. This study compares important measurement properties of these instruments, including reliability and validity [11].

Methods

Study population

The retrospective cohort study included 959 patients who underwent surgical treatment (ORIF) for unstable and closed ankle fractures at two hospitals in SE Norway [12]. Patients were 18 years of age and over and treated in a three year period from January 1, 2009. They received a postal questionnaire that included LEFS, OMAS and SEFAS in January 2015; 299 respondents received a test-retest questionnaire at six weeks. Non-respondents received a reminder at four weeks.

Patient-reported outcome measures

Norwegian translation of the three instruments followed international guidelines [11] including two independent forwards and one independent backwards translations with a meeting to agree on the final Norwegian versions.

The LEFS comprises 20 items relating to physical function and daily activities with a five-point scale from 'extreme difficulty or unable to perform' to 'no difficulty' [8]. Items are summed to give a score from 0 to 80 where 80 is the best possible score. The mean of the completed items is used when up to four items are missing [8, 13] and normative data is available to aid the interpretation of LEFS scores [14]. Two studies have assessed the measurement properties of LEFS in patients with ankle fracture and there is evidence for reliability, validity and responsiveness in Australian patients [15] and in Finnish patients undergoing surgery due to musculoskeletal pathology of the foot and ankle [16].

The OMAS comprises nine items relating to symptoms, physical function and daily activities [9]. The response scales vary from binary to five-points with clinical scoring that reflects the level of disability for individual items. Item responses are summed to give a score from 0 to 100 with higher scores representing the best possible. The instrument has evidence for test-retest reliability and construct validity in patients with ankle fracture in Sweden [17] and Turkey [18].

The SEFAS comprises twelve items relating to pain, limping, swelling, use of orthotics and walking. The five-point scales reflect item content and sum to give a score from 12 to 60 where the former represents normal function [10, 19]. The mean of the completed items is used when one item is missing. The instrument has not been evaluated solely in patients with ankle fracture but has evidence reliability, validity and responsiveness in Swedish patients with foot and ankle disorders undergoing surgery [10, 19]. For purposes of comparison, scores for the LEFS and SEFAS are also presented on a 0 to 100 scale where higher scores represent the best possible.

Two generic instruments were also included in the questionnaire. The EQ-5D-3L includes five items with a three-point response scale which are scored to give a single index [20]. The SF-36 physical function scale comprises ten items with a three-point scale which sum to a 0 to 100 scale where 100 is the best possible health [21].

Statistical analysis

The measurement properties tested and related terminology follow the COSMIN checklist [11]. Levels of missing data were assessed at the item and scale level with the latter also including imputation for missing data where half or more item responses were present. For comparison, all items were recoded from 0 to 4 where 4 is the best possible health.

Confirmatory factor analysis (CFA) with weighted least squares estimation was used to assess structural validity. Model fit was assessed with the comparative fit index (CFI), Tucker-Lewis Index (TLI) and root mean square error of approximation (RMSEA) [22–24]. The CFI and TLI should be greater than 0.90 and RMSEA between 0. 06 and 0.08 for acceptable fit [24, 25]. Internal consistency was assessed using item-total correlation which should exceed 0.4 and Cronbach's alpha, which should exceed 0.7 and 0.9 for use in groups and individual patients, respectively [26]. The intraclass correlation coefficient was used for estimating reliability within a two-way mixed effects model with absolute agreement. Weighted kappa was used for assessing individual item reliability

[27]. The standard error of measurement (SEM) and smallest detectable change (SDC) were calculated. The former is the square root of the total error variance. For individuals the SDC is 1.96 × √2 × SEM and for groups, the SDC for individuals is divided by √n [26].

Hypothesis testing was used to assess the validity of the three ankle instrument scores through comparisons of those for the EQ-5D and SF-36 physical functioning and clinical variables. These instruments were included in previous tests of validity for the LEFS [13] and SEFAS [10] and continue to be the most widely evaluated and applied PROMs [6]. It was hypothesised that scores for the three instruments would be highly correlated over 0. 7. High levels of correlation were expected with SF-36 physical functioning and particularly for the LEFS, given the overlap in content. The three instruments include items that overlap with two or more EQ-5D items and hence high levels of correlation were expected for EQ-5D scores and the EQ-5D mobility item. Moderate levels of correlation in the range 0.5 to 0.7 were expected for the EQ-5D usual activities and pain items. Lower levels of correlation in the range 0.3 to 0.5 were expected for the EQ-5D self-care and anxiety/depression items. Lower levels of correlation under 0.3 were hypothesised for the clinical variables including ASA classification, BMI, duration of operation and fracture classification.

LISREL was used for the CFA and PASW Statistics 18. 0 was used for the remainder of the statistical analysis.

Results

Study population

The questionnaire was returned by 567 (59.1%) patients. Table 1 shows the characteristics of respondents. There were 182 (60.9%) respondents to the test-retest questionnaire.

Statistical analysis

Levels of missing data ranged from 1.2 to 6.2% across the three instruments (Table 2). Levels of missing data were highest for items assessing higher levels of function including ‘hopping’ and ‘running’ for LEFS and ‘jumping’ for OMAS. For the LEFS, the ‘getting in and out of bath’ had the highest level of missing data. Use of mean imputation for missing data increased the number of useable scores by 1.4, 6.9 and 15.7% for the LEFS, SEFAS, and OMAS respectively (Table 2).

Item mean scores were mostly skewed towards the best possible scores across instruments (Table 2). For the LEFS, the lowest scores denoting poorer health were for ‘hopping’ and the highest scores were for ‘walking between rooms’. For the OMAS, the lowest scores were for ‘stiffness’ and the highest scores were for ‘assistive devices’. For the SEFAS the highest scores were for ‘getting up from a chair’ and the lowest scores were for ‘usual pain level’.

Table 1 Characteristics of respondents completing the first questionnaire ($n = 567$)

		%
Age years, mean (range)	57.5 (22.2–91.2)	
Female	322	56.8
Marital status[a]		
Divorced/separated	77	13.6
Cohabitant/married	379	66.8
Single	47	8.3
Widowed	46	8.1
Education		
Under 10 yrs	157	27.7
10–12 yrs	206	36.3
University	181	31.9
Body mass index (kg/m^2), median range	27.4 (14.4–61.0)	
Current smoker	136	25.2
Diabetes	34	6.0
Fracture classification, Weber		
A	15	2.6
B	383	67.5
C	156	27.5
Fracture, clinical features		
Uni-malleolar	294	52.5
Bimalleolar	128	22.9
Trimalleolar	138	24.6
Physical status (ASA classification)		
Completely healthy fit	197	34.7
Mild systemic disease	340	60.0
Severe systemic disease, not incapacitating	30	5.3
Postoperative length of stay in days, median (range)		
Surgery duration in minutes, median (range)	76.0 (7–352)	
Waiting time for surgery in days, median (range)	5.0 (0–68)	

[a]Percentages do not sum to 100 due to missing data

Model fit for the unidimensional SEFAS was good according to all criteria (Table 3). The LEFS and OMAS had a RMSEA that was over the criterion of 0.08. There was support for a bi-dimensional LEFS with scales relating to easy and difficult items. Item-total correlations were over 0.4 for all items with the exceptions of ‘assistive devices’ and ‘use of special innersoles/shoes’ for the OMAS and SEFAS respectively (Table 1). Cronbach’s alpha ranged from 0.82 to 0.96 for the OMAS and LEFS respectively.

Table 4 shows that there were small but insignificant ($p < 0.05$) score improvements across instruments at retest. Weighted kappa for the individual items indicated

Table 2 Descriptive statistics, internal consistency ($n = 567$) and reliability ($n = 182$) where all items are coded[a] 0 to 4 for comparison

Instrument/item	% miss	Mean (SD)	Frequencies %					Cronbach's alpha (scale)/item scale correlation	Test-retest ICC (scores), weighted kappa (items)
			0	1	2	3	4		
Lower Extremity Functional Scale LEFS[b]	4.2	67.20 (15.09)						0.96	0.91
LEFS adjusted[c]	2.8	83.89 (19.01)						–	0.91
1 Usual work, housework, school	2.6	3.51 (0.89)	1.8	2.5	8.2	17.5	70.0	0.81	0.77
2 Hobbies, recreational, sports	4.9	3.22 (1.02)	2.8	5.4	10.2	29.8	51.8	0.78	0.76
3 Getting in and out of bath	5.8	3.54 (0.97)	3.4	3.2	5.1	12.4	75.9	0.72	0.76
4 Walking between rooms	2.8	3.91 (0.40)	0.2	0.5	0.9	5.3	93.1	0.56	0.70
5 Putting on socks or shoes	3.0	3.65 (0.72)	0.9	1.5	4.9	17.3	75.4	0.70	0.71
6 Squatting	3.0	3.03 (1.30)	7.8	9.1	8.0	21.7	53.3	0.73	0.74
7 Lifting things up from floor	2.1	3.82 (0.57)	0.9	0.5	2.2	8.0	88.4	0.61	0.79
8 Light activities in the home	2.5	3.82 (0.54)	0.2	0.9	3.1	8.5	87.3	0.69	0.78
9 Heavy activities in the home	2.5	3.27 (1.05)	2.7	6.5	9.4	23.2	58.1	0.85	0.85
10 Getting in/out of car	2.5	3.72 (0.64)	0.2	1.6	4.4	14.2	79.7	0.67	0.68
11 Walking 2 blocks	3.0	3.69 (0.82)	2.4	1.5	4.4	8.2	83.6	0.74	0.80
12 Walking a mile	3.4	3.42 (1.07)	4.2	3.8	7.9	13.7	70.3	0.82	0.84
13 Going up or down ten stairs	3.2	3.65 (0.78)	1.1	2.4	4.9	13.9	77.7	0.75	0.73
14 Standing 1 h	2.8	3.11 (1.21)	6.0	7.8	8.6	24.0	53.6	0.84	0.85
15 Sitting 1 h	3.4	3.77 (0.65)	0.5	1.8	3.1	9.5	84.8	0.51	0.57
16 Running on even ground	5.1	2.74 (1.46)	13.6	10.3	9.9	20.7	45.5	0.85	0.87
17 Running on uneven ground	4.4	2.46 (1.47)	16.3	12.8	13.0	24.4	33.5	0.83	0.85
18 Sharp turns when running fast	4.9	2.53 (1.52)	17.1	12.5	9.3	22.0	39.1	0.84	0.82
19 Hopping	4.6	2.43 (1.53)	18.2	13.2	12.2	19.9	36.5	0.83	0.83
20 Rolling over in bed	2.7	3.82 (0.54)	0.4	1.1	1.6	10.0	86.7	0.56	0.65
Olerud-Molander Ankle Score OMAS	17.3	74.12 (24.91)						0.82	0.92
OMAS adjusted[c]	1.6	75.62 (24.07)						–	0.91
1 Pain when walking	4.9	3.01 (1.21)	7.3	4.8	13.8	27.6	46.6	0.67	0.76
2 Stiffness (2 pt. scale)	2.7	1.81 (1.99)	54.7				45.3	0.55	0.77
3 Swelling (3 pt. scale)	3.5	2.83 (1.53)	17.1		24.2		58.7	0.51	0.80
4 Use of stairs (2 pt. scale)	1.2	3.25 (1.03)	1.4		35.8		63.8	0.73	0.81
5 Running (2 pt. scale)	2.5	2.66 (1.89)	33.6				66.4	0.66	0.81
6 Jumping (2 pt. scale)	6.2	2.60 (1.91)	34.9				65.1	0.65	0.80
7 Squatting (2 pt. scale)	4.6	2.68 (1.88)	33.0				67.0	0.61	0.68
8 Assistive devices (3 pt. scale)	3.2	3.72 (0.91)	4.4		5.3		90.3	0.37	0.90
			0	*1.33*		*2.67*	*4*		
9 Work and daily activities (4 pt. scale)	2.5	3.27 (1.14)	6.4	5.1		25.8	62.8	0.66	0.77
Self-Reported Foot & Ankle Score SEFAS	8.5	20.78 (9.16)						0.93	0.93
SEFAS adjusted[c]	1.6	81.40 (19.17)						–	0.93
1 Usual pain level	1.6	2.76 (1.51)	2.9	14.9	19.1	29.3	33.8	0.82	0.83
2 Walking time before pain too much	3.7	3.58 (0.83)	0.4	5.0	5.1	14.7	74.8	0.69	0.76
3 Work not done as carefully as usual	2.5	3.27 (0.96)	2.2	3.8	12.0	28.5	53.5	0.69	0.78
4 Use of special innersoles and shoes	1.9	3.54 (1.06)	4.7	4.2	2.7	8.8	79.6	0.35	0.69
5 Usual work, housework, hobbies	2.1	3.29 (0.99)	1.1	6.9	11.0	23.5	57.5	0.87	0.85
6 Limping	1.6	3.02 (1.23)	6.8	4.5	22.7	11.0	55.0	0.75	0.77
7 Staircase	2.3	3.55 (0.80)	0.9	2.0	8.3	18.5	70.3	0.71	0.80

Table 2 Descriptive statistics, internal consistency ($n = 567$) and reliability ($n = 182$) where all items are coded[a] 0 to 4 for comparison *(Continued)*

Instrument/item	% miss	Mean (SD)	Frequencies %					Cronbach's alpha (scale)/item scale correlation	Test-retest ICC (scores), weighted kappa (items)
			0	1	2	3	4		
8 Problem in bed	1.6	3.21 (1.10)	2.5	4.7	22.7	10.1	60.1	0.72	0.70
9 Usual free time activities	1.8	3.11 (1.09)	2.7	9.2	10.6	29.7	47.7	0.86	0.88
10 Swelling	2.1	3.00 (1.20)	7.1	6.9	9.4	32.4	44.3	0.57	0.90
11 Getting up from a chair	1.8	3.60 (0.72)	0.2	1.8	7.0	19.6	71.4	0.77	0.77
12 Sudden strong pain	1.8	3.15 (1.02)	1.3	3.4	27.7	14.2	53.2	0.68	0.77

[a]To aid comparison, all items were coded from 0 to 4 where 4 is the best possible health; OMAS values in italics represent the four scale points for item 9 converted to the 0–4 scale. LEFS and SEFAS have five-point scales for all items. OMAS scaling varies across items which gives the blank spaces for those items with four or less scale categories
[b]Instrument scoring: LEFS 0–80 where 80 is the best possible; LEFS adjusted 0–100 where 100 is the best possible; OMAS 0–100 where 100 is the best possible health; SEFAS 12–60 where 60 is the worst possible; SEFAS adjusted 0–100 where 100 is the best possible health
[c]Mean imputation was used when half or fewer items were missing

good agreement between test and retest (Table 2). Intraclass correlations for the scale scores ranged from 0.91 to 0.93 for the LEFS and SEFAS respectively. The use of alternate scoring had little or no effect on ICC levels (Table 2). The SEMs for the adjusted scores which are comparable, ranged from 5.1 to 7.4 for the SEFAS and OMAS respectively (Table 4). The SDC for comparisons of individual patients ranged from 14.1 to 20.6 for the SEFAS and OMAS respectively. The SDC for comparisons of groups of patients ranged from 0.93 to 1.55 for the SEFAS and OMAS respectively.

Table 5 shows that the hypotheses used in validity testing were largely met but some correlations were higher than expected. The lowest correlation between the three ankle instruments was 0.84 (LEFS and SEFAS) and the highest was 0.89 (SEFAS and OMAS). High levels of correlation were found for SF-36 physical functioning scores, the highest being for the LEFS which were comparable to those between the LEFS and other specific instruments. Moderate to high levels of correlation were found for the EQ-5D mobility and pain/discomfort items. For the three instruments, the correlations with the EQ-5D usual activities item were of a similar moderate level and for the remaining two items of self-care and anxiety/depression, of a similar low level. Correlations with the clinical variables were all of a low level, the lowest were for BMI and the highest were for the duration of operation. The use of adjusted scores had very little effect on the size of the correlations.

Table 3 Confirmatory factor analysis tests and goodness of fit indices ($n = 567$)

Instrument	$\chi 2$	*df*	CFI[a]	TLI[b]	RMSEA[c]
LEFS unidimensional	843.4	171	0.99	0.99	0.091
LEFS bidimensional[d]	604.4	169	1.00	1.00	0.073
SEFAS	165.9	54	0.99	0.99	0.063
OMAS	122.8	27	0.99	0.98	0.087

All $\chi 2$ tests of model fit were significant with the exception of the LEFS ($p < 0.01$)
[a]Comparative fit index
[b]Tucker-Lewis Index
[c]Root mean square error of approximation
[d]LEFS bi-dimensional easy (1,3–5,7,8,10,11,13,15,20) and difficult (2,6,9,12,14,16–19) items

Discussion

There was evidence that the LEFS might be bi-dimensional in this group of patients which contrasts with it is use in applications as a unidimensional measure of lower extremity function. Exploratory factor analysis (data not shown) showed that the items loaded onto two clearly discernible factors relating to easier and more difficult aspects of function which gave better results in the CFA. The LEFS with 20 items, is a good deal longer than the OMAS and SEFAS and such a lengthy instrument that assesses one aspect of health is unusual for PROMs. The OMAS and SEFAS are shorter, have acceptable levels of internal consistency, test-retest reliability and the SEFAS has a lower SEM and hence is more capable of measuring change in individuals and groups of patients.

The current study followed previous studies in treating the LEFS as unidimensional in other aspects of testing but results should be treated with caution until further evidence becomes available. This study is a long-term follow-up of patients and the evidence may be different for patients in the shorter-term post-surgery. LEFS items may differ in their relevance in these patients. For example, more difficult items including 'running', 'squatting' and 'walking a mile' might have greater relevance at follow-up as shown by their much lower ceiling effects compared to the remaining items. The inclusion of easier items in the same scale might mask important effects at follow-up. Eighty percent or more patients had the best possible score on seven LEFS items compared to just one item in each of the OMAS and SEFAS. If long-term outcomes are the focus, then these two instruments might be more responsive to change than the

Table 4 Standard error of measurement (SEM) and smallest detectable change (SDC) for the three instruments[a] ($n = 182$)

Instrument	n	Test mean (SD)	Retest mean (SD)	SEM[b]	SDC[c]individual	SDC[c]group
LEFS (0–80)[c]	179	68.54 (15.03)	69.03 (15.14)	4.50	12.49	0.93
LEFS adjusted	181	85.48 (18.39)	86.19 (18.41)	5.61	15.55	1.16
SEFAS (12–60)[b]	172	19.70 (8.99)	19.49 (9.23)	2.39	6.62	0.50
SEFAS adjusted	182	83.85 (18.52)	84.11 (19.01)	5.09	14.10	0.93
OMAS	140	78.04 (24.44)	79.64 (24.29)	6.87	19.04	0.92
OMAS adjusted	176	77.66 (24.38)	78.85 (23.90)	7.41	20.55	1.55

[a]Instruments scored 0–100 unless otherwise stated
[b]Standard error of measurement
[c]Smallest detectable change
[b]Included for comparison with existing studies that have used the same scoring

unidimensional LEFS. It is recommended that future studies compare the responsiveness to change of these instruments, including treating the LEFS as a bi-dimensional instrument where evidence supports.

There were low levels of missing data at the item level with very few items having more than 5 % missing. These items tended to relate to more difficult activities undertaken less frequently. Hence, the levels of missing data may reflect uncertainty on the part of the patients regarding their performance, or that they may have held back from undertaking such activities due to concerns about the ankle. Such items include running for the LEFS and jumping for the OMAS. The LEFS item 'getting in and out of bath' denotes low levels of function and had relatively high levels of missing data which may because many Norwegians do not have a bathtub at home.

All items with the exception of the assistive devices items for the OMAS and special innersoles/shoes in the SEFAS, had acceptable item-total correlations. This indicates that these two items might not be adequately contributing to the construct being measured. For example, patients might be using assistive devices, innersoles and shoes for reasons other than the severity of their ankle problem or because of other health problems. These items might be considered for removal if future studies also find that they make a limited contribution in a similar patient population. Cronbach's alpha and test-retest correlations were acceptable for the three instruments. Alpha is dependent on the number of items and hence the highest level was expected for the LEFS.

Scores for the three instruments were highly correlated which is evidence that they are assessing very similar aspects of health and have convergent validity. The highest correlations were found between scores for the OMAS and SEFAS which reflects their ankle specific focus compared to the focus on lower extremity function of the

Table 5 Spearman correlations[a] between the ankle instrument scores, those for generic instruments and clinical variables ($n = 567$)

Instrument	LEFS	LEFS Adjusted[b]	OMAS	OMAS Adjusted	SEFAS	SEFAS Adjusted
OMAS	0.86	0.86				
OMAS Adjusted	0.86	0.86				
SEFAS	−0.84	−0.84	− 0.89	−0.89		
SEFAS Adjusted	−0.84	−0.84	− 0.88	−0.88		
SF-36 physical function	0.85	0.86	0.76	0.77	−0.74	−0.73
EQ-5D index	0.73	0.73	0.79	0.79	−0.80	−0.79
Mobility	−0.65	−0.64	− 0.66	−0.67	0.66	0.66
Self-care	−0.35	−0.36	− 0.32	−0.33	0.34	0.34
Usual activities	−0.60	−0.61	− 0.59	−0.60	0.62	0.62
Pain/discomfort	−0.64	−0.64	− 0.73	−0.73	0.76	0.75
Anxiety/depression	−0.30	−0.31	− 0.30	−0.31	0.31	0.30
ASA classification	−0.26	−0.26	− 0.19	−0.21	0.21	0.20
Body Mass Index	−0.15	−0.16	− 0.21	−0.19	0.14	0.15
Duration of operation	−0.24	−0.23	− 0.25	−0.26	0.24	0.22
Uni-, bi-, tri-malleolar	−0.23	−0.22	− 0.21	−0.23	0.21	0.19

[a]All correlations are significant ($p < 0.01$)
[b]Adjusted scores where mean imputation is used for missing data when half or more items are completed

LEFS. These two instruments also had slightly higher correlations with the EQ-5D, including individual EQ-5D items. The LEFS had the highest correlations with SF-36 physical functioning scores and several LEFS items that are not covered by the OMAS and SEFAS, have similar content to this SF-36 scale.

For the LEFS, Cronbach's alpha, test-retest reliability correlation coefficient and the SEM were similar to those previously reported [16]. The OMAS had a slightly higher Cronbach's alpha than in the previous study [17]. The test-retest reliability correlation coefficient was slightly lower and SEM slightly higher than those previously reported [17]. It follows that the smallest detectable change was larger; 19–20 compared to 16 [17]. The SEFAS had a higher alpha and similar level of test-retest reliability compared to the Swedish study that included patients with hind foot and ankle disorders [10]. The SEM and SDC were not reported in this study.

Recommendations for handling missing data were not available for the OMAS. The conventional approach is mean imputation when half or less items are missing. Compared to the approach that has been recommended for the SEFAS [10], this form of imputation increases the number of patients with final scores by 7%. This reduces sample sizes required in evaluative studies including clinical trials. Mean scores and the results of testing were very similar irrespective of the methods of handling missing data. For example, levels of correlation with the EQ-5D scores were virtually unchanged. The conventional approach will reduce sample size requirements in clinical trials and based on these study findings, will increase useable scores by up to 16% for the OMAS.

Clinicians and researchers selecting PROMs for this group of patients should consider using the SEFAS in preference to the LEFS and OMAS. There is uncertainty surrounding the structural validity of the LEFS, it has greater respondent burden and a broader focus on lower limbs rather than the foot and ankle. The broader focus was reflected in correlations between the LEFS and SF-36 physical function scores which were higher than those between the LEFS, OMAS and SEFAS scores. The OMAS has more complex scoring, performed less satisfactorily than the SEFAS in terms of structural validity and had a higher SEM. The use of mean imputation where half or more items are completed, reduces the number of patients needed for recruitment with negligible effects on measurement properties.

Study limitations

Important limitations include the follow-up period, potential respondent bias, choice of instruments and lack of testing for other measurement properties. The median time between surgery and questionnaire completion was 4.3 (IQR 3.9–5.1) years [12], and it is important that the measurement properties of the three instruments are assessed at other clinically important follow-up periods. This limitation means that it was not possible to recommend modifications to the instruments including the use of a bi-dimensional LEFS and removal of items across the instruments. The 59% response rate to the questionnaire is acceptable for this type of study but there were some statistically significant differences between respondents and non-respondents to the questionnaire [12]. Other instruments are available that have undergone limited testing in patients with ankle fracture [5], but respondent burden meant that only three instruments could be included in this study. The design of the study also meant that instrument responsiveness to change could not be assessed. This is an important criterion which further aids the selection of instruments for evaluative studies including clinical trials [11].

Assessment of the SEM and SDC followed the COSMIN checklist [11] and have been previously reported for the LEFS and OMAS [16, 17]. The SDC is the level of change that can be considered real change above measurement error and does not consider whether the change is important. The minimal clinically important difference (MCID) or minimal important change (MIC), are levels of change that patients consider important and further help score interpretation [11]. The MIC has not been reported for the study instruments in this patient population and assessment was not possible within the current study design. It is recommended that the MIC be reported in future studies.

Conclusion

This is the first study that has concurrently evaluated these instruments in patients following surgery for ankle fracture. Moreover, the LEFS and SEFAS have not been previously evaluated solely in patients with ankle fracture. The three instruments have acceptable evidence for internal consistency, test-retest reliability and construct validity. However, there are some doubts about the unidimensionality of the LEFS in this population and it has a relatively large number of items with the largest ceiling effects representing the highest level of functioning. Further testing of these instruments is recommended in patients with ankle fracture including shorter-term follow-up following surgery. Responsiveness to changes in health should also be assessed with instrument completion taking place before and after an intervention of known efficacy. Instrument content should be carefully considered when choosing between these three instruments. The LEFS is specific to the lower extremities and includes a relatively large number of items. The OMAS is designed to be ankle fracture specific and includes clinical weightings whereas the other two instruments are based on simple summed scales. The SEFAS is designed for a range of foot disorders including ankle fractures and has the best measurement properties in this population. Finally, it is recommended that mean imputation is used for missing responses when half or more items are completed by patients.

Abbreviations

BMI: Body Mass Index; CFA: Confirmatory factor analysis; CFI: Comparative fit index; ICC: Intraclass correlation coefficient; LEFS: Lower Extremity Function Scale; MIC: Minimal Important Change; OMAS: Olerud Molander Ankle Score; ORIF: Open reduction internal fixation; PROMs: Patient reported outcome measures; RMSEA: Root mean square error of approximation; SDC: Smallest detectable change; SEFAS: Self-Reported Foot and Ankle Score; SEM: Standard error of measurement; TLI: Tucker-Lewis Index

Acknowledgements

The authors thank Meetali Kakad for back-translation of the questionnaires to English.

Funding

The project was partially funded by The Sophies Minde Foundation and Østfold Hospital. The sponsors had no involvement in study planning, collection, analysis, or interpretation of the data, or in the preparation, or approval of the manuscript.

Authors' contributions

MGN, US, SEU and KS designed the retrospective cohort study and were responsible for data collection. AMG and KS were responsible for the patient reported outcomes component of the study. AMG performed the statistical analysis and drafted the manuscript. All authors read and approved the final manuscript.

Competing interests

The authors declare that they have no competing interests.

Author details

[1]Division for Health Services, Norwegian Institute of Public Health, Oslo, Norway. [2]Department of Orthopaedics, Østfold Hospital, Oslo, Norway. [3]Department of Orthopaedics, Akershus University Hospital, Lørenskog, Norway. [4]Institute of Clinical Medicine, University of Oslo, Oslo, Norway. [5]Department of Pulmonary Medicine, Medical Division, Akershus University Hospital, Lørenskog, Norway. [6]Health Services Research Unit, Akershus University Hospital, Lørenskog, Norway.

References

1. Donken CC, Al-Khateeb H, Verhofstad MH, van Laarhoven CJ. Surgical versus conservative interventions for treating ankle fractures in adults. Cochrane Database Syst Rev. 2012;15(8):CD008470.
2. Somersalo A, Paloneva J, Kautiainen H, Lönnroos E, Heinänen M, Kiviranta I. Incidence of fractures requiring inpatient care. Acta Orthop. 2014;85:525–30.
3. Ma X, Wang X, Huang J, Zhang C, Chen L. Internal fixation of distal tibiofibular syndesmotic injuries: a systematic review with meta-analysis. Int Orthop. 2013;37:1755–63.
4. Van Son MA, De Vries J, Roukema JA, Den Oudsten BL. Health status, health-related quality of life, and quality of life following ankle fractures: a systematic review. Injury. 2013;44:1391–402.
5. Jia Y, Huang H, Gagnier JJ. A Systematic review of measurement properties of patient-reported outcome measures for use in patients with foot or ankle diseases. Qual Life Res 2017; https://doi.org/10.1007/s11136-017-1542-4. [Epub ahead of print].
6. Garratt AM, Schmidt L, Mackintosh A, Fitzpatrick R. Quality of life measurement: bibliographic study of patient assessed health outcome measures. Br Med J. 2002;324:1417–9.
7. Haywood KL, Hargreaves J, Lamb SE. Multi-item outcome measures for lateral ligament injury of the ankle: a structured review. J Eval Clin Pract. 2004;10:339–52.
8. Binkley JM, Stratford PW, Lott SA, Riddle DL. The lower extremity functional scale (LEFS): scale development, measurement properties, and clinical application. North American Orthopaedic Rehabilitation Research Network Phys Ther. 1999;79:371–83.
9. Olerud C, Molander H. A scoring scale for symptom evaluation after ankle fracture. Arch Orthop Trauma Surg. 1984;103:190–4.
10. Cöster MC, Bremander A, Rosengren BE, Magnusson H, Carlsson Å, Karlsson MK. Validity, reliability, and responsiveness of the self-reported foot and ankle score (SEFAS) in forefoot, hindfoot, and ankle disorders. Acta Orthop. 2014;85:187–94.
11. Mokkink LB, Terwee CB, Patrick DL, Alonso J, Stratford PW, Knol DL, et al. The COSMIN checklist for assessing the methodological quality of studies on measurement properties of health status instruments: an international Delphi study. Qual Life Res. 2010;19:539–49.
12. Naumann MG, Sigurdsen U, Utvåg SE, Stavem K. Associations of timing of surgery with postoperative length of stay, complications, and functional outcomes 3-6 years after operative fixation of closed ankle fractures. Injury 2017;48:1662–9.
13. Hoogeboom TJ, de Bie RA, den Broeder AA, van den Ende CHM. The Dutch lower extremity functional scale was highly reliable, valid and responsive in individuals with hip/knee osteoarthrtitis: a validation study. BMC Musculoskeletal Disord. 2012;13:117.
14. Dingemans SA, Kleipool SC, Mulders MAM, Winkelhagen J, Schep NWL, et al. Normative data for the lower extremity functional scale (LEFS). Acta Orthop. 2017;88:422–6.
15. Lin CW, Moseley AM, Refshauge KM, Bundy AC. The lower extremity functional scale has good clinimetric properties in people with ankle fracture. Phys Ther. 2009;89:580–8.
16. Repo JP, Tukiainen EJ, Roine RP, Ilves O, Järvenpää S, Häkkinen A. Reliability and validity of the Finnish version of the lower extremity functional scale (LEFS). Disabil Rehabil. 2016;6:1–7.
17. Nilsson GM, Eneroth M, Ekdahl CS. The Swedish version of OMAS is a reliable and valid outcome measure for patients with ankle fractures. BMC Musculoskelet Disord. 2013;14:109.
18. Turhan E, Demirel M, Daylak A, Huri G, Doral MN, Çelik D. Translation, cross-cultural adaptation, reliability and validity of the Turkish version of the Olerud-Molander ankle score (OMAS). Acta Orthop Traumatol Turc. 2017;51:60–4.
19. Cöster MC, Rosengren BE, Bremander A, Brudin L, Karlsson MK. Comparison of the self-reported foot and ankle score (SEFAS) and the American orthopedic foot and ankle society score (AOFAS). Foot Ankle Int. 2014;35:1031–6.
20. Dolan P. Modelling valuations for EuroQol health states. Med Care. 1997;35:1095–108.
21. Ware JE, Sherbourne CD. The MOS 36-item short-form health survey (SF-36) I: conceptual framework and item selection. Med Care. 1992;30:473–83.
22. Bentler P. Comparative fit indexes in structural models. Psychol Bull. 1990;107:238–46.
23. Tucker L, Lewis CA. Reliability coefficient for maximum likelihood factor analysis. Psychometrika. 1973;38:1–10.
24. Browne MW, Cudeck R. Alternative ways of assessing model fit. In KA Bollen & JS Long (Eds.). Testing structural equation models (pp. 136–162). Newbury Park, CA: Sage, 1993.

Comparison between absorbable pins and mini-screw fixations for the treatment of radial head fractures Mason type II-III

Luigi Tarallo[1*], Raffaele Mugnai[1], Martina Rocchi[1], Francesco Capra[2] and Fabio Catani[1]

Abstract

Background: The treatment of comminuted radial head fractures can include prosthetic replacement or open reduction and internal fixation. The purpose of this study is to evaluate the results of two different internal fixation systems for Mason type II-III radial head fractures.

Methods: Between 2005 and 2015, 82 patients were treated using pins and 65 patients by mini-screws. The follow-up protocol included: a clinical evaluation 15 days after surgery, and clinical and radiographic evaluations performed at 30 and 60 day intervals, unless any complications were reported by the patient. Over a period of at least 12-months of follow-up, patients were checked and interviewed. Clinical examinations included elbow range of motion (ROM), arm, shoulder and hand Disabilities, (DASH), and the Mayo Elbow Performance Score (MEPS).

Results: Sixty-one subjects who had been treated with mini-screws were clinically reviewed at a mean 47.3 ± 35. 8 month of follow-up; all patients who had been treated using absorbable pins were evaluated at a mean 82.5 ± 20. 6 month of follow-up. No significant statistically differences were observed between the two groups in the mean ROM, DASH, and MEPS scores. Residual pain was reported in 15.8%of the patients treated by pins and 9.2% patients treated by mini-screws. Secondary displacement of fracture fragments was observed in 8.5% patients treated by pins and 1.6% using mini-screws.

Conclusions: Both absorbable pins and mini-screws provided adequate strength and rigidity, allowing good clinical and functional scores at a mid-term follow-up. However, a higher rate of secondary displacement of the fracture fragments was reported among subjects who had been treated using absorbable pins.

Keywords: Radial head fracture, Mason, Pin, Mini-screws, Complications, Fixation

Background

The treatment of radial head fractures, for a long time was treated with excision of the fracture fragments. This kind of treatment could lead to instability, proximal migration of the radius, joint stiffness and a mismatch at the radio-ulnar joint [1, 2].

Recently the radial head be fixed and the reduction can be maintained thanks to the new techniques obtained in open-reduction and internal fixation (ORIF) [3].

Recent studies comparing ORIF to alternative treatments (resection or replacement) have shown that fixation provides very favourable results in terms of function in fractures characterized by only a few fragments, while very comminute patterns appear to be best managed with arthroplasty or resection [4–7].

The most commonly employed systems for classifying radial head fractures is the Mason classification [8], originally introduced in the 1950s, and recently modified by Hotchkiss [5]. Type I includes non-displaced or minimally displaced (< 2 mm) fracture of the radial head or neck, or marginal lip fracture. Type II partial articular fractures with displacement > 2 mm. Type III severely comminuted fractures involving the entire radial head. Type IV fractures associated with elbow displacement [9].

The aim of this study is to evaluate the results of two different kinds of internal fixations (absorbable pins and

* Correspondence: tarallo.luigi@policlinico.mo.it
[1]Department of Orthopaedics and Traumatology, University of Modena and Reggio Emilia, Policlinico di Modena, Modena, Italy

mini-screws) in patients with Mason type II and III radial head fracture.

Methods

Patients

This retrospective research was approved by the local institutional ethics committee and was carried out following the guidelines of the ethical standards of the 1964 Declaration of Helsinki as revised in 2000. Between 2005 and 2015, 147 patients (age > 18 years) with radial head fracture Mason type II-III were treated using absorbable pins or mini-screws at the authors' institute, which is a referred trauma and hand surgery center. The only criteria of exclusion to our study is age < 18 years old.

Surgical technique

With the patient placed in the supine position, Kocher's lateral technique was used to expose the radial head between the anconeus and extensor carpi ulnaris. Once reduced, the fracture fragments were fixed with absorbable pins (Fig. 1) or mini-screws (Fig. 2). The choice of the internal fixation system for osteosynthesis was determined by time criterion and independent from subjective characterization: before 2010 only pins were used; later mini-screws became the choice of fixation. In particular the 2 fixation systems employed were:

- Resorbable pins diameter 2.0 mm Orthosorb LS (Lactosorb), composed of 82% Poly-L-lactic acid and 18% Poly-glycolic acid (Zimmer, Biomet).
- Headless compression screws Acutrak mini diameter 3.2 mm (Acumed, Hillsboro, OR).

All procedures were performed by or under the direct supervision of one senior surgeon.

When present, concomitant LCL injuries were treated primarily with bone anchor or trans-osseous bone tunnel. More complex lesions were also repaired at the same time to achieve a complete articular stabilization. A long-arm splint was applied with the elbow in 90° of flexion.

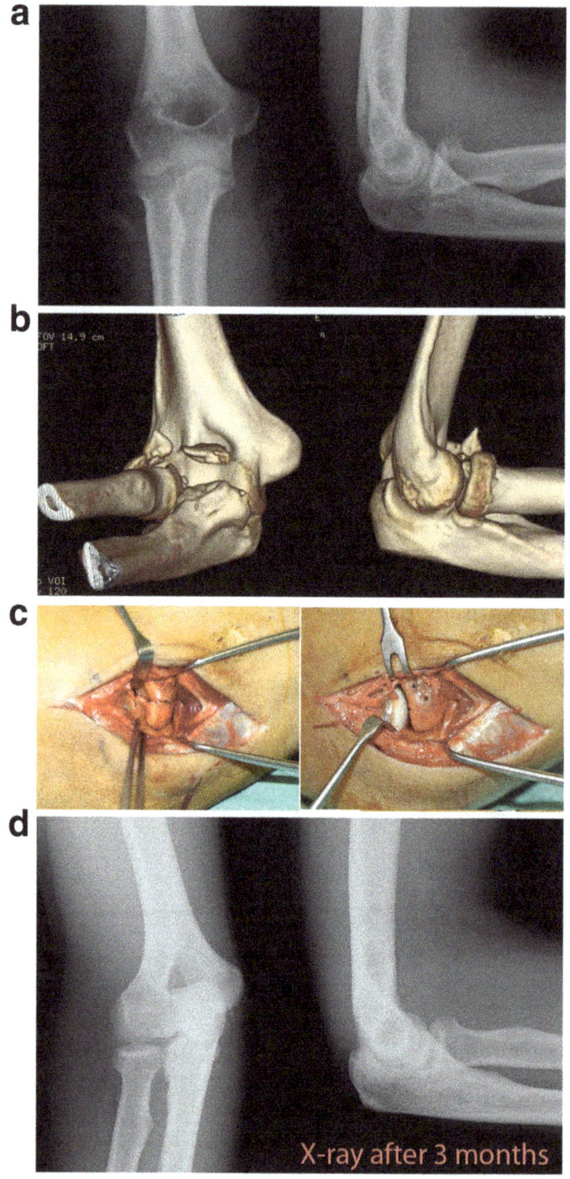

Fig. 1 **a** X-rays showing a Mason type II fracture. **b** 3D-computed tomography evaluation confirming a partial articular fracture with high displacement of the fractured fragments. **c** Intra-operative view showing the reduction and fixation using 2 absorbable pins. **d** X-rays performed after 3 months showing healing of the fracture without signs of secondary displacement of the fragments

Outcomes

The post-operative protocol included a clinical evaluation 15 days after surgery, during which the stitches were removed and in the mini-screws group the long-arm splint was substituted with an articulated elbow brace to allow early mobilization, whereas patients treated by pins were maintained immobilized for about one month, according to the Hirvensalo E. and Pelto K. technique [17, 18]. A clinical and radiographic evaluation was also performed after 30 days and 60 days, unless any complications occurred .

Each patient was finally re-evaluated at a minimum of 12-month follow-up (respectively at a mean 82.5 ± 20.6 month for patients treated using pins, and 47.3 ± 35.8 month using mini-screws) by one of the authors, including elbow Range of Motion (ROM) and the following questionnaires: Arm, Shoulder and Hand Disabilities, (DASH) score, and the Mayo Elbow Performance Score (MEPS) [10, 11].

Any possible adverse reactions including residual pain, symptoms of instability of the elbow, early or late occurrence of clinically evident seroma formation, osteolytic changes of the radial head, non-unions,

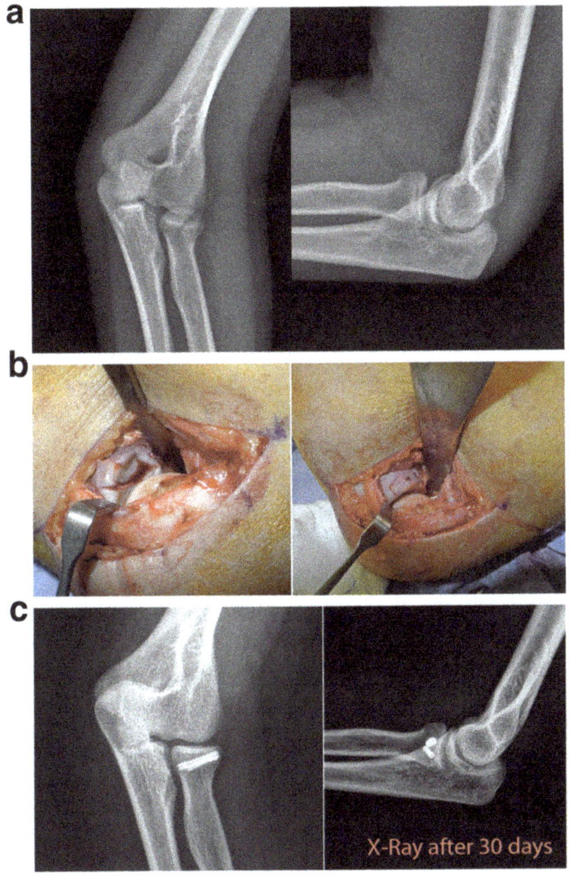

Fig. 2 a X-rays showing a Mason type II fracture. **b** Intra-operative view showing the reduction and fixation using 2 mini-screws. **c** X-rays performed after 30-days with signs of fracture healing and reduction maintenance

infection or loss of fracture reduction were evaluated, and recorded. In particular, the secondary possible displacement using the hospital X-ray program was measured by the author. In the case of displacement, three different points of the fragment had been selected to take the measurement from the articular surface and the mean value was also taken in consideration. The assessments of radiographic outcomes and clinical outcomes were not blinded.

Statistical analysis

A summary and statistical analysis is shown in Table 2 (continuous data were expressed as mean ± standard deviation).

The T-test method was followed to define the two-sided probability of statistical significance in Age comparison due to the F-test more than 0.05 (the variances of the two samples can be assumed to be equal). The other analysis has not presented parametric distribution so the Mann-Whitney test for independent samples was carried out. Post-hoc power calculator was introduced to evaluate the statistical strength of the trial. Statistical analysis was monitored using MedCalc for Windows, version 12.2.1 (MedCalc Software, Mariakerke, Belgium).

Results

The study of population was composed of 74 men and 73 women. The left elbow was affected in 75 patients (7 dominant), whereas the right elbow in 72 patients (69 dominant). The mean age of the subjects treated by mini-screws and pins was 47.2 ± 15.4 and 45.4 ± 13. 1 years, respectively. Absorbable pins were used in 82 patients, mini-screws in 65 subjects. Pin population was composed of 61 Mason II and 21 Mason III fractures, while mini-screw group included 47 Mason II and 18 Mason III fractures. A complex injury pattern was present in 20 patients: a concomitant olecranon fracture in 5 cases, coronoid fracture in 10 cases, lateral column distal humerus fracture in 4 patients, and 1 patients had a complex arm injury (concomitant fractures of the scaphoid and scapho-lunate dissociation). The lateral collateral ligament (LCL) was treated in 12 patients. Table 1 lists the concomitant injuries of both fixation methods, mini-screws and pins, and their statistical comparison showed that there were no significant differences between the two study groups.

Sixty-one of the 65 subjects treated by mini-screws were clinically evaluated at a mean 47.3 ± 35.8 month follow-up, as it was not possible to contact 4 of the patients for the last clinical control. None of the patients treated using absorbable pins were absent at an average 82.5 ± 20.6 month of follow-up. The mean elbow ROM for the pin group was: flexion 138.2° ± 5.5, extension

Table 1 Associated injuries

Concomitant Injury	PIN ($n = 82$) N (%)	Mini-screws ($n = 65$) N (%)	p-value
Olecranon fractures	2 (2.4)	3 (4.6)	0.6551[a]
Coronoid fractures	6 (7.3)	4 (6.1)	1.0000 [a]
Lateral column humerus fractures	4 (4.9)	0 (0.0)	0.1299 [a]
Scaphoid fracture	0 (0.0)	1 (1.5)	0.4422 [a]
LCL	5 (6.1)	7 (10.8)	0.3699 [a]

[a] Fisher test

deficit 5.5° ± 11.7, pronation 73.1° ± 3.4, and supination 82.3° ± 6.0, whereas, the mean ROM for the patients treated using mini-screw was: flexion 139.5° ± 2.2, extension deficit 2.0° ± 7.0, pronation 73.6° ± 2.3, and supination 81.7° ± 5.4 (Table 2).

The mean DASH score was 0.8 ± 2.0 for patients treated using pins, and 0.3 ± 0.5 for the mini-screw group. Considering the MEPS, a mean score of 97.3 ± 5.8 was reported in the pin group, and 98.3 ± 5.7 for the patients treated using mini-screws. Comparing the ROM, DASH, and MEPS scores between the two groups no significant differences were observed (Table 2). No cases of symptoms of elbow instability, early or late occurrence of clinically evident seroma formation, osteolytic changes of the radial head, non-union, or infection was observed in either group. Residual pain was reported in 13 (15.8%) patients treated using pins, and in 6 (9.2%) patients treated using mini-screws. Radiological anatomical reduction was achieved intraoperatively in all cases; however, 7 (8.5%) patients treated using pins presented a secondary displacement of the fracture fragments of more than 1 mm (range 1–3 mm) in the postoperative radiographs (Fig. 3) vs. 1 case (1.6%) among the patients treated with mini-screws (Fig. 4). At the final clinical evaluation, no functional limitation which could influence social day to day life was highlighted in all subjects. Post-hoc power analysis is 8.2%; the minimum number of subjects for adequate study power is 3252 (1626 patients for each group – alpha error rate 0.05, beta error 0.2 and power of 80%). There are no significant differences for complications such as pain or fragments displacement (Table 2).

Discussion

The properties of an ideal fixation for articular fractures include adequate strength and rigidity, lack of adverse side effects, any interference with bone healing and avoidance of an implant removal operation. Griffin et al. demonstrated that cross-cannulated 3 mm screws offered better rigidity than conventional T-plates in a cadaveric non-comminuted radial neck fracture model [12]. Koslowsky et al. performed a biomechanical study using radius saw bone models in Mason type III fractures comparing the quality of reduction, the failure load and the displacement of the reconstructed radial head at 50 N between fine threaded wires, T-mini-plates, 2 mm mini-screws and 2 mm K-wires [13]. The authors achieved a much better quality of reduction using fine threaded wires, followed by mini-screws and k-wires, and poor results with mini-plates. The ultimate failure load was similar for fine threaded wires, mini-screws and K-wires, but poor for mini-plates. The mean displacement at 50 N was significantly greater for plate fixation, than for fine threaded wires, mini-screws and k-wires [13]. Recently, absorbable pins have been proposed and tested in several studies [14-16, 20].

Hirvensalo et al., prospectively evaluated 24 patients treated with 2.0 mm absorbable polyglycolide pins for displaced radial head fracture, obtaining, at a mean 28 months of follow-up, excellent or good functional results in 22 patients (91%). Complications were represented by postoperative displacement of fractured fragments (range 1–3 mm) reported in 4 (16.7%) patients with severely comminuted fractures, and transient inflammatory reaction around the implants occurred in 2 (8.3%) cases 8–12 weeks postoperatively [17]. Pelto et al., reviewed, at an average 27 months of follow-up, 38 patients were treated with absorbable polyglycolide pins for Mason type II-III radial head fractures, reporting excellent or very positive functional results in 36 patients (95%), with 1 case of postoperative re-displacement and no adverse side effects from the implant [18].

Table 2 Clinical results and statistical analysis

	PIN (mean ± SD) n = 82	Mini-screw (mean ± SD) *n* = 61	*p*-value	Post-hoc analysis of power[c]
Patient's age (years)	45.4 ± 13.1	47.2 ± 15.4	0.459[a]	
Follow-up (months)	82.5 ± 20.6	47.3 ± 35.8	< 0.001[b]	
Flexion (°)	138.2 ± 5.5	139.5 ± 2.2	0.217[b]	58.2%
Extension deficit (°)	5.5 ± 11.7	2.0 ± 7.0	0.085[b]	49.7%
Pronation (°)	73.1 ± 3.4	73.6 ± 2.3	0.623[b]	18.7%
Supination (°)	82.3 ± 6.0	81.7 ± 5.4	0.290[b]	8%
DASH	0.8 ± 2.0	0.3 ± 0.5	0.554[b]	72.9%
MEPS	97.3 ± 5.8	98.3 ± 5.7	0.072[b]	17.8%
Comparison of displacement of the fragments			1.000[c]	
Comparison of residual pain			0.109[c]	

[a] T-test
[b] Mann-Whitney test
[c] Fisher's test

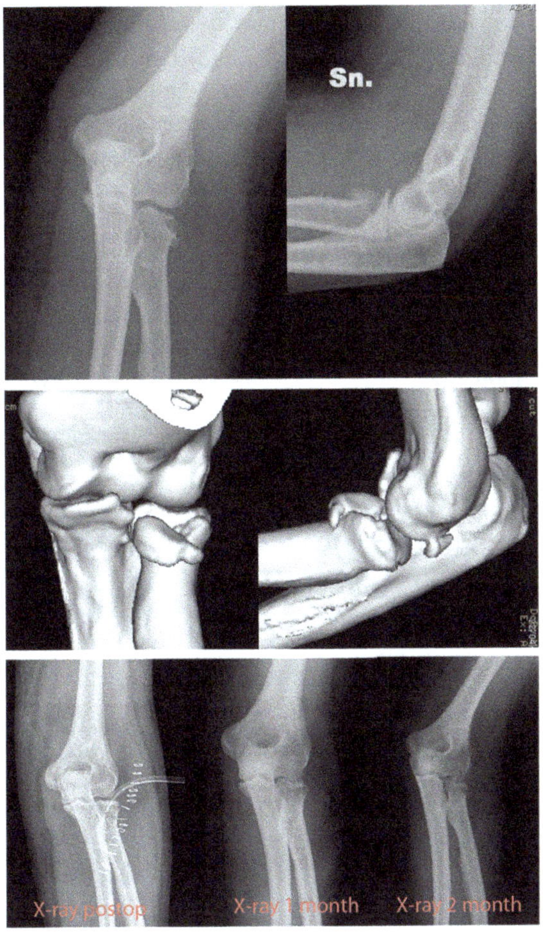

Fig. 3 a Severely displaced Mason type II fracture. **b** 3D-computed tomography study. **c** X-rays follow-up with secondary displacement of fracture fragments of about 3 mm observed 2 months after surgery

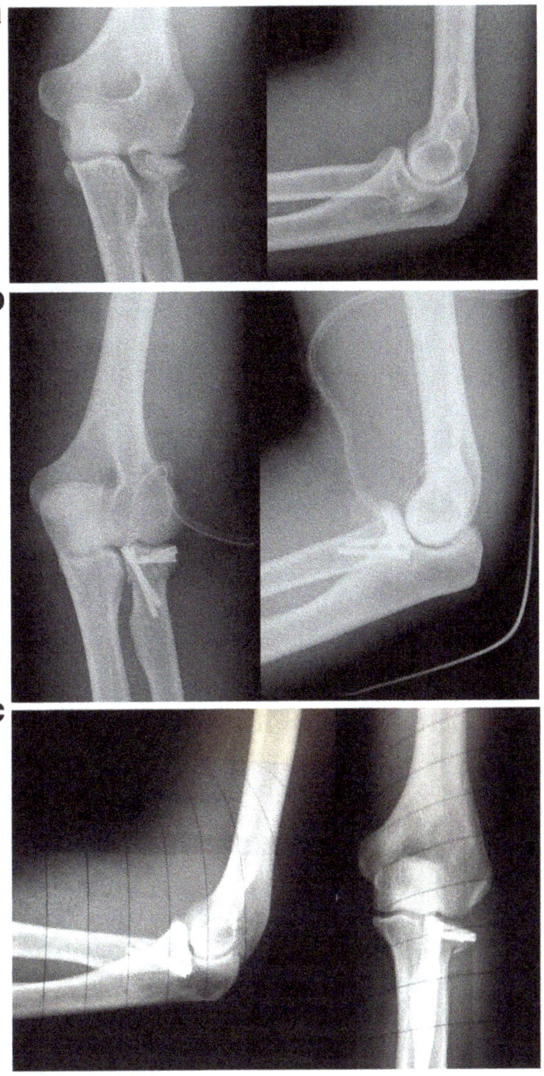

Fig. 4 a X-rays showing a Mason type III fracture. **b** Post-operative x-rays with acceptable reduction using mini-screws. **c** X-rays showing secondary displacement of fracture fragments of about 4 mm observed 1 months after surgery

Helling et al., published in 2006 a prospective, randomized, controlled multicentre study comparing standard mini-fragment metal implants (mini-screws, k-wires, mini-fragment plates) with biodegradable polylactide implants in 164 subjects with AO type B2.1, B2.2 and B2.2 radial head fractures [19]. At a mean 2-years follow-up, 96% of the polylactide patients and 92% of the control patients had excellent or good results, with an average Bromberg and Morrey Elbow Score of 93.3 in the polylactide group, and 90.9 in the control group (differences not statistically significant). Sixty-nine of the polylactide patients (84.1%) and 66 of the control patients (80.4%) were completely complication-free. Complications were represented by secondary fragment displacement in 5 cases in polylactide group and in 2 control patients, and osteolysis in 1 case for each group [19].

Givissis et al., retrospectively reviewed 21 patients with Mason type II-III-IV fractures treated with absorbable pins, reporting at a mean 81 months of follow-up (range, 36–136 months). The study reported good fracture healing with no radiographic signs of osteolysis in every case, no material-related adverse reactions, mean MEPS score of 93.8 (range, 20–100), and mean elbow ROM of 9°-132° in flexion, 79° pronation, and 77° supination [20]. These results are comparable in terms of functional score and ROM with those obtained in the present research using absorbable pins and mini-screws (Table 2).

The authors reported the same satisfactory clinical results for both methods: the means MEPS score is 97.3 +/- 5.8 in pin population and 98.3 +/- 5.7 in screws population, the mean DASH score is respectively 0.8 +/- 2 and 0.3 +/- 0.5. Different studies recorded higher DASH score [21], we believe that such poor results could be down to different pattern of fractures. The trend of better results in terms of outcomes for patients treated by mini-screws is not statistically significant. The minimal limitation of excursion and moderate pain, that had been registered did not influence day to day life and each patient expressed great satisfaction for their surgical treatment (Table 2). It is of importance to note that the residual pain and limitation of excursion, are not related to secondary displacement. This factor, could possibly be linked to a different post-operative protocol of immobilization that could lead to stiffness. However, we preferred to immobilize the patients who we had treated with pins, according to literature [17, 18] because of minor axial strength [19]. The lack of detailed clinical data regarding functional outcomes of two groups at 30 and 60 days after surgery limited our thoughts regarding the range of motion recovery.

Limitation

A possible limitation of this study is represented by the different follow-up duration of the 2 groups, respectively 82.5 ± 20.6 for the pin group vs. 47.3 ± 35.8 for the mini-screw group. This is due to replacement of the surgical practice using pins in the last five years in our institute. This technical decision was based on the surgeon's personal preference. The collection of data, over a long period of time, is a significant area of potential study bias as the surgeon could have possibly experienced substantial technical improvement. Furthermore, the measurements regardless of the final results of the clinical check up carried out by one of the authors, could also affect our study. It is important to note that the post-operative protocol has not changed and the classification of fracture pattern, was carried out by the same author.

Unfortunately, it was impossible for the author to find any clinical data, regarding functional results between the two groups at 30 and 60 days in our records. The possible late recovery of range of motion could be an important factor influencing the choice of treatment.

Another limitation is the absence of a long-term radiological evaluation to assess possible delayed adverse effects of the bio-absorbable material used for pins and the onset of radio-humeral arthrosis.

A further limitation of the study is the low statistical power. Although Post-Hoc Analysis was discussed as a post-hoc method, analysis would require a larger sample of patients to achieve results with greater power. Finally, post-hoc analysis of power is poor possibly due to the restricted sample size. For any further studies, it may be helpful to increase the sample size to avoid the risk of type II error that could affect our work and results.

Conclusions

Both absorbable pins and mini-screws provide good clinical and functional scores at a mid-term follow-up. However, a higher rate (8.5% of cases) of secondary displacement of the fracture fragments was reported among those subjects treated using absorbable pins.

On the other hand, little incongruence of the articular surface could not determine major complications in term of function and pain after an average follow-up of 10 years, as we have shown in our study. We suggest adopting a post-operative protocol including longer immobilization, perhaps a further twenty days, in a cast or elbow brace and at the same time to start physiotherapy treatment taking into consideration cautious mobilization to avoid any stiffness.

Abbreviations

DASH: Disabilities of the arm, shoulder and hand; LCL: Lateral collateral ligament; MEPS: Mayo elbow performance score; ORIF: Open-reduction and internal fixation; ROM: Range of motion

Acknowledgements

Not applicable.

Funding

This research received no specific grant or financing from any public, private, profit or non profit agencies or sectors.

Authors' contributions

LT and RM set up and carried out the study. MR was responsible for data collection. FC was responsible for data analysis. FC contributed to interpretation of data. RM and MR drafted the manuscript. All authors critically revised the manuscript. All authors read and approved the final manuscript.

Consent for publication

Not applicable.

Competing interests

The authors declare that they have no competing interests.

Author details

[1]Department of Orthopaedics and Traumatology, University of Modena and Reggio Emilia, Policlinico di Modena, Modena, Italy. [2]Private Practitioner, Rimini, Italy.

References

1. Hall JA, McKee MD. Posterolateral rotatory instability of the elbow following radial head resection. J Bone Joint Surg Am. 2005;87:1571–9.
2. Geel CW, Palmer A. Radial head fractures and their effect on the distal radioulnar joint. A rationale for treatment. Clin Orthop Relat Res. 1992;275:79–84.
3. Ikeda M, Sugiyama K, Kang C, Takagaki T, Oka Y. Comminuted fractures of the radial head: comparison of resection and internal fixation. Surgical technique. J Bone Joint Surg Am. 2006;88(suppl 1 pt 1):11–23.
4. Sanders RA, French HG. Open reduction and internal fixation of comminuted radial head fractures. Am J Sports Med. 1986;14:130–5.
5. Ring D, Quintero J, Jupiter J. Open reduction and internal fixation of fractures of the radial head. J Bone Joint Surg Am. 2002;84:1811–5.

6. Leigh WB, Ball CM. Radial head reconstruction versus replacement in the treatment of terrible triad injuries of the elbow. J Shoulder Elb Surg. 2012; 21(10):1336–41.
7. Pike JM, Grewal R, Athwal GS, Faber KJ, King GJ. Open reduction and internal fixation of radial head fractures: do outcomes differ between simple and complex injuries? Clin Orthop Relat Res. 2014 Jul;472(7):2120–7.
8. Mason M. Some observations on fractures of the head of the radius with a review of one hundred cases. Br J Surg. 1959;42:123–32.
9. Hotchkiss RN. Displaced fractures of the radial head: internal fixation or excision? J Am Acad Orthop Surg. 1997;5:1–10.
10. Hudak PL, Amadio PC, Bombardier C. Development of an upper extremity outcome measure: the DASH (disabilities of the arm, shoulder and hand) [corrected]. The upper extremity collaborative group (UECG). Am J Ind Med. 1996;29(6):602–8.
11. Morrey BF, An KN, Chao EYS. Functional evaluation of the elbow. In: Morrey BF, editor. The elbow and its disorders. Philadelphia: WB Saunders; 1993. p. 86–9.
12. Giffin JR, King GJ, Patterson SD, Johnson JA. Internal fixation of radial neck fractures: an in vitro biomechanical analysis. Clin Biomech. 2004;19:358–61.
13. Koslowsky TC, Mader K, Dargel J, Koebke J, Hellmich M, Pennig D. Reconstruction of a Mason type-III fracture of the radial head using four different fixation techniques. An experimental study. J Bone Joint Surg Br. 2007;89(11):1545–50.
14. Claes L, Burri C, Kiefer H, Mutschler W. Resorbierbare Implantate zur Refixierung von osteochondralen Fragmenten in Gelenkflächen. Aktuel Traumatol. 1986;16:74–7.
15. Vasenius J, Vainionpää S, Vihtonen K, Mero M, Mikkola J, Rokkanen P, Törmälä P. Biodegradable self-reinforced polyglycolide (SR-PGA) composite rods coated with slowly biodegradable polymers for fracture fixation. Strength and strength retention in vitro and in vivo. Clin Materials. 1989;4: 307–17.
16. Vihtonen K. Fixation of rabbit osteotomies with biodegradable polyglycolic acid thread. Acta Orthop Scand. 1988;59:279–83.
17. Hirvensalo E, Böstman O, Rokkanen P. Absorbable polyglycolide pins in fixation of displaced fractures of the radial head. Arch Orthop Trauma Surg. 1990;109(5):258–61.
18. Pelto K, Hirvensalo E, Bostman O, Rokkanen P. Treatment of radial head fractures with absorbable polyglycolide pins: a study on the security of the fixation in 38 cases. J Orthop Trauma. 1994;8(2):94–8.
19. Helling HJ, Prokop A, Schmid HU, Nagel M, Lilienthal J, Rehm KE. Biodegradable implants versus standard metal fixation for displaced radial head fractures. A prospective, randomized, multicenter study. J Shoulder Elb Surg. 2006;15(4):479–85.
20. Givissis PK, Symeonidis PD, Ditsios KT, Dionellis PS, Christodoulou AG. Late results of absorbable pin fixation in the treatment of radial head fractures. Clin Orthop Relat Res. 2008;466(5):1217–24.
21. Al-Burdeni S, Abuodeh Y, Ibrahim T, Ahmed G. Open reduction and internal fixation versus radial head arthroplasty in the treatment of adult closed comminuted radial head fractures (modified Mason type III and IV). Int Orthop. 2015;39(8):1659-64.

Permissions

All chapters in this book were first published in MD, by BioMed Central; hereby published with permission under the Creative Commons Attribution License or equivalent. Every chapter published in this book has been scrutinized by our experts. Their significance has been extensively debated. The topics covered herein carry significant findings which will fuel the growth of the discipline. They may even be implemented as practical applications or may be referred to as a beginning point for another development.

The contributors of this book come from diverse backgrounds, making this book a truly international effort. This book will bring forth new frontiers with its revolutionizing research information and detailed analysis of the nascent developments around the world.

We would like to thank all the contributing authors for lending their expertise to make the book truly unique. They have played a crucial role in the development of this book. Without their invaluable contributions this book wouldn't have been possible. They have made vital efforts to compile up to date information on the varied aspects of this subject to make this book a valuable addition to the collection of many professionals and students.

This book was conceptualized with the vision of imparting up-to-date information and advanced data in this field. To ensure the same, a matchless editorial board was set up. Every individual on the board went through rigorous rounds of assessment to prove their worth. After which they invested a large part of their time researching and compiling the most relevant data for our readers.

The editorial board has been involved in producing this book since its inception. They have spent rigorous hours researching and exploring the diverse topics which have resulted in the successful publishing of this book. They have passed on their knowledge of decades through this book. To expedite this challenging task, the publisher supported the team at every step. A small team of assistant editors was also appointed to further simplify the editing procedure and attain best results for the readers.

Apart from the editorial board, the designing team has also invested a significant amount of their time in understanding the subject and creating the most relevant covers. They scrutinized every image to scout for the most suitable representation of the subject and create an appropriate cover for the book.

The publishing team has been an ardent support to the editorial, designing and production team. Their endless efforts to recruit the best for this project, has resulted in the accomplishment of this book. They are a veteran in the field of academics and their pool of knowledge is as vast as their experience in printing. Their expertise and guidance has proved useful at every step. Their uncompromising quality standards have made this book an exceptional effort. Their encouragement from time to time has been an inspiration for everyone.

The publisher and the editorial board hope that this book will prove to be a valuable piece of knowledge for researchers, students, practitioners and scholars across the globe.

List of Contributors

Liang Yan, Baorong He, Jijun Liu and Dingjun Hao
Department of Spinal Surgery, Hong Hui Hospital, Xi'an Jiaotong University College of Medicine, 555 Friendship East Road, Xi'an 710054, Shaanxi, China

Zhenguo Luo
Department of Anesthesiology, Hong Hui Hospital, Xi'an Jiaotong University College of Medicine, 555 Friendship East Road, Xi'an 710054, Shaanxi, China

Sung-Hee Oh
National Evidence-based Healthcare Collaborating Agency, Seoul, Republic of Korea
Social and Administrative Pharmacy, College of Pharmacy, Yonsei University, Incheon, Republic of Korea

Dam Kim and Sang-Cheol Bae and Yoon-Kyoung Sung
Department of Rheumatology, Hanyang University Hospital for Rheumatic Diseases, 222-1 wangsimni-ro, Seoundong-gu, Seoul 133-792, Republic of Korea

Young Eun Lee
National Evidence-based Healthcare Collaborating Agency, Seoul, Republic of Korea
Department of Biostatistics and Epidemiology, Graduate School of Public Health, Seoul National University, Seoul, Republic of Korea

Deog-Yoon Kim
Department of Nuclear Medicine, Kyung Hee University Hospital, Seoul, Republic of Korea

Yu Kyung Lee
National Evidence-based Healthcare Collaborating Agency, Seoul, Republic of Korea

Joo-Hyun Lee
Department of Rheumatology, Inje University Ilsan Paik Hospital, Goyang, Republic of Korea

Yun Young Choi
Department of Nuclear Medicine, Hanyang University Hospital, Seoul, Republic of Korea

Junhee Pyo
WHO Collaborating Centre for Pharmaceutical Policy and Regulation, Department of Pharmaceutical Science, Utrecht University, Utrecht, Netherlands

Jeonghoon Ahn
National Evidence-based Healthcare Collaborating Agency, Seoul, Republic of Korea
Department of Health Convergence, Ewha Womans University, 52 Ewhayeodae-gil, Seodaemun-gu, Seoul 03760, Republic of Korea

Soo Beom Choi and Deok Won Kim
Department of Medical Engineering, Yonsei University College of Medicine, Seoul, Korea
Graduate Program in Biomedical Engineering, Yonsei University, Seoul, Korea

Il Suk Lyu
Department of Medicine, Yonsei University College of Medicine, Seoul, Korea

Wanhyung Lee
Graduate School of Public Health, Yonsei University College of Medicine, Seoul, Korea

Axel Gamulin, Anne Lübbeke, Patrick Belinga, Pierre Hoffmeyer, Matthieu Zingg and Gregory Cunningham
Department of Surgery, Division of Orthopaedic and Trauma Surgery, University Hospitals of Geneva, 4 Rue Gabrielle-Perret-Gentil, CH-1211 Geneva 14, Switzerland

Thomas V. Perneger
Division of Clinical Epidemiology, University Hospitals of Geneva, 4 Rue Gabrielle-Perret-Gentil, CH-1211 Geneva 14, Switzerland

Michiaki Miura, Junichi Nakamura, Yusuke Matsuura, Yasushi Wako, Takane Suzuki, Shigeo Hagiwara, Sumihisa Orita, Kazuhide Inage, Yuya Kawarai, Masahiko Sugano, Kento Nawata and Seiji Ohtori
Department of Orthopedic Surgery, Graduate School of Medicine, Chiba University, 1-8-1 Inohana, Chuo-ku, Chiba city, Chiba 260-8677, Japan

Hong-fei Shi, Jin Xiong, Yi-xin Chen, Jun-fei Wang, Xu-Sheng Qiu and Yin-he Wang
Department of Orthopaedics, Nanjing Drum Tower Hospital, The Affiliated Hospital of Nanjing University Medical School, No. 321 Zhongshan Road, Nanjing, China

Jie Huang and Xue-yang Gui
Nanjing Medical University, Nanjing, China

Si-yuan Wen
Nanjing University Medical School, Nanjing, China

Young Yi
Seoul Foot and Ankle Center, Inje University Seoul Paik Hospital, Seoul, Republic of Korea

Dong-Il Chun and Sung Hun Won
Department of Orthopedic Surgery, Seoul Hospital, Soonchunhyang University College of Medicine, Seoul, Republic of Korea

Suyeon Park
Department of Biostatistics, Seoul Hospital, Soonchunhyang University College of Medicine, Seoul, Republic of Korea

Sanghyeon Lee and Jaeho Cho
Department of Orthopaedic Surgery, Chuncheon Sacred Heart Hospital, Hallym University, 77, Sakju-ro, Chuncheoni-si, Gangwon-do 200-704, Republic of Korea

Ping-Jui Tsai, Kuo-Feng Fan, Lih-Huei Chen, Chia-Wei Yu, Po-Liang Lai, Chi-Chien Niu, Tsung-Ting Tsai and Wen-Jer Chen
Department of Orthopedic Surgery, Chang Gung Memorial Hospital and Chang Gung University, Taoyuan, Taiwan
5, Fu-Hsin Street, Kweishan Shiang, Taoyuan, 333, Linkou, Taiwan
Bone and Joint Research Center, Chang Gung Memorial Hospital, Linkou, Taiwan

Ming-Kai Hsieh
Bone and Joint Research Center, Chang Gung Memorial Hospital, Linkou, Taiwan

Zhipeng Huang, Wenjun Xie, Xiang Li, Xiaodong Qin and Jun Hu
Department of Orthopedics, The First Affiliated Hospital of Nanjing Medical University, Nanjing 210029, China

Yuan Liu
Department of Infectious Diseases, The First Affiliated Hospital of Nanjing Medical University, Nanjing 210029, China

Mikk Jürisson and Mait Raag
Institute of Family Medicine and Public Health, University of Tartu, Ravila st 19, 50411 Tartu, Estonia

Riina Kallikorm and Margus Lember
Institute of Clinical Medicine, University of Tartu, L. Puusepa st 8, 51014 Tartu, Estonia
Internal Medicine Clinic, Tartu University Hospital, L. Puusepa st 8, 51014 Tartu, Estonia

Caroline Kihlström, Katarina Lönn and Olof Wolf
Department of Orthopaedics, Institute of Surgical Sciences, Uppsala University Hospital, SE-751 85 Uppsala, Sweden

Michael Möller
Department of Orthopaedics, Sahlgrenska University Hospital Gothenburg/ Mölndal, SE-431 80 Mölndal, Sweden

Adeel Anwar, Zhen Zhang, Decheng Lv and Ming Lu
Department of Orthopaedic Surgery, The First Affiliated Hospital of Dalian Medical University, 222 Zhongshan road, 116011 Dalian, Liaoning, People's Republic of China

Gang Lv and Yanfeng Wang
Department of Orthopaedic Surgery, The First Affiliated Hospital of China Medical University, 155 Nanjing north street, 110001 Shenyang, Liaoning, People's Republic of China

Zhi Zhao
Department of Orthopaedic Surgery, The Second Affiliated Hospital of Dalian Medical University, 456 Zhongshan road, 116027 Dalian, Liaoning, People's Republic of China

Yue Cai
Department of Automation, School of Electrical Engineering, Dalian Jiaotong University, 794 Huanghe road, 116028 Dalian, Liaoning, People's Republic of China

Wasim Qasim
Department of General Surgery, The Second Affiliated Hospital of Dalian Medical University, 456 Zhongshan road, 116027 Dalian, Liaoning, People's Republic of China

Muhammad Umar Nazir
Department of Respiratory Medicine, The Second Affiliated Hospital of Dalian Medical University, 456 Zhongshan road, 116027 Dalian, Liaoning, People's Republic of China

Jen-Chung Liao
Department of Orthopedic Surgery, Bone and Joint Research Center, Chang Gung Memorial Hospital, Chang Gung University, Taoyuan, Taiwan

Weng-Pin Chen and Hao Wang
Department of Mechanical Engineering, National Taipei University of Technology, 1, Sec. 3, Chung-Hsiao E. Rd, Taipei 10608, Taiwan

Chun Xu, Jaques Reifman and Ginu Unnikrishnan
Department of Defense Biotechnology High Performance Computing Software Applications Institute, Telemedicine and Advanced Technology Research Center, United States Army Medical Research and Materiel Command, Fort Detrick, Maryland, USA

Amy Silder
Department of Bioengineering, Stanford University, Stanford, California, USA

Ju Zhang
Auckland Bioengineering Institute, University of Auckland, Auckland, New Zealand

Tobias Helfen, Georg Siebenbürger, Wolfgang Böcker and Ben Ockert
Department General, Trauma and Reconstructive Surgery, Ludwig Maximilians University, Munich University Hospital, Nußbaumstr. 20, 80336 Munich, Germany

Florian Haasters
Department Knee, Hip and Shoulder Surgery, Schön Klinik Munich-Harlaching, Harlachinger Str. 51, 54817 Munich, Germany

Kazuhiko Arima, Yasuyo Abe, Takayuki Nishimura and Kiyoshi Aoyagi
Department of Public Health, Nagasaki University Graduate School of Biomedical Sciences, 1-12-4 Sakamoto, Nagasaki 852-8523, Japan

Takuhiro Okabe, Yoshihito Tomita, Satoshi Mizukami and Mitsuo Kanagae
Department of Public Health, Nagasaki University Graduate School of Biomedical Sciences, 1-12-4 Sakamoto, Nagasaki 852-8523, Japan
Department of Rehabilitation, Nishi-Isahaya Hospital, Isahaya, Japan

Jen-Ta Shih, Chun-Lin Kuo, Tsu-Te Yeh, Hsain-Chung Shen, Ru-Yu Pan and Chia-Chun Wu
Department of Orthopaedic Surgery, Tri-Service General Hospital, National Defense Medical Center, No. 325, Sec. 2, Chenggong Rd., Neihu Dist, Taipei City 11472, Taiwan, Republic of China
Peter Michael Prodinger, Rüdiger v. Eisenhart-Rothe and Rainer Burgkart Klinik für Orthopädie und Sportorthopädie, Klinikum rechts der Isar der Technischen Universität München, Ismaninger Straße 22, 81675 Munich, Germany

Dominik Bürklein
Abteilung für Fuß-und Sprunggelenkchirurgie, Klinik Volkach, Volkach, Germany

Peter Foehr
Abteilung für Biomechanik, Klinik für Orthopädie und Sportorthopädie, Klinikum rechts der Isar der Technischen Universität München, Munich, Germany

Kilian Kreutzer
Klinik für Mund-, Kiefer-und Gesichtschirurgie, Universitätsklinikum Hamburg Eppendorf, Hamburg, Germany

Hakan Pilge
Orthopädische Klinik, Universitätsklinikum Düsseldorf, Heinrich-Heine Universität, Düsseldorf, Germany

Andreas Schmitt
Abteilung für Sportorthopädie, Klinik für Orthopädie und Sportorthopädie, Klinikum rechts der Isar der Technischen Universität München, Munich, Germany

Oliver Bissinger
Klinik für Mund-, Kiefer- und Gesichtschirurgie, Klinikum rechts der Isar der Technischen Universität München, Munich, Germany

Thomas Tischer
Orthopädische Klinik und Poliklinik der Universität Rostock, Rostock, Germany

Jae-Man Kwak
Department of Orthopaedic Surgery, Asan Medical Center, University of Ulsan, Seoul, Republic of Korea

Gu-Hee Jung
Department of orthopaedic surgery, Gyeongsang national university, college of medicine and Gyeongsang national university Changwon hospital, 555 Samjungja-Dong, Changwon-si 642-160, Republic of Korea

Zixian Yang and Peggy Poh Hoon Lim
Department of Occupational Therapy, Singapore General Hospital, Singapore, Singapore

Sing Hwee Teo
Department of Occupational Therapy, Tan Tock Seng Hospital, Singapore, Singapore

Huiwen Chen
Department of Occupational Therapy, Changi General Hospital, Singapore, Singapore

Huaying Qiu
Department of Occupational Therapy, Ng Teng Fong General Hospital, Singapore, Singapore

Yong Hao Pua
Department of Physiotherapy, Singapore General Hospital, Singapore, Singapore

Leif Mattisson and Lasse J. Lapidus
Department of Clinical Science and Education, Stockholm South General Hospital, Karolinska Institutet, Unit of Orthopaedics, S-118 83 Stockholm, Sweden

Anders Enocson
Department of Clinical Science and Education, Stockholm South General Hospital, Karolinska Institutet, Unit of Orthopaedics, S-118 83 Stockholm, Sweden
Department of Molecular Medicine and Surgery, Karolinska University Hospital, Karolinska Institutet, Stockholm, Sweden

Teemu P. Hevonkorpi and Lauri Raittio
School of Medicine, University of Tampere, 33014 Tampere, Finland

Antti P. Launonen, Bakir O. Sumrein and Minna K. Laitinen
Department of Orthopaedics, Unit of Musculoskeletal Surgery, Tampere University Hospital, Teiskontie 35, PL2000, 33521 Tampere, Finland

Toni Luokkala and Aleksi Reito
Central Finland Central Hospital, Keskussairaalantie 19, 40620 Jyväskylä, Finland

Juha Kukkonen
Satakunta Central Hospital, Sairaalantie 3, 28500 Pori, Finland

Ville M. Mattila
School of Medicine, University of Tampere, 33014 Tampere, Finland
Department of Orthopaedics, Unit of Musculoskeletal Surgery, Tampere University Hospital, Teiskontie 35, PL2000, 33521 Tampere, Finland

Guanyi Liu
Department of Orthopedics, Ningbo NO.6 Hospital, 1059 Zhongsandong Road, Ningbo, Zhejiang 315040, People's Republic of China
Department of Orthopedics, the Second Affiliated Hospital, School of Medicine, Zhejiang University 88 Jiefang RoadHangzhou, Zhejiang 310009, People's Republic of China

Erman Chen and Zhijun Pan
Department of Orthopedics, the Second Affiliated Hospital, School of Medicine, Zhejiang University 88 Jiefang RoadHangzhou, Zhejiang 310009, People's Republic of China

Dingli Xu, Weihu Ma, Leijie Zhou and Jianming Chen
Department of Orthopedics, Ningbo NO.6 Hospital, 1059 Zhongsandong Road, Ningbo, Zhejiang 315040, People's Republic of China

Hong-Wei Chen
Department of Orthopedic Surgery, Yiwu Central Hospital, the Affiliated Yiwu Hospital of Wenzhou Medical University, Yiwu 322000, People's Republic of China

Hong-Hui He
Department of Joint Surgery and Sports Medicine, the Affiliated Nanhua Hospital, University of South China, Hengyang 421002, People's Republic of China

Bin-Li Gao
Department of Orthopedics, the Affiliated Hospital of Inner Mongolia Medical University, No. 1, Tongdao North Road, Hohhot 010050, The Inner Mongolia Autonomous Region, People's Republic of China

Zhen Jian, Rongguang Ao, Jianhua Zhou, Xinhua Jiang and Baoqing Yu
Department of Orthopaedics, Shanghai Pudong Hospital, Shanghai Fudan Univercity Pudong Medical Center, Shanghai 201399, China

Dianying Zhang
Department of Orthopedics, Peking University People's Hospital, Beijing 100044, China

Andrew M. Garratt
Division for Health Services, Norwegian Institute of Public Health, Oslo, Norway

Markus G. Naumann
Department of Orthopaedics, Østfold Hospital, Oslo, Norway

Ulf Sigurdsen
Department of Orthopaedics, Akershus University Hospital, Lørenskog, Norway

Stein Erik Utvåg
Department of Orthopaedics, Akershus University Hospital, Lørenskog, Norway
Institute of Clinical Medicine, University of Oslo, Oslo, Norway

Knut Stavem
Institute of Clinical Medicine, University of Oslo, Oslo, Norway
Department of Pulmonary Medicine, Medical Division, Akershus University Hospital, Lørenskog, Norway
Health Services Research Unit, Akershus University Hospital, Lørenskog, Norway

Luigi Tarallo, Raffaele Mugnai, Martina Rocchi and Fabio Catani
Department of Orthopaedics and Traumatology, University of Modena and Reggio Emilia, Policlinico di Modena, Modena, Italy

Francesco Capra
Private Practitioner, Rimini, Italy

Hans Juto, Helena Nilsson and Per Morberg
Sunderby Research Unit, Department of Surgical and Perioperative Sciences (orthopaedics), Umeå University, Umeå, Sweden

Index

www.ingramcontent.com/pod-product-compliance
Lightning Source LLC
LaVergne TN
LVHW080710210926
848485LV00003B/444
* 9 7 8 1 6 3 9 2 7 3 9 4 2 *